BONE—CERTAIN ASPECTS OF NEOPLASIA

Previous volumes in the Colston Papers are:

Vol. I. 1948 *Cosmic Radiation*—Editor, Professor F. C. Frank (out of print)

Vol. II. 1949 *Engineering Structures*—Editor, Professor A. G. Pugsley (out of print)

Vol. III. 1950 *Colonial Administration*—Editor, Professor C. M. MacInnes (out of print)

Vol. IV. 1951 *The Universities and the Theatre*—Editor, Professor D. G. James (out of print).

Vol. V. 1952 *The Suprarenal Cortex*—Editor, Professor J. M. Yoffey

Vol. VI. 1953 *Insecticides and Colonial Agricultural Development*—Editors, Professor T. Wallace and Dr. J. T. Martin (out of print)

Vol. VII. 1954 *Recent Developments in Cell Physiology*—Editor, Dr. J. A. Kitching (out of print)

1955 No symposium held this year

Vol. VIII. 1956 *The Neurohypophysis*—Editor, Professor H. Heller (out of print)

Vol. IX. 1957 *Observation and Interpretation*—Editor, Professor S. Körner (out of print)

Vol. X. 1958 *The Structure and Properties of Porous Materials*—Editors, Professor D. H. Everett and Dr. F. S. Stone (out of print)

Vol. XI. 1959 *Hypersonic Flow*—Editors, Professor A. R. Collar and Dr. J. Tinkler

Vol. XII. 1960 *Metaphor and Symbol*—Editors, Professor L. C. Knights and Basil Cottle

Vol. XIII. 1961 *Animal Health and Production*—Editors, Professor C. S. Grunsell and A. I. Wright

Vol. XIV. 1962 *Music and Education*—Editor, Professor Willis Grant (out of print)

Vol. XV. 1963 *Reality and Creative Vision in German Lyrical Poetry*—Editor, Professor A. Closs

Vol. XVI. 1964 *Economic Analysis for National Economic Planning*—Editors, P. E. Hart, G. Mills and J. K. Whitaker (out of print).

Vol. XVII. 1965 *Submarine Geology and Geophysics*—Editors, Professor W. F. Whittard and R. Bradshaw

Vol. XVIII. 1966 *The Fungus Spore*—Editor, M. F. Madelin

Vol. XIX. 1967 *The Liver*—Editor, A. E. Read

Vol. XX. 1968 *Towards a Policy for the Education of Teachers*—Editor, Professor William Taylor (out of print).

Vol. XXI. 1969 *Communication and Energy in Changing Urban Environments*—Editor, Professor D. Jones

Vol. XXII. 1970 *Regional Forecasting*—Editors, M. Chisholm, A. E. Frey and Professor P. Haggett

Vol. XXIII. 1971 *Marine Archaeology*—Editor, D. J. Blackman.

BONE—CERTAIN ASPECTS OF NEOPLASIA

Edited by

C. H. G. PRICE and F. G. M. ROSS

with the assistance of

A. L. EYRE-BROOK, B. T. HALE
and J. H. MIDDLEMISS

*Proceedings of the
Twentyfourth Symposium of the Colston Research Society
held in the University of Bristol
April 5th to 8th, 1972*

LONDON

BUTTERWORTHS

THE BUTTERWORTH GROUP

ENGLAND: BUTTERWORTH & CO. (PUBLISHERS) LTD.
LONDON: 88 Kingsway, WC2B 6AB

AUSTRALIA: BUTTERWORTHS PTY. LTD.
SYDNEY: 586 Pacific Highway, NSW 2067
MELBOURNE: 343 Little Collins Street, 3000
BRISBANE: 240 Queen Street, 4000

CANADA: BUTTERWORTH & CO. (CANADA) LTD.
TORONTO: 14 Curity Avenue, 374

NEW ZEALAND: BUTTERWORTHS OF NEW ZEALAND LTD.
WELLINGTON: 26/28 Waring Taylor Street, 1

SOUTH AFRICA: BUTTERWORTH & CO. (SOUTH AFRICA) (PTY)
LTD.
DURBAN: 152/154 Gale Street

August 1973

ISBN 0 408 70530 2

Made and Printed in England by
J. W. Arrowsmith Ltd., Bristol BS3 2NT and Bound by Webb, Son & Co. Ltd., London

Key to Symposium Photograph

1. V. R. McCready
2. M. P. Finkel
3. J. Roylance
4. R. C. Marcove
5. W. F. Enreking
6. P. Kossey
7. R. D. T. Jenkin
8. J. F. Loutt
9. J. Ball
10. B. T. Hale
11. N. C. D. Fizey
12. D. C. Dahiin
13. G. S. Lodwick
14. J. M. Vaughan
15. R. J. Burwood
16. D. H. Mackenzie
17. H. D. Suit
18. B. Stener
19. U. Nilsonne
20. A. J. Webb
21. A. H. C. Ratliff
22. M. E. H. Halford
23. N. P. G. Edling
24. D. R. Sweetnam
25. R. Barnes
26. H. N. Hadders
27. J. C. Mulier
28. H. A. Sissons
29. L. V. Ackerman
30. M. Bonfiglio
31. R. B. Duthie
32. C. J. Campbell
33. J. Vermeij
34. J. T. Makley
35. J. R. von Ronnen
36. B. Friedman
37. M. P. McCormack
38. R. C. Tudway
39. F. H. Doyle
40. Th. G. van Rijssel
41. F. G. M. Ross
42. F. Schajowicz
43. E. Spira
44. I. O. Brennhovd
45. W. Frommhold
46. J. N. Wilson
47. P. Jacobs
48. E. P. Cortes
49. G. M. Jeffree
50. J. H. Middlemiss
51. R. O. van der Heul
52. S. Perry
53. H. K. Lucas
54. D. E. Truscott
55. A. L. Eyre-Brook
56. C. H. G. Price

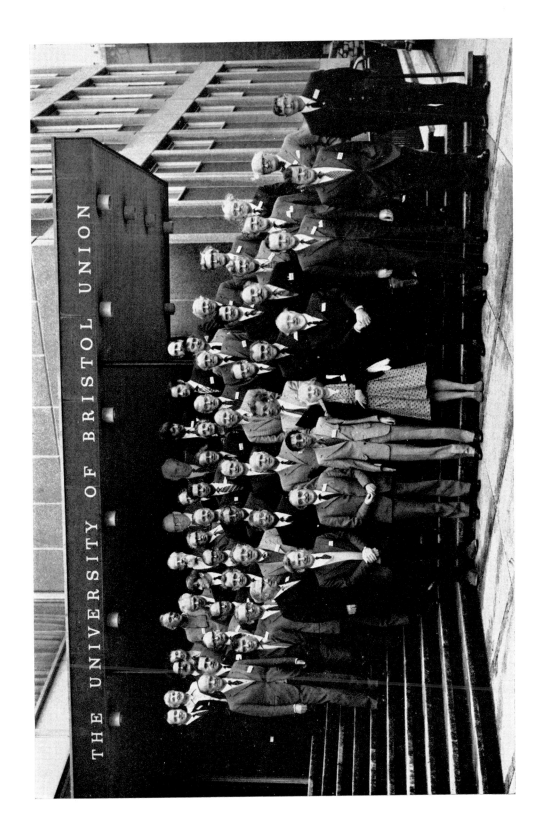

Foreword

THE NAME of Edward Colston, the great seventeenth-century philanthropist and educationalist, is associated in Bristol with a number of scholastic and charitable institutions. It was adopted by a group of public-spirited citizens when, in 1899, they established the "University College Colston Society", with the aim of fostering the young and struggling University College. For a decade it played a part in the movement which culminated in the institution of the University of Bristol in 1909.

The Society then changed its name and made its object more precise: it became the "Colston Research Society" and devoted itself to the encouragement of original work in the University. It made grants for the purchase of apparatus and for other expenses of research. As resources increased, activities expanded and, notably, in the later 'thirties the Society financed a full-scale Social Survey of Bristol.

After the war, a new reconsideration of policy led to the decision to devote the major part of the Society's efforts to the promotion of an annual symposium, the first being held in 1948. The rapid growth of the symposium as a means for the advancement of knowledge is one of the remarkable features of the intellectual life of recent years. Usually, such meetings are fostered by bodies interested in one particular field of learning. As the list of titles (on the page opposite) shows, no such limitation applies to the symposia of the Colston Research Society. That the subject should be one at an interesting and active stage of development is the main factor in making a choice. The fact that the symposium is held in one of the younger seats of learning, with its home in an historic city, is a stimulus not only to the University but also, we believe, to the visiting guests who have come from many countries. The publication of the proceedings ensures the communication of the papers and discussions to wider circles.

It was my privilege to be President of the Colston Research Society for the year 1971–1972, during which the twentyfourth symposium was promoted by the Society. The subject was "Bone—Certain Aspects of Neoplasia" and the proceedings are printed here as the twentyfourth volume of the Colston Papers.

R. H. BROWN

A*

Members of the Symposium

President
Prof. J. H. Middlemiss, Department of Radiodiagnosis, The Medical School, University of Bristol, Bristol BS8 1TD (Diagnostic Radiologist)

Vice-President
Mr. A. L. Eyre-Brook, Department of Orthopaedic Surgery, Bristol Royal Infirmary, Bristol BS2 8HW (Surgeon)

Secretaries
Dr. C. H. G. Price, Bone Tumour Registry, Pathology Research Laboratory, Phase I Building, Royal Infirmary, Bristol, BS2 8HW (Pathologist)

Dr. F. G. M. Ross, Department of Radiodiagnosis, Bristol Royal Infirmary, Bristol BS2 8HW (Diagnostic Radiologist)

Assistant Secretaries
Dr. R. J. Burwood, Department of Radiodiagnosis, The Medical School, University of Bristol, Bristol BS8 1TD (Diagnostic Radiologist)

Mr. M. O'Driscoll, Department of Orthopaedic Surgery, Bristol Royal Infirmary, Bristol BS2 8HW (Surgeon)

Treasurer
Dr. J. Roylance, Department of Radiodiagnosis, Bristol Royal Infirmary, Bristol BS2 8HW (Diagnostic Radiologist)

Members of Bone Tumour Registry Panel
Mr. J. R. Clough, Department of Surgery, Frenchay Hospital, Bristol BS16 1LE (Surgeon)

Dr. B. T. Hale, Radiotherapy Centre, Bristol Royal Infirmary, Bristol BS2 8HW (Radiotherapist)

Dr. E. W. Hall, Area Central Laboratory, Royal United Hospital (North), Bath BA1 3NN (Pathologist)

Dr. F. J. W. Lewis, Department of Pathology, Southmead General Hospital, Bristol BS10 5NB (Pathologist)

Dr. O. C. Lloyd, Department of Pathology, The Medical School, University of Bristol, Bristol BS8 1TD (Pathologist)

Mr. H. K. Lucas, Department of Orthopaedic Surgery, Bristol Royal Infirmary, Bristol BS2 8HW (Surgeon)

Mr. M. P. McCormack, Department of Orthopaedic Surgery, Bristol Royal Infirmary, Bristol BS2 8HW (Surgeon)

Dr. N. C. D. Pizey, Radiotherapy Centre, Bristol Royal Infirmary, Bristol BS2 8HW (Radiotherapist)

Dr. C. D. Thomson, X-ray Department, Royal United Hospital, Bath BA1 3NN (Diagnostic Radiologist)

Dr. R. C. Tudway, Radiotherapy Centre, Bristol Royal Infirmary, Bristol BS2 8HW (Radiotherapist)

Mr. A. J. Webb, Department of Surgery, Bristol Royal Infirmary, Bristol BS2 8HW (Surgeon)

Mr. P. Yeoman, Bath and Wessex Orthopaedic Hospital, Bath BA1 3NN (Surgeon)

Participants

Prof. L. V. Ackerman, Division of Surgical Pathology, Washington University School of Medicine, Barnes Hospital Plaza, St. Louis, Missouri 63110, United States of America (Pathologist)

Dr. J. Ball, Department of Rheumatism Research, Clinical Sciences Building, York Place, Manchester M13 0JJ (Pathologist)

Prof. R. Barnes, Department of Orthopaedic Surgery, Western Infirmary, Glasgow G11 6NT (Surgeon)

Prof. M. Bonfiglio, Department of Orthopaedic Surgery, University of Iowa, Iowa City, Iowa 52240, United States of America (Surgeon)

Dr. I. O. Brennhovd, Norwegian Radium Hospital, Montebello, Oslo 3, Norway (Surgeon)

Dr. H. J. Brenner, The Chaim Sheba Medical Centre, Tel Hashomer, Israel (Radiotherapist)

Dr. P. D. Byers, Dept., of Morbid Anatomy, Institute of Orthopaedics, Royal National Orthopaedic Hospital, 234 Great Portland Street, London W1N 6AD (Pathologist)

Prof. C. J. Campbell, Division of Orthopaedic Surgery, Albany Medical College of Union University, Albany, New York 12208, United States of America (Surgeon)

Dr. M. Catto, Department of Pathology, Western Infirmary, Glasgow G11 6NT (Pathologist)

Dr. E. P. Cortes, Department of Medicine, Long Island Jewish Medical Center, 82–68, 164 St., Jamaica, N.Y. 11432, United States of America (Physician)

Prof. D. C. Dahlin, Department of Surgical Pathology, Mayo Clinic, Rochester, Minnesota 55901, United States of America (Pathologist)

Dr. F. H. Doyle, Diagnostic X-ray Department, Hammersmith Hospital, Ducane Road, London W12 0HS (Diagnostic Radiologist)

Prof. R. B. Duthie, Department of Orthopaedic Surgery, Nuffield Orthopaedic Centre, Headington, Oxford OX3 7LD (Surgeon)

Prof. N. P. G. Edling, Karolinska Sjukhuset, Stockholm 60, S–10401, Sweden (Diagnostic Radiologist)

Prof. W. F. Enneking, Division of Orthopaedic Surgery, University of Florida, Gainesville, Florida 32601, United States of America (Surgeon)

Prof. M. A. Epstein, Department of Pathology, The Medical School, University of Bristol, Bristol BS8 1TD (Pathologist)

Dr. M. P. Finkel, Experimental Radiation Pathology Group, Argonne National Laboratory, Argonne, Illinois 60439, United States of America (Experimental Biologist)

Mr. J. M. Fitton, Department of Orthopaedic Surgery, Leeds University (St. James') Hospital, Leeds LS9 7TF (Surgeon)

Dr. B. Friedman, Severance Medical Arts Building, 5 Severance Circle, Cleveland Heights, Ohio 44118, United States of America (Surgeon)

Prof. W. Frommhold, Medizinisches Strahleninstitut der Universität, Rontgenweg 11, 74 Federal Republic of Germany (Diagnostic Radiologist)

Dr. I. R. S. Gordon, Department of Radiodiagnosis, Bristol Royal Hospital for Sick Children, Bristol BS2 8BJ (Diagnostic Radiologist)

Prof. H. N. Hadders, Pathologisch-Anatomisch Laboratorium, Oostersingel 63, Groningen, Netherlands (Pathologist)

Prof. R. O. van de Heul, Medical Faculty of Rotterdam. Pathology 1. Hougboon, Rotterdam, Netherlands (Pathologist)

Dr. P. Jacobs, The White Cottage, 19 Aldlerbrook Road, Solihull, Warwickshire (Diagnostic Radiologist)

Prof. R. D. T. Jenkin, Department of Radiotherapy, Princess Margaret Hospital, Toronto 5, Ontario, Canada (Radiotherapist)

Dr. P. Kossey, Cancer Research Institute, ul. Čs. Armády 17, Bratislava, Czechoslovakia (Pathologist)

Mr. E. Stanley Lee, Department of Surgery, Westminster Hospital, London SW1P 2AP (Surgeon)

Prof. G. S. Lodwick, Department of Radiology, University of Missouri, Columbia, Missouri 65201, United States of America (Diagnostic Radiologist)

Dr. J. F. Loutit, Medical Research Council Radiobiology Unit, Harwell, Didcot, Berks. (Radiobiologist)

Prof. D. H. Mackenzie, Department of Pathology, Westminster Hospital, London SW1P 2AP (Pathologist)

Dr. J. T. Makley, Division of Orthopaedic Surgery, Case Western Reserve University, 2065 Adelbert Road, Cleveland, Ohio 44106, United States of America (Surgeon)

Dr. R. C. Marcove, 517 East 71st Street, New York, New York 10021, United States of America (Surgeon)

Dr. B. Marsh, Division of Orthopaedic Surgery, University of Florida, Gainesville, Florida 32601, United States of America (Surgeon)

Dr. V. R. McCready, Department of Nuclear Medicine, Royal Marsden Hospital, Downs Road, Sutton, Surrey (Diagnostic Radiologist)

Prof. R. Méary, 158 bis Avenue de Suffren (XVe), Paris, France (Surgeon)

Dr. M. Moore, Robert Jones and Agnes Hunt Orthopaedic Hospital, Oswestry, Shropshire, SY10 7AG (Immunologist)

Prof. J. C. Mulier, Department of Orthopaedic Surgery, Pellenberg 3041, St. Barbara Klinik, Leuven, Belgium (Surgeon)

Dr. R. O. Murray, Institute of Orthopaedics, Royal National Orthopaedic Hospital, 234 Great Portland Street, London W1N 6AP (Diagnostic Radiologist)

Dr. K. A. Newton, Department of Radiotherapy, Westminster Hospital, London SW1P 2AP (Radiotherapist)

Dr. U. Nilsonne, Department of Orthopaedic Surgery, Karolinska Institute, Norrbackain-stitutet, P.O. Box 6403, 113 82 Stockholm 6, Sweden (Surgeon)

Dr. L. N. Owen, Department of Animal Pathology, School of Veterinary Medicine, Madingley Road, Cambridge CB3 0ES (Veterinary Pathologist)

Dr. W. M. Park, Robert Jones and Agnes Hunt Orthopaedic Hospital, Oswestry, Shropshire, SY10 7AG (Diagnostic Radiologist)

Dr. J. F. Patton, X-ray Department, Manchester Royal Infirmary, Oxford Road, Manchester M13 9WL (Diagnostic Radiologist)

Dr. S. Perry, Department of Health, Education and Welfare, National Institute of Health, Bethesda, Maryland 21104, United States of America (Experimental Biologist)

Prof. Th. G. van Rijssel, Pathologisch Laboratorium, Boerhaavekwartien, Leiden, Netherlands (Pathologist)

Prof. J. R. von Ronnen, Academisch Ziekenhuis, Leiden, Netherlands (Diagnostic Radiologist)

Prof. F. Schajowicz, Hospital Italiano, Gasçon, 450 Buenos Aires, Argentina (Pathologist)

Prof. H. A. Sissons, Department of Morbid Anatomy, Institute of Orthopaedics, Royal National Orthopaedic Hospital, 234 Great Portland Street, London W1N 6AD (Pathologist)

Prof. E. Spira, Rehabilitation Centre, Tel Hashomer Hospital, Tel Hashomer, Israel (Surgeon)

Prof. B. Stener, Department of Orthopaedic Surgery II, University of Göteborg, Göteborg 41345, Sweden (Surgeon)

Dr. H. D. Suit, Department of Radiation Medicine, Massachusetts General Hospital, Boston Massachusetts, United States of America (Radiotherapist)

Mr. D. R. Sweetnam, Department of Orthopaedic Surgery, Middlesex Hospital, London W1P 7PN (Surgeon)

Prof. J. M. Thomine, Centre Hospitalier Universitaire, Rouen, France (Surgeon)

Prof. A. Trifaud, Hôpital de la Conception, 144 rue de St. Pierre, Marseille 13, France (Surgeon)

Dame Janet Vaughan, 1 Fairlawn End, First Turn, Wolvercote, Oxford OX2 8AR (Radiobiologist)

Dr. J. Vermeij, Department of Radiology, University Hospital, Leiden, Netherlands (Diagnostic Radiologist)

Mr. J. N. Wilson, Institute of Orthopaedics, Royal National Orthopaedic Hospital, 234 Great Portland Street, London W1N 6AD (Surgeon)

Day Members

Dr. F. L. Cole, Department of Radiology, Gloucestershire Royal Hospital, Gloucester GL1 3NN (Diagnostic Radiologist)

Dr. A. B. Dew, Department of Radiology, Gloucestershire Royal Hospital, Gloucester GL1 3NN (Diagnostic Radiologist)

Dr. G. Evison, Department of Radiology, Royal United Hospital, Bath BA1 3NN (Diagnostic Radiologist)

Miss C. Gibbs, Department of Veterinary Surgery, University of Bristol, Bristol BS8 1TD (Veterinary Diagnostic Radiologist)

Dr. M. J. Gibson, Department of Radiology, Frenchay Hospital, Bristol BS16 1LE (Diagnostic Radiologist)

Dr. R. C. M. Hadden, Department of Radiotherapy, Royal Devon and Exeter Hospital, Exeter EX1 1PQ (Radiotherapist)

Dr. M. E. H. Halford, Department of Pathology, Weston-super-Mare General Hospital, Weston-super-Mare BS23 1PH (Pathologist)

Dr. G. M. Jeffree, Pathology Research Laboratory, Royal Infirmary, Bristol BS2 8HW (Histochemist)

Mr. J. R. Kirkup, Bath and Wessex Orthopaedic Hospital, Bath BA1 3NN (Surgeon)

Dr. M. S. F. McLachlan, Department of Radiology, Cardiff Royal Infirmary, Cardiff (Diagnostic Radiologist)

Mr. R. Merryweather, Department of Orthopaedic Surgery, Gloucestershire Royal Hospital, Gloucester GL1 3NN (Surgeon)

Mrs. L. N. Owen, Cambridge CB3 0ES

Dr. J. Pizey, Radiotherapy Centre, Bristol Royal Infirmary, Bristol BS2 8HW (Radiotherapist)

Mr. A. H. C. Ratliff, Department of Orthopaedic Surgery, Bristol Royal Infirmary, Bristol BS2 8HW (Surgeon)

Mr. P. H. Roberts, Department of Orthopaedic Surgery, Weston-super-Mare General Hospital, Weston-super-Mare BS23 1PH (Surgeon)

Mr. R. H. C. Robbins, Department of Orthopaedic Surgery, Royal Cornwall Hospital, Truro (Surgeon)

Dr. G. Stewart Smith, 413 Topsham Road, Exeter (Pathologist)

Dr. D. E. Truscott, Department of Radiology, West Cornwall Hospital, Penzance (Diagnostic Radiologist)

Mr. J. J. Yeats, Department of Veterinary Surgery, University of Bristol BS8 1TD (Veterinary Surgeon)

Dr. W. B. Young, Department of Radiology, Royal Free Hospital, London WC1X 8LF (Diagnostic Radiologist)

Contents

Where there are several co-authors, the name of the member of the Symposium who presented the paper is given first.

Session I—Giant-cell Tumour: Paget's Sarcoma: New Techniques of Treatment: Tumour Progression

Chairman: Mr. A. L. Eyre-Brook

Session II—Tumour Diagnosis

Chairman Prof. J. H. Middlemiss

Session III—Malignant Round-cell Tumours in Bone

Chairman: Prof. Lauren V. Ackerman

Session IV—Metastatic and Residual Sarcoma

Chairman: Dr. Brendan T. Hale

Session V—Experimental Studies

Chairman: Prof. M. Bonfiglio

Session VI—Immunology: Chondrosarcoma

Chairman: Prof. R. Barnes

xix

Preface

TOO OFTEN communication between scientists is uncritical or is distant. Too often papers are read in public to large gatherings without adequate opportunity for public discussion. Alternatively, ideas may be discussed among peers in a department or school without there being sufficient critical discussion among persons of like experience.

The Colston Symposia, until now provided for the University of Bristol, England, by a prominent and significant group of Bristol citizens, has given University departments an opportunity to gather together persons of similar or parallel experience in different environments to discuss their common experience and problems, and so to provide a forum for discussion, the exchange of ideas and the comparison of research methods and research approach to similar problems.

In the quarter century during which the Colston Symposia have been held, a symposium has previously been allocated to a department in the Faculty of Medicine on three occasions. When the opportunity came to the University Department of Radiodiagnosis to conduct a Symposium it was decided to hold a meeting based on the work of the Bristol Bone Tumour Registry, inviting radiologists, radiotherapists, orthopaedic surgeons, pathologists and experimental workers in the chosen field to participate. The generous provision of the Colston Research Society permits the President of the Symposium to invite sixty or seventy professional men from within Europe to participate in the meeting at no cost to themselves. Persons from outside Europe may also be invited to participate at no cost to themselves once they have reached Europe. On this occasion, in addition to 58 persons from the U.K. and Europe, 18 persons from outside Europe, including Israel, Argentina, the United States of America and Canada, were invited and all accepted.

The Bristol Bone Tumour Registry was started in 1946. The Panel consists of a group of orthopaedic surgeons, pathologists, radiologists, radiotherapists, and other scientists interested in this field, most of whom have now worked together for much of the 25 years. The Registry has had more than 3,000 cases referred to it—albeit not all neoplastic —and now has fully documented records of over 1,500 cases of neoplastic disease in bone spread over more than a quarter of a century. In the U.K. this is a unique registry, though it is recognized that in the United States, records of this type of clinical problem may extend over a greater period and may be more fully documented. It seemed to the Bristol workers however that we had grounds, based on our own experience and records, for trying to get together the world's most experienced scientists in this field to exchange ideas. We limited presentation and discussion to "Sarcoma in Bone" but within these confines made no restriction as to whether the presentation was of experimental work, analytical, basic, diagnostic, therapeutic or peripheral.

It is no secret that this project succeeded. The 76 members lived together, fed together, spent their spare moments talking together, and listened to each other in the formal presentations, knew each other by this experience well enough to bring out in discussion areas of agreement or disagreement without worry of offence to each other. It was in fact a unique experience.

These Proceedings present most of the formal presentations and most of the discussion though naturally the latter has been edited. As President of the Symposium I commend these published Proceedings to any reader interested in this field of work. Here he will find not only the most up-to-date work being undertaken in this realm, but also explanations of the exploratory research work being undertaken in many departments and discussion of the problems still facing us. The thoughts, fumblings, stretchings out into research realms, some controlled, others merely inspired, are all here. In a field of medicine affecting predominantly young persons, relatively rare in occurrence, mainly poor in prognosis, here is the 1970's assessment of the present and the immediate future situation.

For the Bristolians the experience of this Symposium was a privilege. For the other participants it was agreed by them to have been an unusual and highly successful scientific meeting. For readers of these Proceedings it is hoped that the spirit, scientific level and sense of probing that infused and enthused this meeting may strike them.

To the sponsors of the meeting, the Bristol Colston Research Society, we are all grateful.

J. H. MIDDLEMISS
President, Colston Symposium 1972
Professor of Radiodiagnosis
University of Bristol

Editorial Note

THIRTY-SEVEN papers were delivered at this Symposium by speakers from nine countries, each in his own personal style. In preparing these Proceedings for publication, the Editors have considered it important to preserve the individual character of each contribution and have therefore made no effort to achieve uniformity in presentation including the references. The one exception to the rule has been the Editors' efforts to achieve reproduction throughout of radiographs in negative form, and this has been almost completely achieved. All the papers and discussions were recorded on tape and every care has been taken to ensure verbal accuracy. Wherever possible any inadvertent ambiguity has been eliminated. This has only occasionally been a serious problem, and its occurrence has been almost entirely restricted to the discussions following the papers, the tape recordings of which have sometimes been anomalous or obscured by background noises. If any real uncertainty ultimately existed, the transcribed oral version has been referred to the speaker for elucidation. Nevertheless, some editorial abbreviation has been deemed necessary both in the papers and discussion. The majority of the summaries of papers have been written by the Editors and subsequently approved by the author. All this has caused some unavoidable delay in the publication of the Proceedings. It has been assumed that none of the tables and illustrations have been previously published, or if they have been, permission for their reproduction here has already been obtained by the authors. Where this is not so, due acknowledgement has been made in this volume.

The use of abbreviations in the text and tables has been reduced to a minimum and where they occur, they have been explained in the text. However, certain abbreviations have been accepted as in common use.

The Editors emphasize that the opinions expressed in these Proceedings are the views of the individual authors of the papers and that they are not necessarily those of the Editors nor the Panel of the Bristol Bone Tumour Registry.

We wish to record our thanks to Mrs. Joan Nutt and Miss Angela Sainsbury for their varied and invaluable services at the reception desk during the Symposium, also for their willing secretarial assistance together with Mrs. E. M. Doyle, Miss M. Mitchell, Miss C. Phillips, Miss G. Pocock and Mrs. V. Young. Likewise, it is a pleasure to acknowledge the unfailing courtesy and advice given by Mr. F. A. Keedwell who supervises the printing of the Colston Papers by Messrs. J. W. Arrowsmith Ltd. of Bristol.

C. H. G. PRICE
F. G. M. ROSS

Acknowledgments

THE FOLLOWING generously contributed financial or other assistance towards the cost of the Symposium. These gifts are gratefully acknowledged by the Organizing Committee:

Agfa Geveart Limited
Bristol Evening Post
Bryan Adams Trust Fund
Charities Aid Fund
Down Bros., Meyer & Phelps Limited
Ilford Limited
Imperial Chemical Industries Limited
John Harvey & Sons Limited
Organon Laboratories Limited
Philips Electrical Systems Limited
Swan-Morton (Sales) Limited
Tenovus
Upjohn Limited
Warner, Mr. & Mrs. of Derby

Thanks are also due to the Director of the University of Bristol Audio Visual Aids Unit, and the Head of the University of Bristol Department of Medical Illustration for their valuable services during the Symposium.

Giant-cell tumour: Paget's sarcoma: New techniques of treatment: Tumour progression

Chairman: MR. A. L. EYRE-BROOK

Malignant giant-cell tumours of bone

by

P. KOSSEY and J. ČERVEŇANSKÝ

SUMMARY

The histological picture and clinical course of 10 clinically malignant giant-cell tumours of bone are presented. Five tumours were histologically benign but with clinically malignant behaviour—three amputations, two deaths. In one of these patients metastases were demonstrated as pulmonary opacities, but she survived 22 years. A recent woman patient was observed with a tumour of the sacrum which although radiographically benign was shown to be histologically malignant and followed a malignant clinical course.

The tumours of four patients had originally a benign histological structure, which later changed to frank malignancy—to fibrosarcoma[3] and to osteogenic sarcoma.[1] In three cases the transition took place after a remarkably long period of time.

Our Department of surgical pathology covers the entire field of oncology with the exception of brain tumours, the bone tumour pathology being only one part of our work. This latter material we receive from several institutions—mostly from the University Department of Orthopaedics in Bratislava since 1955. We encounter about 80 new cases of bone tumours or allied lesions annually, and amongst these, those which are most interesting are the giant-cell tumours—notably the malignant ones. Therefore, I would like to present our cases of such giant-cell tumours, some being only clinically malignant, others both clinically and histologically.

Case 1. The first example is one of our oldest cases, the histological specimens being received from the University Institute of Pathology in 1955. The patient was a 23-year-old woman with a tumour of the sacrum. Surgical excision was done and biopsy revealed a giant-cell tumour with hypercellular stroma and large giant cells. One year later the tumour recurred, but unfortunately it was not possible to obtain tissue from the recurrence for microscopy. One year later, i.e., 2 years from the original diagnosis of giant-cell tumour, she died with generalized metastases and no autopsy was carried out.

Case 2. In our next patient, a woman of 21 years, the natural course of the disease is very unusual and not completely clear. The specimens again came from the University Institute of Pathology. In February 1950 a tumour of the fibula head was found: 2 months later this was resected and giant-cell tumour histologically diagnosed (Fig. 1). Some months later recurrence was noted in the operation scar which was irradiated, but the lesion progressed and the skin became ulcerated. Re-excision was performed again revealing the histological picture of giant-cell tumour with some mitoses (Fig. 2). The leg was amputated and for 2 years the patient was well, but subsequent chest radiographs

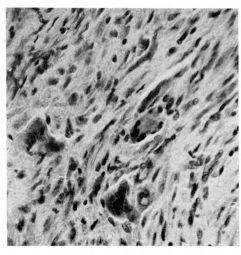

Fig. 1. H & E × 200. Primary giant-cell tumour of fibula head (Case 2).

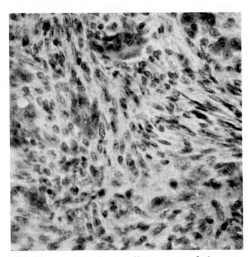

Fig. 2. H & E × 200. Recurrent giant-cell tumour of the same patient. There are some mitoses in this field.

showed a shadow in the lung (Fig. 3). This was regarded by several radiodiagnosticians as a metastasis and for several years the shadow grew, later to become stationary. This woman is alive and well, and works as a clerk at the Medical School in Bratislava. It is now 22 years since the original diagnosis of giant-cell tumour.

Case 3. In our next patient, a woman of 23-years-old, osteogenic sarcoma of the distal femur was diagnosed on clinical and radiological grounds. The radiographic picture seemed so clear and unequivocal that the orthopaedic surgeon quite exceptionally amputated the leg without histological proof. Biopsy revealed a quite typical giant-cell

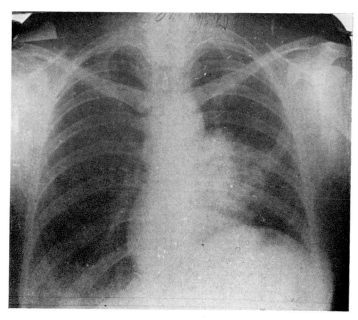

Fig. 3. Chest radiograph showing shadow in the left lung (Case 2).

tumour with some mitoses and a little osteoid formation, but nowhere was there histological evidence of malignancy. There was no histological basis for a diagnosis of osteosarcoma (Fig. 4). The clinicians were very surprised by this report, but 7 months later our own astonishment was greater still, when apparent metastatic nodules were demonstrated in the patient's lung. These remained static for some years, and it was hoped that this patient would follow a similar course as our second case mentioned above. However, 6 years later the woman died at home and no autopsy was carried out.

Case 4. A woman of 33 years presented with a giant-cell tumour of the fibula head in which histology showed some mitoses. Following the resection, the woman became pregnant and there was a recurrence of the tumour. This was not irradiated, and the woman was delivered of a healthy child. Some months later however, the tumour perforated the cortex and invaded the adjacent soft tissues. Although regarded as clinically malignant, further biopsy revealed again giant-cell tumour with some mitotic activity, but no certain evidence of malignancy. However, on clinical evaluation, the leg was amputated and the patient is now alive and well 17 years later.

Case 5. A 30-year-old woman was seen with a swelling of the tibial tubercle which for 9 months had been treated as an inflammatory condition. Following admission to a tuberculosis sanatorium the diagnosis of a bone tumour was made. The first histological examination showed a giant-cell tumour with about one mitosis per low-power field of tumour tissue. Excision was shortly followed by recurrence so that after 5 months a second excision was done. Histological study showed no change from the original specimen. Two months later there was soft tissue spread and the leg was amputated. Sections of the tumour from the amputated limb were similar to the previous material. 15 years later the woman is alive and well.

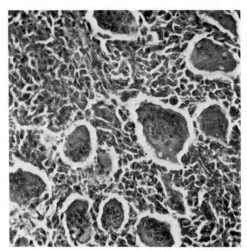

Fig. 4. H & E × 200. Giant-cell tumour of the distal femur. The patient died after 6 years (Case 3).

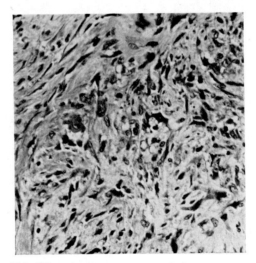

Fig. 5. H & E × 200. Fibrosarcomatous part of the recurrent giant-cell tumour. (Case 6).

Case 6. A 34-year-old woman had a swelling of the proximal tibia, ostensibly following an injury, which proved to be a giant-cell tumour. A resection was performed, the patient remaining quite well for 8 years. In the ninth year, however she complained of pain at the site of the former tumour, with swelling of the knee. The lesion was re-excised; histology showing malignancy, the greater part being fibrosarcomatous (Fig. 5) together with some tumour cartilage (Fig 6); elsewhere there were areas with the structure of non-malignant conventional giant-cell tumour (Fig. 7). The leg was amputated and the patient survives in good health 3 years later.

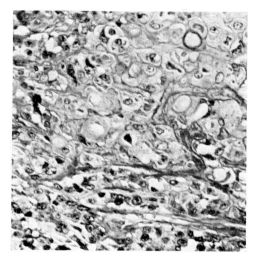

Fig. 6. H & E × 200. Chondrosarcomatous part of the recurrent giant-cell tumour (Case 6).

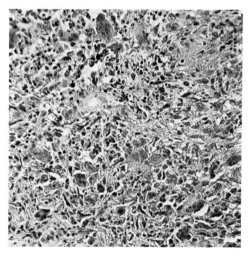

Fig. 7. H & E × 100. Non-malignant conventional giant-cell tumour from the same tumour as Figures 5 and 6.

Case 7. The next patient, a woman of 51 years old, has a very long history. In 1926 when 19 years of age, a diagnosis of "brown tumour" of the distal tibia was made by Professor Lorenz in Vienna. The tumour was curetted. The patient had no hyperparathyroidism. At that time the giant cell tumours often were called "brown tumours" and there was no clear distinction between these two entities. Until 1958—for 32 years—she was well; then, at the site of the previous tumour, she had pain and a further swelling. Histology showed this to be a fibrosarcoma (Fig. 8) and the leg was amputated. Unfortunately, she died 2 years later with metastases.

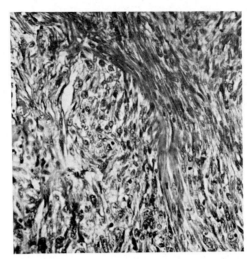

Fig. 8. H & E × 200. Fibrosarcoma of the distal tibia. At the site of this tumour a giant-cell tumour was diagnosed 32 years ago (Case 7).

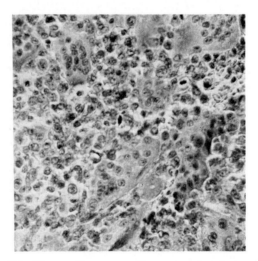

Fig. 9. H & E × 200. Giant-cell tumour of sacrum; showing several mitoses. The tumour was considered as histologically malignant. The patient died (Case 10).

Case 8. A somewhat similar case, but with a much shorter history, was a man aged 54 years. In 1947 a giant cell tumour of the distal femur was diagnosed; this was excised, the man remaining well for 10 years. The pain recurred at the former tumour site and 4 years later he died of metastases. The recurrent tumour histologically was a fibrosarcoma.

Case 9. In a small country hospital a 52-year-old man was seen with a giant-cell tumour of the proximal tibia. Six months after treatment there was a recurrence, histologically a fibrosarcoma but with a few giant cells in some areas. The patient died 1 year after ablation of the leg.

10. The last patient was a woman aged 21 years with a tumour of the sacrum which radiographically and at operation simulated an aneurysmal bone cyst. Histologically it was giant-cell tumour with rather frequent mitoses and atypical stroma cells (Fig. 9). After some deliberation the sections were interpreted as being malignant. The tumour recurred with metastases which caused the death of the patient.

Details of these cases are summarized in two tables. In Table 1 are our cases with clinical malignancy only, in Table 2 are the cases with clinical as well as with histological malignancy.

TABLE 1

GIANT-CELL TUMOUR—CLINICAL MALIGNANCY ONLY

	Age	Sex	Location	Clincial course
1	23	Fe	Sacrum	After 1Y. R., 2Y. Later D.
2	21	Fe	Proximal Fibula	After some months R., Irradiation, A. 2Y. Later lung M., 22Y. Alive
3	23	Fe	Distal Femur	A., 7 months later lung M. 6Y. Later D.
4	33	Fe	Proximal Fibula	Excision, Pregnancy, R., A., 17Y., Alive
5	33	Fe	Proximal Tibia	Excision, R., Infiltration of soft tissues, A., 15Y. Alive

R = Recurrence   M = Metastases   A = Amputation   D = Death
Y = Year

TABLE 2

GIANT-CELL TUMOUR—CLINICAL AND HISTOLOGICAL MALIGNANCY

	Age	Sex	Location	Clinical course
1	34	Fe	Proximal Tibia	Resection, 9Y. Later R., Osteosarcoma, A., 3Y Alive
2	51	Fe	Distal Tibia	1926, "Brown Tumour", 1938 R., Fibrosarcoma, A., 1960 D
3	54	M	Distal Femur	1947 G.C.T., 1957 R., Fibrosarcoma, 1961 D.
4	52	M	Proximal Tibia	G.C.T. 6 months later R., Fibrosarcoma. A., 1Y. Later D
5	21	Fe	Sacrum	Primary Malignant G.C.T., 6 months R., M., After 1Y. D

R = Recurrence   M = Metastases   A = Amputation   D = Death
Y = Year   G.C.T. = Giant-cell tumour

B

COMMENT

We have in our files about 35 examples of conventional giant-cell tumour. Our percentage of malignancy is high, but our series is to some extent selective, three cases being included only by reason of clinical malignancy.

It seems important to stress that none of these patients were primarily (i.e. before recurrence) irradiated.

From a practical point of view it is important to answer the question—What is a malignant giant-cell tumour of bone? In certain cases, where the original tumour was benign, later to change to fibrosarcoma or osteogenic sarcoma, the practical answer is quite simple. We had four such cases, our cases Nos. 6, 7, 8 and 9 (the first four cases in Table 2).

The diagnosis of the so-called "primary malignant giant-cell tumour" is often questionable, but, without any doubt, such cases do exist. The last case in our series, (Table 2, tumour of the sacrum) is an example of this variant. In practically all series of giant-cell tumours there are very disturbing cases for the surgical pathologist—the so-called "benign giant-cell tumour with a clinically malignant course", or the "benign metastasising giant-cell tumour". Such anomalous lesions are reported by several authors, [1-7] the best known being those of Jaffe,[4] Ackerman,[3,5] and Dahlin.[6] Sometimes, long survival has been reported following surgical removal of pulmonary metastases. Spontaneous regression of histologically proven metastases is also recorded.[7] There is no satisfactory explanation for these curious and puzzling cases. One may speculate on the variable host response of tumour metastases which may reach a state of stable equilibrium with the environment and lose their aggressive character. The pulmonary lesions of the second patient mentioned above (Table 1, case 2) were not histologically proven, but the clinical course of 22 years survival probably indicates that the lesion of the fibula should be assigned to this rare group of giant-cell tumours. The third patient (Table 1, case 3) with a "benign metastasising giant-cell tumour" died after 6 years; who can say whether excision of her pulmonary metastases would have been successful in saving her life?

The other peculiar and troublesome sort of giant cell tumour is the aggressive recurrent, but histologically benign group. In our series this is represented by two patients with several recurrences and soft tissue spread. What would be their fate without amputation? Is amputation always really necessary? Where and how do we discern the borderline between the aggressive recurrent benign giant-cell tumour and the malignant form? This difficult area of bone tumour pathology merits full consideration and discussion.

REFERENCES

1. Finch, E. P. & Gleave, H. H. A Case of Osteoclastoma (Mycloid Sarcoma, Benign Giant-cell Tumour) with Pulmonary Metastases. *J. Path. Bact.*, **29**, 399, 1926.
2. Dyke, S. C. Metastasis of the "Benign" Giant-cell Tumour of Bone. *J. Path. Bact.*, **34**, 259, 1931.
3. Murphy, W. R. & Ackerman, L. V. Benign and Malignant Giant-cell Tumors of Bone. A Clinico-Pathological Evaluation of Thirty-one Cases. *Cancer*, **9**, 317, 1956.
4. Jaffe, H. L. *Tumors and Tumorous Conditions of the Bones and Joints.* Lea and Febiger, Philadelphia, 1958.

5. Ackerman, L. V. & Spjut, H. J. *Tumors of Bone and Cartilage, Atlas of Tumor Pathology*, Section II, Fascicle 4. Armed Forces Institute of Pathology, Washington, 1962.
6. Dahlin, D. C. *Bone Tumors*, Second Edition, *General Aspects and Data on 3987 Cases*. Charles C. Thomas, Springfield, Illinois, 1967.
7. Stargardter, F. L. & Cooperman, L. R. Giant-cell Tumour of Sacrum with Multiple Pulmonary Metastases and Long-term Survival. *British J. Radiol.*, **44**, 976, 1971.

Discussion

Dr. Brenner   I want to ask Dr. Kossey whether any of his cases had any form of irradiation at any stage previous to the diagnosis of malignancy, because there are a number of surgeons and radiotherapists who believe that irradiation of a benign giant-cell tumour can produce or pre-dispose to malignancy as such?

Dr. Kossey   None of these were primarily irradiated. One patient was irradiated for a recurrence of giant-cell tumour, and patients who were thought to have recurrences were irradiated, but the new ones were not.

Dr. Byers   I think that as pathologists we would all be very interested to know what sort of criteria were used first of all to make the diagnosis of giant-cell tumour, and secondly to distinguish those thought to be malignant.

Dr. Kossey   The decision is quite difficult going by the features as described in the text books and in particular we only consider the number of mitoses. Where only one or two were seen in a microscopic field we diagnosed the tumour as a benign one; when mitoses were often seen, as in the last patient's tumour, we diagnosed a primary malignant tumour after some deliberation. Such primary malignant tumours were one only in the series.

Dr. Ball   May I just point that up by asking a more specific question. I wonder whether in fact you attempted to assess the frequency distribution of mitoses in your cases? It is very difficult to know what it means when they say there is one mitosis per field or high-power field. We have just been doing a little preliminary study on these lines and my impression at the moment is that in most of these giant-cell tumours there are mitoses, and that these will be between say one and seven mitotic figures per square millimetre of tumour tissue, and there is another group of cases with a much higher rate in the region of over 20. I also wonder whether you have looked into the problem of mitotic rate in relation to the clinical course of your cases?

Dr. Kossey   Well, in all tumours we have seen some mitoses, but they were not frequent. The one with many mitoses was the last case and this we diagnosed as a malignant giant-cell tumour. Otherwise, where there was only one mitosis to a field we regarded the tumour as benign.

Dr. Ball   I must make it clear that when this sort of thing is being discussed it would be I feel a very good idea if people would express the numbers of mitoses with reference to some definite area of tumour tissue. It would be an immense help to those who read descriptions to know what precisely the numbers refer to in terms of any area of tumour tissue.

Dr. Price Regarding the number of mitoses to be found in giant-cell tumours, I have studied about sixty from this point of view. Firstly, counting mitoses is a time consuming and rather tedious occupation. I found that in examining undamaged well-preserved tumour tissue that the mode for the number of mitoses was of the order of 1 to 5 per square millimetre of tumour. The range of those that I regarded as histologically benign ran from 1 to 10 mitoses per square millimetre, and when mitoses were more than this the histological appearance was obviously malignant.

Professor van Rijssel I cannot see the difference between the number of mitoses in just a microscopic field and per square millimetre. It just depends upon the magnification used, and you search as many fields as you want so fixing the number examined to what is needed. Somehow you have to adopt a base-line. Is it possible for Dr. Kossey to say how many microscopic fields you had to go through to find on the average one mitosis? If I understood you correctly you said that every microscopic field showed one mitosis? Was that so, and what was the magnification used?

Dr. Kossey I used the objective × 10.

Professor Lodwick I am wondering if you have any certain X-ray criteria which you use for your diagnosis of giant-cell tumour or whether you make the diagnosis on purely histologic grounds.

Dr. Kossey Yes, when the picture is not quite certain I see the X-ray films and consult the surgeon and radiologist for their opinions. I see the X-rays myself, but I do not make a diagnosis based upon them.

Dr. Lloyd It is all very well for Dr. Price to say "obviously malignant" giant-cell tumour, but this is just the one thing that I find difficult with these tumours. Clearly, one can't go only by numbers of mitoses, otherwise we will spend all night and half the next day counting mitoses. Therefore, one has to decide on other criteria which I find very difficult. Will somebody please tell us how to tell the difference between a benign and malignant giant-cell tumour.

Professor Bonfiglio My question is a similar one. Can one predict *a priori* which tumour will metastasize and kill the patient; and which one is going to metastasize and not kill the patient, and which one will not metastasize at all?

Mr. Eyre-Brook—Chairman A very difficult question.

Professor Schajowicz You cannot predict which tumours will act as benign or malignant for this reason. It has been agreed by many pathologists in America, including my friend Professor Ackerman that it is hopeless and useless to try grading giant-cell tumours. You cannot get beyond a general diagnosis of giant-cell tumour. You cannot do this also for there many tumours which look like giant-cell tumours and I think that some are not giant-cell tumours at all. You cannot decide this to say which are genuine giant-cell tumours; I think that in fact some are sarcomas. So, it is enough for us to say that this is a giant-cell tumour—a genuine giant-cell tumour, not to grade it. In the last 50 cases we have never had a recurrence or a metastasis of a giant-cell tumour. This is our opinion generally, and I hope to hear the paper by Bonfiglio and Campbell and to discuss this point further. After the paper of Dr. Kossey there is a lot of confusion in my mind and in the minds of others, because he said to us that there was only one thoroughly malignant giant-cell tumour amongst his cases—what were the others? We have heard ten or twelve times of malignant behaviour of a giant-cell tumour—What were these? Was there some malignant transformation or were these all similar cases? And amongst 45 cases in all there were 12 with malignant behaviour. This proportion is too much.

Dr. Kossey   In this series we had 10 cases of malignant giant-cell tumour (Tables 1 and 2). Half of them (Table 1) were histologically benign although clinically they behaved as malignant. The second half of the patients (Table 2) were malignant both clinically and histologically. The first four cases in Table 2 were patients in whom primarily benign giant-cell tumour altered to fibrosarcoma or to osteosarcoma. The last case of the series was a primarily malignant giant-cell tumour.

Aggressiveness and malignancy in Giant-cell tumors of bone

by

CRAWFORD J. CAMPBELL and MICHAEL BONFIGLIO

SUMMARY

The authors show some of the difficulties they encountered in trying to prognosticate the malignant potential in giant-cell tumors of bone. Cases are used to illustrate examples of frankly malignant giant-cell tumor when first treated, malignant transformation following curettage or radiation therapy, and radiation sarcoma occurring many years following treatment. It is impossible to make an exact prognosis in any individual case, but a careful study of the clinical manifestations, course, roentgenography and histology were often an aid in the choice of therapy to be instituted. Ablation of the tumor by local resection or amputation gives the best results but is not always practicable.

THERE ARE many reports of small and large series of giant-cell tumors. [8,9,17,22,44,52] Although these have been helpful in defining this rather rare tumor, much remains to be learned about the significance of the pathological findings, factors influencing the incidence of recurrence and occasionally metastases, and the indications for different types of therapy. Whether potentially benign or malignant, they have various features in common. They can be defined as neoplasms composed of spindle-shaped or ovoid stromal cells in which giant cells are regularly interspersed. They are usually found in the end of a tubular long bone of a young adult between the ages of 15 and 40. The clinical signs and symptoms are similar to those found in many bone tumors; pain, tenderness, and enlarging mass, limp and atrophy. The duration of complaints may range from a few weeks to many months.

Giant-cell tumors usually appear in roentgenograms as an expanding radiolucent lesion in the epiphyseal end of a long bone (Fig. 1). Trabeculations when present should suggest the possibility of either a recurrence, particularly when curettage or X-ray therapy had been employed, or of spontaneous regression. Although the roentgenograms may suggest the possibility of a giant-cell tumor, they are not diagnostic since other benign and malignant tumors may simulate these findings. An adequate open biopsy is necessary to confirm the diagnosis prior to the initiation of treatment.

Giant-cell tumors vary in their biological behavior from benign to extremely malignant. The word "malignancy" when discussing giant-cell tumor has not been well defined. Jaffe[30] considers it a tumor which, if a substantial amount of tumor tissue is examined

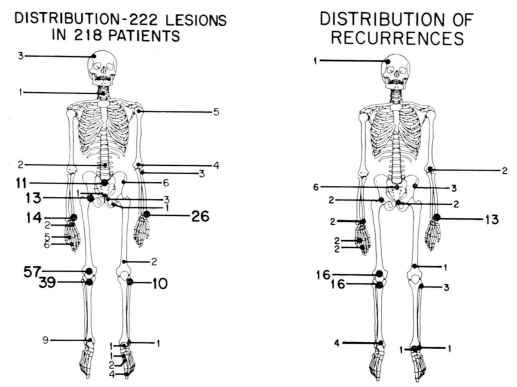

Chart 1. Distributions of Primary Lesions and Recurrences.

shows consistently the characteristic pattern of giant cells and stromal cells, but in which the appearance of the stromal cells is such as to give the tissue a sarcomatous cast. He includes some cases which he considers potentially malignant from the start and which maintain their giant-cell tumor appearance histologically, and also those cases which originally had the typical histological appearance of giant-cell tumor but showed progressive cytological changes so that the metastases appear entirely different. He split off a group of tumors as "post-irradiation sarcoma" in which a sarcoma develops years later (usually 5 to 8 years) at the site of a proven giant-cell tumor treated by irradiation. Dahlin[17] includes this latter group which had irradiation therapy. Out of a total of 156 cases he had four cases which initially appeared sarcomatous, two which subsequently became sarcomatous which had not had previous X-ray therapy (one of these 22 years and again 15 years) following curettage and bone grafting developed a fibrosarcoma, and nine followed treatment which included irradiation. Hutter *et al.*[26] found evidence of obvious fibrosarcoma in 21 of 23 cases classified as malignant giant-cell tumor in a series of 75 giant-cell tumors. These included tumors that were malignant at the time of the initial biopsy, malignant transformation following either surgery or radiation therapy, and suggestive radiation sarcomas. There are also occasional cases which have been called "benign giant-cell tumor with pulmonary metastases".[30,31]. We have included them as malignant giant-cell tumors.

The purpose of this study is to show some of the problems in the classification, recognition, and treatment of the more aggressive and frankly malignant giant-cell tumors. It is based on cases pulled from our previous analysis[22] of 222 giant-cell tumors in 218 patients (Chart 1) and an additional 10 cases seen subsequently. We are particularly concerned with the problems of recognition of malignancy in the previously untreated case, the transformation of histological type and biological behavior to a more aggressive and frankly malignant tumor following various modalities of treatment, and the development of sarcoma in the primary site many years following therapy.

HISTOLOGICAL GRADING: QUESTION OF PROGNOSTIC VALUE

Although the attempt to grade giant-cell tumors by Jaffe and Lichtenstein[28,30,36] has not been particularly helpful as a classification, it has alerted pathologists to the need for a careful study of all the tissue removed at biopsy for manifestations of malignancy such as abundant and closely compacted stromal cells, tendency to irregular whorled arrangement, atypism with the tendency of the cells to be large, and anaplasia. The giant cells usually tend to be dwarfed and to contain only a few nuclei. Hutter *et al.*,[26] although not using specific grades, used criteria similar to Jaffe's Grade III in determining malignancy in giant-cell tumors. In our study[22] we did an independent evaluation using the grading of Jaffe (Grades I to III), of the original tissue section in each of the 222 tumors without any knowledge of the clinical or roentgenographic findings. Although there was a slight difference of opinion between Grades I and II, there was unanimity of initial opinions in those cases considered frankly malignant (Grade III). Our histological grading was of no prognostic aid in predicting recurrence (Grade I, recurrence rate of 39%, Grade I–II, recurrence rate of 19%, Grade II, recurrence rate 34%, Grade III, recurrence rate of 24%). However, the recognition of manifestations of malignancy as shown by our placing them in Grade III was meaningful. Of the 29 patients whose primary tumor we classified as Grade III, nine died of the disease, seven had recurrences, and 13 were alive and well 6 to 14 years after the diagnosis was first established. Of the 14 patients who died of their tumors (Chart 2), nine were Grade III.

Unsuccessful attempts have also been made by other authors to correlate the roentgenographic features with the subsequent behavior of giant-cell tumor. Fractures and extension of the tumor outside the cortex often influenced the surgeon to undertake a radical excision or amputation.

RECURRENCE AND METASTASES

It is of interest that 12 of the 14 patients whose death was clearly related to giant-cell tumor had a local recurrence. These are included in the 77 (35% of the 218 patients) with recurrence (Charts 1 and 2). All but two of the recurrences occurred within 2 years following diagnosis (Table 1). Thirteen patients had known metastases. These were to the lungs in 11 patients, to the brain in one, and to the lymph nodes in one. One patient had metastases to both lungs and the mediastinum. Histological sections from the primary tumor were available for each of the 13 patients with metastases. The histological grades of these tumors were Grade I in two, Grade II in five, and Grade III in

B*

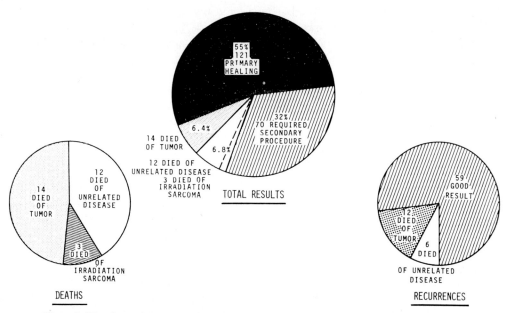

Chart 2. Total results, recurrences, and deaths in 218 cases of giant-cell tumors.

six. At the time of this study, eight of the 13 patients with metastases had died: five, within 1 year of the time that the primary diagnosis was made and three, 2 to 5 years after diagnosis.

It is generally believed that patients with giant-cell tumors whose roentgenograms show a metastatic pulmonary focus will die within 6 to 12 months of wide-spread metastases. The successful result in five of the six patients who were treated by surgery for metastases to the lungs in this series indicates the value of lobectomy in the treatment of giant-cell tumors (Table 2).

TABLE 1.

Time Interval Between Diagnosis and Recurrence

Time	No. of Cases
2– 6 months	19
7–12 months	39
13–24 months	17
3 years	1
12 years	1
Total	77

TABLE 2.

Pulmononary Metastases—13

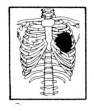

	Number	Survival (6 yrs. +)
Resection	6	5
Untreated	7	0

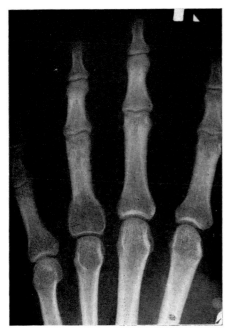

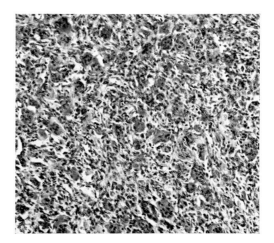

Fig. 1–A. Roentgenogram shows an expanding lytic lesion in the proximal phalanx of the ring finger in a twenty-two year old male who had complained of pain and swelling since a twisting injury three months previously. An attempt to resect the affected portion of bone was unsuccessful because the tumor was broken into. Amputation of the entire digit and a portion of the related metacarpal bone was performed.

Fig. 1–B. The initial photomicrograph (× 75) was reported as Grade II. Further perusal of the tissue showed more ominous signs of malignancy. The histology of the original biopsy revealed evidence of malignancy, although it was originally classified "borderline".

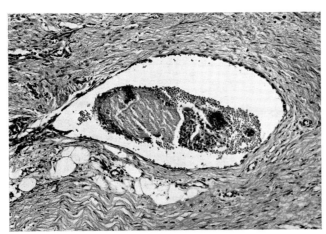

Fig. 1–C. Photomicrograph (× 105) shows tumor cells in a vein adjacent to the tumor. Although this finding indicates a malignant grading of giant-cell tumor, some cases in this study with this finding have survived many years without recurrence or metastases. This patient developed a local recurrence requiring an amputation of half the hand eleven months after the initial surgery.

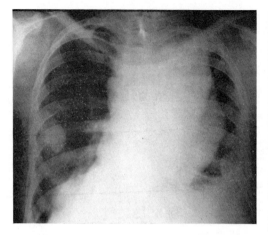

Fig. 1–D. Roentgenogram shows metastases to the lungs 3 years after the initial surgery. There was no further local recurrence in the remaining portion of the hand. The patient died one month later.

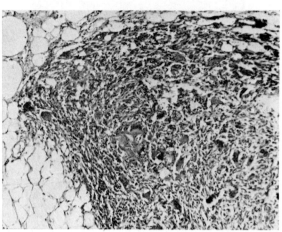

Fig. 1–E. Photomicrograph ($\times 75$) shows the histology of the tumor in the metastasis to be similar to that found at the time of resection.

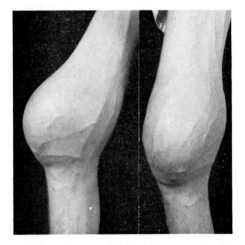

Fig. 2–A. Photographs of the right thigh show a large swelling which extends into the knee joint of this 25 year old white male. He had continued dull aching pain for a period of three months despite the application of a cast by his physician. He had lost 30 pounds in weight.

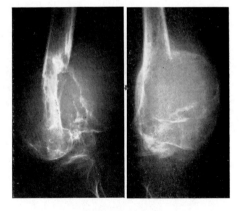

Fig. 2–B. Roentgenograms show a lytic lesion which is eccentrically located in the lower end of the femur. It extends well out into the soft tissues and although a thin osseous border can be defined along its margins, in other areas it cannot. Pathological fractures extend into the knee joint.

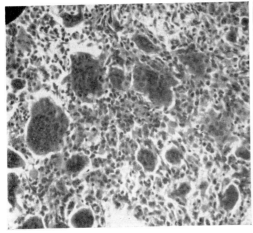

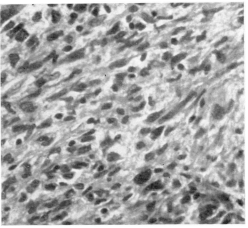

Fig. 2–C. Photomicrograph (× 100) shows numerous multinucleated giant cells, densely packed spindle cell stroma lacking collagenization.

Fig. 2–D. Photomicrograph (× 150) shows mitotic figures in another area of the same tumor which resembles a fibrosarcoma. On the basis of the pathology, aggressive behavior, and location, an amputation was performed as the primary treatment.

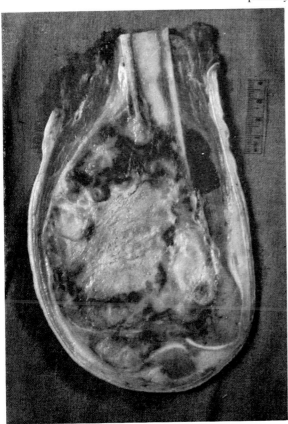

Fig. 2–E. The specimen shows a firm white tissue in the center, surrounded by white, yellow, and tan friable tissue. There are some cystic hemorrhagic areas. The patient is living and well with no evidence of recurrence or metastases 8 years following his amputation.

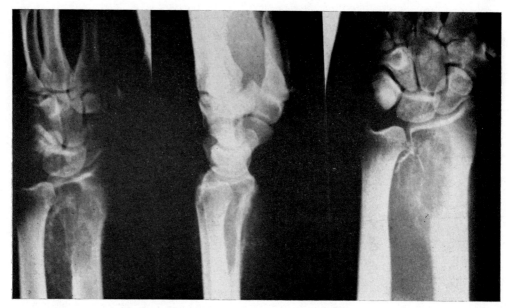

Fig. 3.–A. Roentgenograms of the left wrist of this 23 year old white male who had the complaints of increasing pain and swelling for 3 months show an eccentrically placed lesion in the lower end of the radius which has destroyed the center and extends into the surrounding soft tissue toward the ulna and volarward. There was no clearcut margin and the possibility of a malignant tumor was entertained.

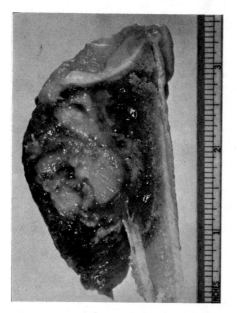

Fig. 3–B. A biopsy excision was done. To avoid entering the tumor, the periosteum of the ulna and interosseous membrane was excised with the tumor. The center of the tumor was white, firm and gritty and the outer border red and rust colored and friable.

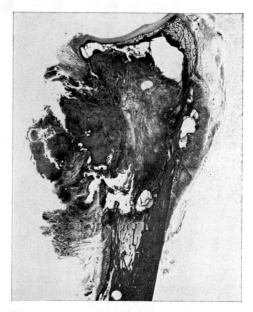

Fig. 3–C. A sagittal section shows finger-like projections into the surrounding tissue.

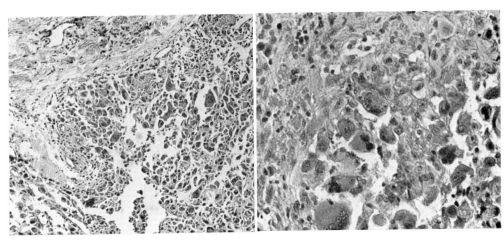

Fig. 3–D.   Photomicrograph (×75) shows the pattern of the cellular arrangement along the border of the tumor. There are irregularly shaped giant cells with marked anisocytosis of both stomal and giant cells.

Fig. 3–E.   Photomicrograph (×125) shows the obvious findings of a very malignant giant-cell tumor.

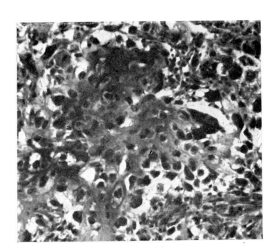

Fig. 3–F.   Photomicrograph (×125) shows metaplastic bone formation. Foci of malignant tumor bone were found in the center of the lesion. Hyperchromasia with marked variation in size and shape of the nuclei was found throughout the lesion.

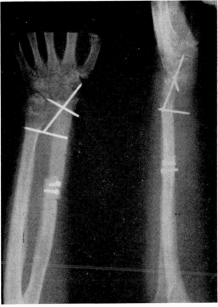

Fig. 3–G.   Roentgenogram shows the autogenous graft from the postero-medial area of the upper tibia. It was placed between the remaining fragment of radius and the navicular and lunate.

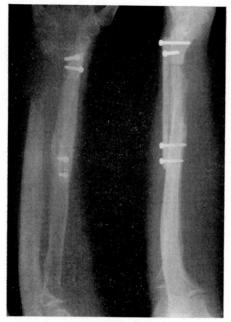

Fig. 3–H. The patient sustained many accidents, breaking casts and grafts. This roentgenogram shows a second graft 6 months following his initial treatment.

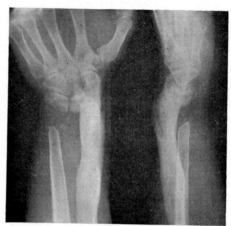

Fig. 3–I. Roentgenogram taken 6 years after his initial treatment. The patient works at heavy labor and it is now 8 years following the resection with no evidence of tumor.

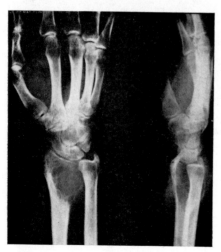

Fig. 4–A. Roentgenogram of the right wrist in 1952 shows a lytic lesion in the distal radius of a thirty-three year old white male (Case 5) after several episodes of pain following minor traumata. There is perforation of the cortex medially and dorsally.

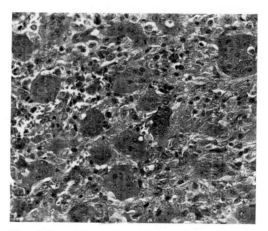

Fig. 4–B. Photomicrograph (× 125) of tissue removed at biopsy shows the features of a giant cell tumor. There are abundant, large, multi-nucleated giant cells. The stroma is very benign in appearance.

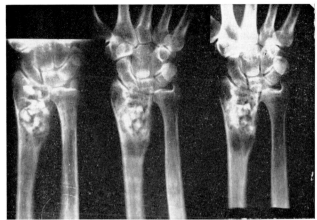

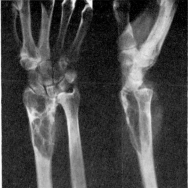

Fig. 4-C. Roentgenograms three, six, and nine months following a curettage and insertion of autogenous iliac bone chips show a recurrence which was unrecognized despite the complaint of increasing pain.

Fig. 4-D. Roentgenogram 15 months following the curettage and bone graft shows a massive recurrence. The patient was referred to one of the authors for amputation because of an extensive soft tissue mass which involved the previous operative scar.

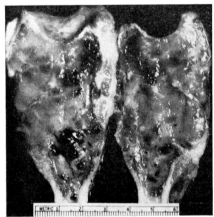

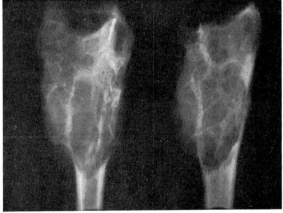

Fig. 4-E. Photograph shows the sectioned tumor specimen removed by block resection without entering the tumor tissue.

Fig. 4-F. Roentgenogram shows the extensive destruction of cortical and cancellous bone in the distal radius.

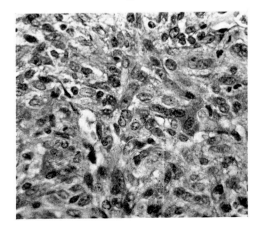

Fig. 4-G. Photomicrograph ($\times 200$) shows a change in histological appearance to a more aggressive sarcoma. The appearance is that of a fibrosarcoma. There was transformation from a benign to a more aggressive or malignant tumor.

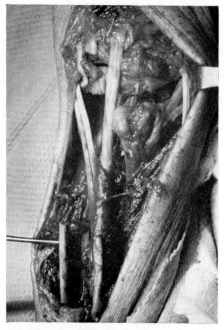

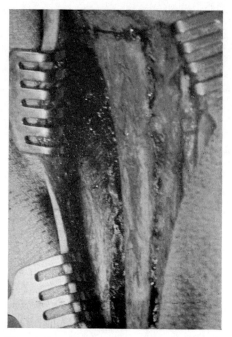

Fig. 4–H. Photograph shows the defect in the radius following the local resection. The original operative scar with tumor in it and all muscles adherent to the mass along with the joint capsule and periosteum of the ulna were excised "en masse".

Fig. 4–I. A graft was taken from the upper tibia along its postero-medial surface. It must be taken from the contra-lateral tibia to take advantage of the natural flare and abundant cancellous bone.

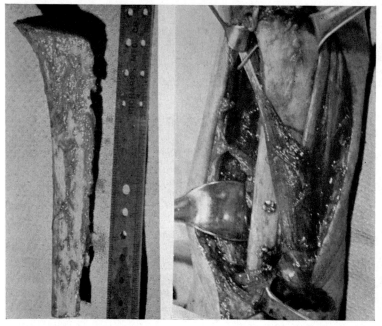

Fig. 4–K. The graft in situ. The cancellous bone fits snugly against the prepared cancellous bed of the navicular and lunate bones. Cancellous chips can be placed in the area of the step-cut attachment to the radius. The endosteal surface of the graft should face volarward to take advantage of the better blood supply. A similar graft to replace the tibia should be placed up against the fibula with the endosteal surface posterior.

Fig. 4–J. The graft ready to insert.

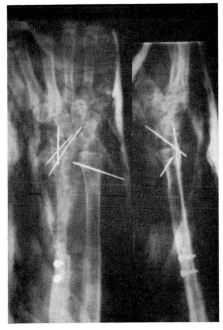

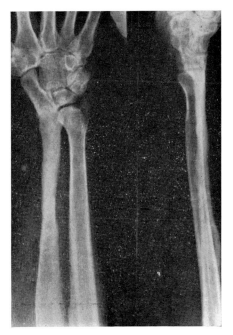

Fig. 4–L. Roentgenogram shows details of the reconstruction done at the time of the block excision in 1953, using a large autogenous graft taken from the postero-medial aspect of the proximal tibia. Immobilization was continued for one year.

Fig. 4–M. Roentgenograms four years after operation. The graft has firmly united to the navicular and lunate bones.

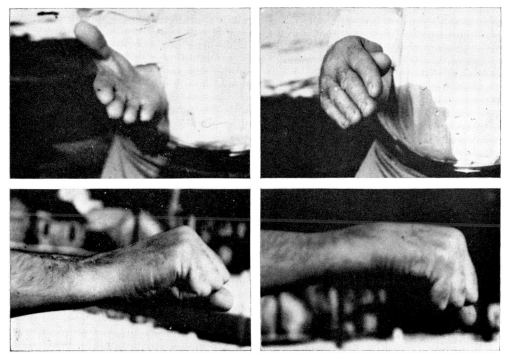

Fig. 4–N. Photograph shows the functional result sixteen years after the operation.

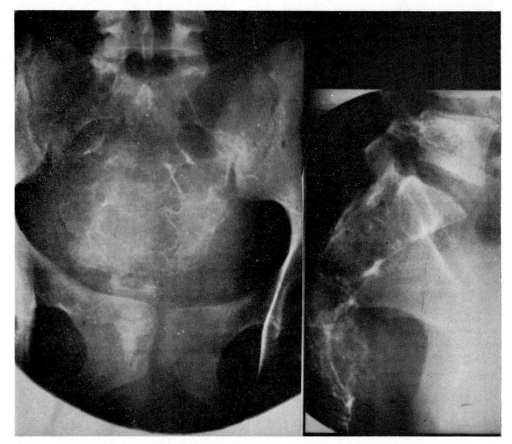

Fig. 5–A. Roentgenograms taken in 1955 show a destructive lesion of the sacrum in a twenty-one year old white female (Case 6) who had complained of increasing pain in the lower abdomen and low back for eleven months. There was a large mass extending anteriorly from the sacrum.

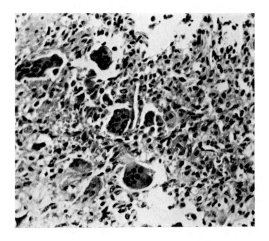

Fig. 5–B. Photomicrograph ($\times 125$) is representative of the histology at biopsy. There is an aggressive vascular stroma.

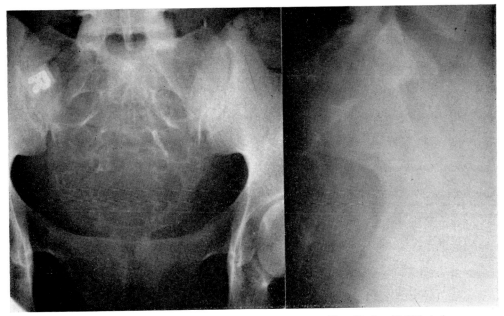

Fig. 5–C.   Roentgenograms six months after a course of irradiation (3,600 r) show a progressive extension of the lesion.

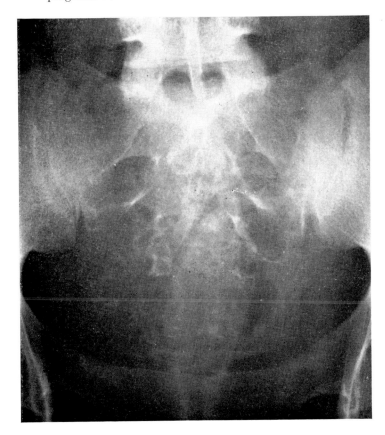

Fig. 5–D.   Roentgenogram following an attempt to curette the lesion through a posterior approach shows an iliac graft inserted into the defect. The posterior wall of the rectum was involved by the tumor.

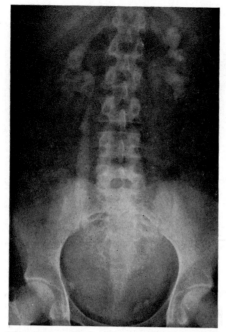

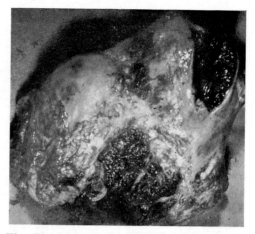

Fig. 5–F.   Photograph shows the tumor mass excised in September 1956 which was 12 cms in diameter. This required an abdomino-perineal resection, thorough curettement of the sacrum intra-abdominally, transplantation of the involved ureter into the bladder, and colostomy.

Fig. 5–E.   Roentgenogram five months after curettage shows a large grape-fruit size mass causing an obstruction of one ureter. It also obstructed the rectum.

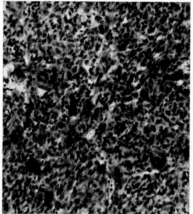

Fig. 5–G. Photomicrograph (× 75) shows the same aggressive histology as the initial biopsy.

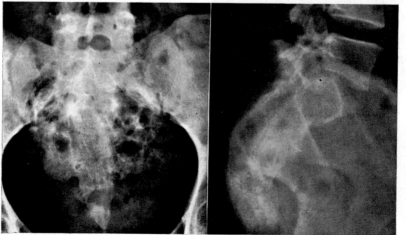

Fig. 5–H. Roentgenograms three years following excision shows the incorporation of the bone graft. There has been no recurrence during the subsequent 17 years. The patient has normal bladder control and gave birth to 2 children.

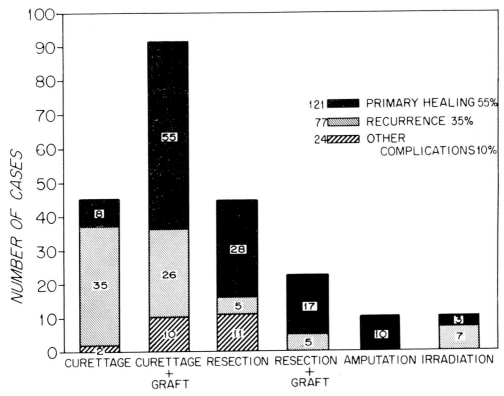

Chart **3.** This Bar Graph shows the results of primary treatment in total series of 218 giant-cell tumors.

Although the cases in which there were metastases and death can be considered malignant, there remains a sizeable group which were potentially malignant. As one can note in some of our illustrative cases (Figs. 2, 3, 4 and 5) the nature of the tumor histologically and clinically suggested a malignant potential but following ablation by extensive local resection or amputation there was no recurrence or metastases. It is our belief that the incidence of such cases is probably higher than the often-stated 10%. The question arises as to whether the specific treatment employed cured the patient of his sarcoma, or was the tumor really a benign lesion from the start despite its ominous histological appearance and aggressive behavior.

TREATMENT

An adequate open biopsy should be the initial surgical procedure. In two of our cases a needle biopsy was attempted unsuccessfully so that another open biopsy was subsequently performed. In eight cases an excisional biopsy was performed. Several of these were in the fibula and ulna, sites where the bone could be dispensed with, without loss of function. The others were in the lower end of the radius and lower end of the tibia when the joint was irreparably damaged by the tumor and some form of reconstruction was necessary to rehabilitate the extremity.

TABLE 3

SURGICAL PROCEDURES USUALLY PREFERRED BY AUTHORS

Location	Treatment
Phalanx (finger)	Amputation
Metacarpal	Resection with bone graft or amputation of affected ray
Carpal bones	Resection of carpal bones and fusion of wrist
Radius—distal end	Resection and replacement with autogenous tibial graft (postero medial, proximal end of tibia—contralateral)
Ulna—distal end	Resection
Radius—head and neck	Resection
Humerus	Resection and replacement with iliac bone graft or resection and arthroplasty or resection and arthrodesis
Humerus—Proximal end	Resection and replacement with fibula graft
Pelvis	Resection
Femur—proximal	Curettage + cancellous bone grafts and if recurrence— Resection and prosthetic replacement or arthrodesis of hip
Femur—distal end	Curettage + cancellous bone grafts and if recurrence— resection, bone graft, and arthrodesis of knee
Tibia—proximal end	Curettage + cancellous bone grafts and if recurrence— resection, bone graft, and arthrodesis of knee
Fibula—proximal end	Resection
Tibia—distal end	Resection and replacement with bone graft (postero-medial tibia—proximal end—contralateral)
Tarsal bone	Resection and arthrodesis (bone grafts)
Metatarsal	Resection—amputation if ray or bone graft
Phalanx (toe)	Amputation

Once the diagnosis is established of giant-cell tumor each case must be carefully studied as to the extent of the lesion, its biological behavior up to that time, its location relative to feasible surgical procedures, functional gains or losses anticipated, and the time and expense of a very extensive reconstruction versus a simpler procedure with a higher risk of recurrence. In our series (Chart 3) the results of the primary treatment correlated very well with the thoroughness of removal of the tumor. The authors prefer ablation when feasible, especially in the frankly malignant or aggressive case (Table 3). This is not a problem when the part affected is one which can be dispensed with such as the patella, portions of the pelvis, the upper end of the fibula, the lower end of the ulna, metacarpal bones and phalanges. Resection of the tumor-bearing portion of a bone and reconstruction with an autogenous graft is our procedure of choice in the upper or lower ends of the humerus, the lower end of the radius, and the lower ends of the tibia and fibula.

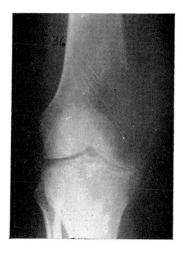

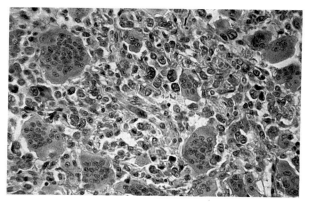

Fig. 6–B. Photomicrograph (×150) shows some hyperchromatic nuclei and mitoses in the stroma. The giant cells are diffusely arranged throughout the tumor. The lesion was classified as a giant-cell tumor, benign.

Fig. 6–A. Roentgenogram of the lower end of the right femur of a 36 year old white female shows an eccentric area of radiolucency approximately 8 cm in diameter. It extends to the subchondral cortex of the medial condyle, and has destroyed the medial cortex of the femur.

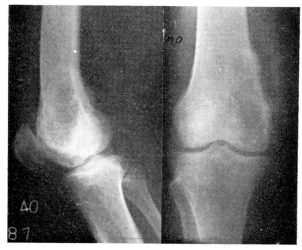

Fig. 6–C. Roentgenograms show good healing with abundant ossification 4 months following radiation therapy of 1,000 r.

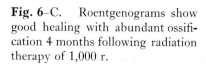

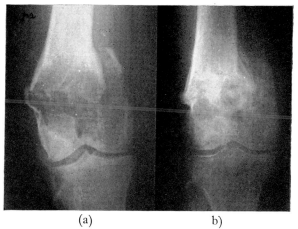

Fig. 6–D. Roentgenograms 2½ years (a) later show a pathological fracture in the tumor which has increased in size. By six months following radiation therapy (900 r) there is considerable healing-in (b). There was no pain and no evidence of progression for the next 7 years.

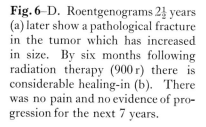

(a)   b)

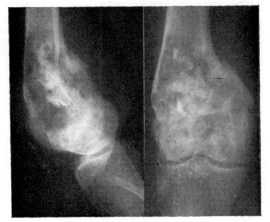

Fig. 6–E.   Roentgenograms 10 years following the time of initial biopsy show further destructive changes in the lower femur. At this time the patient had onset of severe pain.

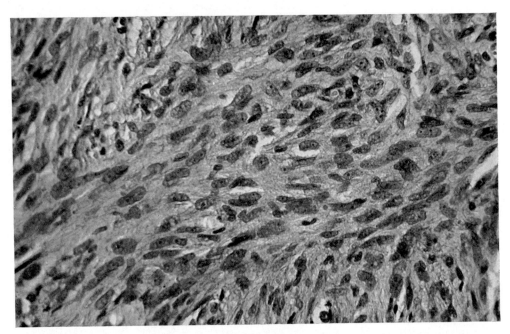

Fig. 6.–F.   Photomicrograph (×250) of the tissue show the typical characteristics of a fibrosarcoma. A mid-thigh amputation was done but the patient developed metastases and died 13 years after the onset. This case is considered to be a postradiation sarcoma, although the possibility of transformation to a more malignant lesion of foci of the original tumor cannot be ruled out.

Table 4.

RESULTS OF IRRADIATION THERAPY

	Number of Cases	Dose Range	Follow-up (Average)
Ineffective	29	1200-5320	8 yrs. (1/3 to 21)
Questionable	9	1600-4450	11 yrs. (5 to 22)
Effective	8	1400-5000	10 yrs. (3 to 27)

An aggressive or frankly malignant giant-cell tumor presents a very difficult problem in treatment when located in the proximal end of the femur and proximal end of the tibia. These locations involve the two major weight bearing joints, the hip and knee. It is in an attempt to preserve the function in these joints that the authors often prefer to do a curettage and packing with cancellous bone chips even though the risk of recurrence is higher than in doing a resection or amputation (Chart 3). The risk indicates that in a series of 91 cases treated by a large number of surgeons, many of whom were not particularly adept at this type of procedure, 55 healed primarily. To be effective curettage must remove all visible tumor tissue and must extend well beyond the tumor in all directions. This can be accomplished by using gouges and coarse-cut burrs. It can then be filled with bone chips. If there is a recurrence in the proximal femur we prefer to do a local excision and prosthetic replacement or arthrodesis. In the area of the knee joint we prefer to do a local excision and replacement with an autogenous bone graft and arthrodesis. Attempts to preserve some function of the knee by using homograft joint transplantation[40] and prosthetic appliances have occasionally been successful. Radiation therapy has at times been effective.[6,36,52] In cases of massive recurrence, infection, hemorrhage, or joint destruction amputation was necessary. In our series of 212 patients, although amputation was done as the primary treatment in only 10 patients, it was done as a secondary procedure in 46. Of 96 lesions located in the lower femur or upper tibia, 4 were amputated as the primary and 31 as secondary procedures.

Although roentgentherapy has been used successfully in some cases, its use must be counterbalanced by the danger of inducing malignant changes in the neoplasm or a postradiation sarcoma in the surrounding bone. Neither the indications for radiotherapy nor the optimum time dose relationship are well established. Generally a tumor dose of 2,500 to 3,000 r delivered over a period of 2 to 3 weeks is recommended. Occasionally second or third courses have been given.

Roentgentherapy was not particularly successful as a primary or secondary form of treatment in 46 cases in our series (Table 4). Ten patients were treated by preliminary biopsy followed by irradiation. Three of these 10, one with a tumor located in the proximal end of the femur and two whose tumor was in a lumbar vertebra, had primary healing, and they were alive and well with no evidence of recurrence 8, 5, and 8, years respectively, after diagnosis. A fourth patient with polyostotic Paget's disease and a giant-cell tumor located in the skull had primary healing of the initial tumor following irradiation, but subsequently had recurrent giant-cell tumor in various parts of the skull face, and axial skeleton. The results of radiation therapy were difficult to evaluate in the remaining 6 cases since it was given in conjunction with other therapy.

In the 46 cases irradiation was thought to be ineffective in 29 cases, possibly effective in nine, and effective in eight. We correlated the dosage of radiation therapy with the result obtained. In the ineffective group, the dosage ranged from 1,200 to 5,320 r; in the possibly effective group, it was from 1,600 to 4,450 r; and in the effective group, from 1,400 to 5,000 r. The follow-up after irradiation in these three groups was as follows: in the ineffective group, the average was 8 years and the range from 4 months to 21 years; in the possibly effective group, the average was 11 years and the range from 5 to 22 years; and in the effective group, the average was 10 years and the range from 3 to 27 years. The term "ineffective" was used to designate the radiation therapy of patients whose course after irradiation, either as primary or secondary therapy, was characterized by recurrence, metastasis, or death. "Effective" was used to designate the therapy of patients who, after primary or secondary irradiation, had healing of their tumor without complications after a follow-up of more than 3 years. "Possibly effective" designated the therapy of patients who after primary or secondary irradiation, had apparent healing of the tumor but there was insufficient evidence to determine whether the apparent cure was the result of the irradiation or of the other forms of therapy.

POSTRADIATION SARCOMA

We believe that the following criteria must be established before a case can be classified as a postradiation sarcoma following giant-cell tumor: that there should be microscopic evidence of giant-cell tumor in the primary tumor: that irradiation must have been given and that the sarcoma that subsequently developed was in the area included within the therapeutic beam: a relatively long asymptomatic latent period must have elapsed after irradiation before the clinical manifestations of sarcoma: and the sarcomatous nature of the postradiation lesion is established histologically.

In Dahlin's series of 195 giant-cell tumors, sarcomas developed in seven (19%) of the 37 patients treated by irradiation and in one of the patients treated surgically. Five of the 12 postradiation sarcomas reported by Steiner[48] occurred from 4 to 30 years following the radiation treatment of giant-cell tumors.

In our series three patients died of postradiation sarcomas, 9, 13, and 31 years after the diagnosis of giant-cell tumors was established. The primary tumor was located in the proximal end of a femur in one patient, and in the distal end of the femur in the other two (Fig. 6). The radiation dosages administered were 6,300, 13,400, and 7,400 r, respectively. Longer follow-up may increase the incidence of postradiation sarcoma in the patients reported here. Considering these factors the authors recommend radiation therapy for giant-cell tumors of the spine and sarcoma when they are inaccessible for good surgical ablation.

REFERENCES AND BIBLIOGRAPHY

1. Aegerter, E. E. Giant-cell Tumor of Bone. A Critical Survey. *Amer. J. Path.*, **23**, 283–297, 1947.
2. Barry, H. C. Sarcoma in Paget's Disease of Bone in Australia. *J. Bone Jt. Surg.*, **43-A**, 1122–1134, 1961.
3. Bloodgood, J. C. Benign Giant-cell Tumor of Bone. Its Diagnosis and Conservative Treatment. *Amer. J. Surg.*, **37**, 105–112, 1923.
4. Bloodgood, J. C. The Giant-cell Tumor of Bone and the Specter of the Metastasizing Giant-cell Tumor. *Surg., Gynec., and Obstet.*, **38**, 784–789, 1924.
5. Bullock, W. K. & Luck, J. V. Giant-cell Tumor-like Lesions of Bone. A Preliminary Report of a Pathological Entity. *Calif. Med.*, **87**, 32–36, 1957.
6. Buschke, F. & Cantril, S. T. Roentgen Therapy of Benign Giant-cell Tumor of Bone. *Cancer* **2**, 293–315, 1949.
7. Cahan, W. G., Woodward, H. Q., Higinbotham, N. L., Stewart, F. W. & Coley, B. L. Sarcoma Arising in Irradiated Bone. Report of Eleven Cases. *Cancer*, **1**, 3–29, 1948.
8. Christensen, F. C. Bone Tumors. Analysis of One Thousand Cases with Special Reference to Location, Age and Sex. *Ann. Surg.*, **81**, 1074–1092, 1925.
9. Coley, B. L. *Neoplasms of Bone and Related Conditions. Their Etiology, Pathogenesis, Diagnosis and Treatment.* Paul B. Hoeber, Inc., New York, 1949.
10. Coley, B. L. & Higinbotham, N. L. Giant-cell Tumor of Bone. *J. Bone Jt. Surg.*, **20**, 870–884, 1938.
11. Coley, W. B. Prognosis in Giant-cell Sarcoma of the Long Bones. Based Upon the End-results in a Series of 50 Cases. *Ann. Surg.*, **79**, 321–357, 1924.
12. Coley, W. B. Malignant Changes in the So-called Benign Giant-cell Tumor. *Amer. J. Surg.*, **28**, 768–820, 1935.
13. Compere, E. L. The Diagnosis and Treatment of Giant-cell Tumors of Bone. *J. Bone Jt. Surg.*, **35-A**, 822–830, 1953.
14. Cooper, Astley & Travers, B. *Surgical Essays*, Vol. 1, pp. 186–208. Cox and Son and Longman and Co., London, 1818.
15. Cruz, Miguel, Coley, B. L. & Stewart, F. W. Postradiation Bone Sarcoma. Report of Eleven Cases. *Cancer*, **10**, 72–88, 1957.
16. Dahlin, D. C., Ghormley, R. K. & Pugh, D. G. Giant-cell Tumor of Bone: Differential Diagnosis. *Proc. Mayo Clinic*, **31**, 31–42, 1956.
17. Dahlin, D. C. *Bone Tumors.* Charles C. Thomas, Springfield, Illinois, 1957.
18. Gilmer, W. S. Segmental Resection or Total Excision of Bones, pp. 1246–1248. In *Campbell's Operative Orthopaedics*, 4th Ed., C. V. Mosby, St. Louis, 1963.
19. Gold, A. M. Use of a Prosthesis for the Distal Portion of the Radius Following Resection of a Recurrent Giant-cell Tumor. *J. Bone Jt. Surg.*, **39-A**, 1374–1380, 1957.
20. Gold, A. M. Use of a Prosthesis for the Distal Portion of the Radius Following Resection of a Recurrent Giant-cell Tumor. (Follow-up Note.) *J. Bone Jt. Surg.*, **47-A**, 216–218, 1965.
21. Goldenberg, R. R. Neoplasia in Paget's Disease of Bone. *Bull. Hosp. Jt. Dis.*, **22**, 1–38, 1961.
22. Goldenberg, R. R., Campbell, C. J. & Bonfiglio, M. Giant-cell Tumor of Bone. An Analysis of Two-Hundred and Eighteen Cases. *J. Bone Jt. Surg.*, **52-A**, 519–664, 1970.
23. Goldner, L. J. & Forrest, J. S. Giant-cell Tumor of Bone. *Sth. Med. J.* (Bgham., Ala.), **54**, 121–133, 1961.
24. Haggart, G. E. & Hare, H. F. Combined Roentgen Radiation and Surgical Treatment of Large Benign Giant-cell Tumors of Bone. *Ann. Surg.*, **124**, 228–244, 1946.
25. Hatcher, C. H. The Development of Sarcoma in Bone Subjected to Roentgen or Radium Irradiation. *J. Bone Jt. Surg.*, **27**, 179–195, 1945.
26. Hutter, R. V. P., Worcester, J. N., Jr., Francis, K. C., Foote, F. W., Jr. & Stewart, F. W. Benign and Malignant Giant-cell Tumors of Bone. A Clinicopathological Analysis of the Natural History of the Disease. *Cancer*, **15**, 653–690, 1962.
27. Hutter, R. V. P., Foote, F. W., Jr., Frazell, E. L. & Francis, K. C. Giant-cell Tumors Complicating Paget's Disease of Bone. *Cancer*, **16**, 1044–1056, 1963.

28. Jaffe, H. L., Lichtenstein, Louis & Portis, R. B. Giant-cell Tumor of Bone. Its Pathologic Appearance, Grading, Supposed Variants and Treatment. *Arch. Path.* (Chicago), **30**, 993–1031, 1940.

29. Jaffe, H. L. Giant-cell Tumor (Osteoclastoma) of Bone: Its Pathologic Delimitation and the Inherent Clinical Implications. *Ann. roy. Coll. Surg.*, Engl., **13**, 343–355, 1953.

30. Jaffe, H. L. *Tumors and Tumorous Conditions of the Bones and Joints.* Lea and Febiger, Philadelphia, 1958.

31. Jewell, J. H. & Bush, L. F. "Benign" Giant-cell Tumor of Bone with a Solitary Pulmonary Metastasis. A Case Report. *J. Bone Jt. Surg.*, **46-A**, 848–852, 1964.

32. Johnson, E. W., Jr. & Dahlin, D. C. Treatment of Giant-cell Tumor of Bone. *J. Bone Jt. Surg.*, **41-A**, 895–904, 1959.

33. Kraft, G. L. & Levinthal, D. H. Acrylic Prosthesis Replacing Lower End of the Femur for Benign Giant-cell Tumor, *J. Bone Jt. Surg.*, **36-A**, 368–374, 1954.

34. Lasser, E. C. & Tetewsky, Hyman. Metastasizing Giant-cell Tumor. Report of an Unusual Case with Indolent Bone and Pulmonary Metastases. *Amer. J. Roentgenol.*, **78**, 804–811, 1957.

35. Lebert, H. Traité d'Anatomie Pathologique Générale et Spéciale. *J-B. Bailliére*, Paris, 1845.

36. Lichtenstein, Louis. *Bone Tumors.* C. V. Mosby Co., St. Louis, 1965.

37. Mnaymneh, W. A., Dudley, H. R. & Mnaymneh, L. G. Giant-cell Tumor of Bone. An Analysis and Follow-up Study of the Forty-one Cases Observed at the Massachusetts General Hospital Between 1925 and 1960. *J. Bone Jt. Surg.*, **46-A**, 63–75, 1964.

38. Nélaton, E. D'une nouvelle espéce de tumeurs bénignes des os, ou tumeurs à myéloplaxes. *Advin Delehaye*, Paris, 1860.

39. Paget, J. Lectures on Surgical Pathology, p. 446, Lindsay and Blakeston, Philadelphia, 1854.

40. Parrish, F. F. Treatment of Bone Tumors by Total Excision and Replacement with Massive Autologous and Homologous Grafts. *J. Bone Jt. Surg.*, **48-A**, 968–990, 1966.

41. Pearlman, A. W. & Friedman, Milton. Radiation Therapy of Benign Giant-cell Tumor Arising in Paget's Disease of Bone. *Amer. J. Roentgenol.*, **102**, 645–651, 1968.

42. Riley, L. H., Jr., Hartmann, W. H. & Robinson, R. A. Soft-Tissue Recurrence of Giant-cell Tumor of Bone after Irradiation and Excision. *J. Bone Jt. Surg.*, **49-A**, 365–368, 1967.

43. Russell, D. S. Malignant Osteoclastoma. And the Association of Malignant Osteoclastoma with Paget's Osteitis Deformans. *J. Bone Jt. Surg.*, **31-B**, 281–290, 1949.

44. Schajowicz, Fritz. Giant-cell Tumors of Bone (Osteoclastoma). A Pathological and Histochemical Study. *J. Bone Jt. Surg.*, **43-A**, 1–29, 1961.

45. Schajowicz, Fritz & Slullitel, Isidoro. Giant-cell Tumor Associated with Paget's Disease of Bone. A Case Report. *J. Bone Jt. Surg.*, **48-A**, 1340–1349, 1966.

46. Schurch, O. & Uehlinger, E. Experimentelles Knockensarkom nach Radiumbestrahlung bei einem Kaninchen. *Z. Krebsforsch.*, **33**, 476–484, 1931.

47. Sherman, M. S. Giant-cell Tumor of Bone, pp. 165–177. In *Tumors of Bone and Soft Tissue.* A Collection of Papers Presented at the Eighth Annual Clinical Conference on Cancer, 1963, at The University of Texas M.D. Anderson Hospital and Tumor Institute, Houston, Texas. Year Book Medical Publishers, Inc., Chicago, 1965.

48. Steiner, G. C. Postradiation Sarcoma of Bone. *Cancer*, **18**, 603–612, 1965.

49. Thomson, A. D. & Turner-Warwick, R. T. Skeletal Sarcomata and Giant-cell Tumor. *J. Bone Jt. Surg.*, **37-B**, 266–303, 1955.

50. Toriyama, S. & Abe, M. *Operative Treatment for Giant-cell Tumor—Follow-up Result of 360 Cases.* Presentation at Meeting of the American Orthopaedic Association, Denver, Colorado, 1966.

51. Virchow, R. *Die Krankaften Geschwülste*, **Vol. 2.** Hirschwald, Berlin, 1846–1865.

52. Walter, J. Giant-cell Lesions of Bone. Osteoclastoma and Giant-cell Tumour Variants. Survey of a Radiotherapeutic Series. *Clinical Radiology*, **11**, 114–124, April 1960.

53. Williams, R. R., Dahlin, D. C. & Ghormley, R. K. Giant-cell Tumor of Bone. *Cancer*, **7**, 764–773, 1954.

Discussion

Prof. van Rijssel   If I understood you, you state that out of 14 patients that you have lost from a tumor there were nine which had the suspected histology of malignancy.

Prof. Campbell   Of the 14 patients, the only time it helped us in trying to arrive at a histological classification, Dr. Goldenberg and Dr. Bonfiglio and I each went over the total series separately with all the microscopic slides. We came almost exactly the same on our histological grading, in an attempt to check this. The only time it was of interest was in the extremely malignant group, where of the 14 patients who died of tumors nine we had classified as malignant grades.

Prof. van Rijssel   I think perhaps that makes the point that grading of giant-cell tumors has some sense, and in the discussion after the former lecture someone asked—"Is it possible to see from the microscopy that a giant-cell tumour will metastasize?." I think that you can't expect it from the histology. From histology you can expect that we can predict whether the risk of metastases in a given tumour is a high risk or a very small risk, or no risk of metastases at all. I think that in the giant-cell tumours there are, let's say 10% perhaps, which have more aggressive histology; and you can expect in this group that there is a high risk of metastases. When the tumour is resected or amputated, then of course many of these tumours which could have metastases when untouched will not metastasise when they had been removed completely. So the results of the surgery for your sacral malignant tumours do not prove what the tumour prognosis is in the high risk group. But when more than half of the tumours which had a fatal outcome were placed in the high risk group from histological signs, I think this is in favour of grading of giant-cell tumours as such.

Prof. Campbell   We always look for what we consider manifestations of malignancy like we do with any tumour, and we keep that in the back of our minds along with the roentgenographic picture and biological course to see how things are going. I usually treat all giant-cell tumours rather aggressively in the beginning. By so doing in our city since 1948 we have had 21 giant-cell tumours: we had one death, and the one death was in a sacral lesion where there was pulmonary embolus of nothing but tumour. She died of that pulmonary embolus, but that is the only death we have had.

Mr. Eyre-Brook   There are five cases after all that were given a good prognosis from the pathologists; and they died of malignancy. Do you want to put it the other way around?

Prof. van Rijssel   Yes, but no pathologist pretends that he can make a difference, that he can say the risk in this group is higher than in that group. But no pathologist would say for any giant-cell tumour that this tumour will not metastasise.

Question. Have any cases resected or amputated so far produced metastases or died?

Prof. Campbell So far in our series we have not had a death from giant-cell tumours following radical ablation.

Prof. Bonfiglio Except in an instance of post-radiation sarcoma.

Prof. Schajowicz It is much simpler than we believe. If we make the diagnosis of a giant-cell tumour and have been able to carry out a resection, we have never seen a metastasis nor a recurrence. So the problem is this—to say if it is malignant or not malignant—a genuine giant-cell tumour. In most cases it is easy to do a resection—in the rib or the femur or the upper epiphysis of the tibia. But we don't often scrape it.

Prof. Campbell In closing, I would like to agree with him in every respect and I would like to say one thing which I was unable to say before about these cases. I feel that giant-cell tumour can be easily seeded, and therefore it is imperative either to do your biopsy and excision at the same time, or to do an excisional biopsy initially. If you do a biopsy first, then excision later, then for heavens sake treat the scar as though it is all contami-ted tissue. Be sure to get the initial contaminated area out of there. The second thing is that in following the case in these large grafts, I believe that one should go in about 6 months later and take your hardware out and put in some more graft material in the centre of the graft to keep these fractures from occurring such as I showed in that one case.

Paget's Sarcoma in bone—a radiological study

by

F. G. M. ROSS, J. H. MIDDLEMISS AND J. M. FITTON

SUMMARY

A series of 148 cases of histologically proven sarcomata arising in Paget's disease of bone has been collected from the Bone Tumour Registries in Bristol and Leeds and the Cancer Research Campaign Bone Tumour Panel in London. The sex ratio was 1·9 males to 1 female. The average age at which the tumour developed was 67·4 years with a peak incidence in the two decades between 60–79 years. The sarcomata arose at a slightly earlier age in males than in females, the youngest occurring at 46 years. The sarcomata occurred most frequently in the bones around the knee joint but the incidence was also high in the pelvis. The commonest histological type of tumour was osteosarcoma, the next commonest being fibrosarcoma, then primary malignant bone tumour (sarcoma) unspecified. Small numbers of giant cell sarcoma, chondrosarcoma, reticulosarcoma and malignant round cell tumours were encountered. The radiological appearances of these sarcomata were analysed. Destruction occurred in nearly 90% of the series, soft tissue tumour in 57%, sclerosis in 15%, new bone formation in 32% and fracture in 36%.

BARRY,[1] in his book on Paget's disease of bone, states that "the development of neoplastic changes in Paget's disease is well-known and provides an extraordinary feature which is of great interest to both clinicians and pathologists". It is of course of extreme interest to radiologists as well and it is because of this interest that two radiologists from Bristol and one orthopaedic surgeon from Leeds have combined to study a series of patients in whom sarcoma has supervened on Paget's disease of bone.

SOURCE OF CASES (TABLE 1)

These cases have been obtained from the Bone Tumour Registries at Bristol which has provided 55 cases and at Leeds which has provided 40 cases. The Bone Tumour Panel of the Cancer Research Campaign, who collect cases from all over the United Kingdom, has provided 53 cases. This makes a total of 148 cases which have been collected between the years of 1946 and 1972, and includes those reported by Price and Goldie[2]. It is important to note that in all these patients, the Paget's disease has been proven either histologically or radiologically and the histology of the tumour arising within the bone affected by Paget's disease has been discussed and classified by one of these panels.

41

TABLE 1

SOURCE OF CASES OF PAGET'S SARCOMA OF BONE (1946–1972)

Bone Tumour Registry* at	
Bristol	55
Leeds	40
Cancer Research Campaign Bone Tumour**	
Panel	53
Total	148

Abbreviation to: * B.T.R.
                 ** C.R.C.B.T. Panel.

SEX DISTRIBUTION (TABLE 2)

These tumours have occurred in 97 males and 51 females, giving a sex ratio of 1·9 males to 1 female. The proportion of males to females in the two cities, Bristol and Leeds, and in the Panel material is roughly the same.

TABLE 2

PAGET'S SARCOMA.   SEX DISTRIBUTION (148 CASES)

	Male	Female	Total
Bristol B.T.R.	35	20	55
Leeds B.T.R.	27	13	40
C.R.C.B.T. Panel	35	18	53
Total	97	51	148
Ratio	1·9	: 1	

AVERAGE AGE OF ONSET (TABLE 3)

The average age of the patients when the tumours were first detected in this series was 67·4 years. However, the average age for the males was slightly younger than that of the females. The earliest case occurred at the age of 46 years and the oldest at the age of 91 years. The peak incidence occurred in the two decades between the ages of 60 and 79 years. It is interesting to note that sarcoma in Paget's disease arises at an earlier age in males than in females (average ages, males 66·7 years, females 68·6 years).

TABLE 3

AGE OF ONSET OF PAGET'S SARCOMA IN YEARS (148 CASES)

	Total Series	Males	Females
Average age	67·4	66·7	68·6
Range	46–91	46–91	51–86

SITE OF THE TUMOUR AND THE SEX INCIDENCE (TABLE 4)

In this series, Paget's sarcoma arose most frequently in the femur. There were 57 cases in which the femur was affected—39% of the series. The next most commonly affected single long bone was the humerus with a total of 21 cases—14·5% of the series. The tibia was the next most frequently affected long bone and there were 16 cases in this bone—11% of the series. Of the other bones, Paget's sarcoma originated most frequently in the ilium. There were 22 cases in the ilium representing 15% of the series. In addition there

TABLE 4

PAGET'S SARCOMA. SITE OF TUMOUR AND SEX INCIDENCE (145 CASES)

| | Number of cases | | | Percentage |
	Male	Female	Total	Incidence
Femur	34	23	57	39
Humerus	13	8	21	14·5
Tibia	9	7	16	11
Ulna	1	0	1	0·75
Ilium	18	4	22	15
Skull	4	3	7	5
Scapula	5	0	5	3·5
Ischium	4	1	5	3·5
Calcaneum	3	0	3	2
Talus	1	0	1	0·75
Spine and sacrum	3	4	7	5

Long bones above the line

were small numbers of cases affecting the skull, the scapula, the ischium, the calcaneum, talus, spine and sacrum. It is interesting to note that there were no cases of Paget's sarcoma arising in the pubic bone. The total number of cases occurring in the pelvis was 27 (22 in the ilium and five in the ischium) which is nearly 19% of the series. Therefore the pelvis was the next most common site of origin of a Paget's sarcoma after the femur in this series. Another point of interest is that in the long bones the male to female incidence ratio was about 1·5 to 1, whereas in the pelvis it was 4 to 1 with males predominating.

TABLE 5

PAGET'S SARCOMA. SITE INCIDENCE WITHIN 81 LONG BONES

| | Number of cases in | | | |
	Upper third	Middle third	Lower third	Total
Femur	19	7	23	49
Tibia	9	3	3	15
Humerus	8	1	7	16
Ulna	1	0	0	1

SITE OF ORIGIN OF THE PAGET'S SARCOMA IN THE LONG BONES
(TABLE 5)

The long bones were divided into equal upper, middle and lower thirds and the site of origin of the tumour within these divisions was analysed for each bone. In the femur the commonest sites were at the upper and lower ends. In the tibia the commonest site was at the upper end and in the humerus, like the femur, the commonest sites were at the upper and lower ends. The most frequent site of origin was thus around the knee joint, in common with so many other tumours.

TABLE 6

HISTOLOGICAL TYPES OF PAGET'S SARCOMA (148 CASES)

Histological types of tumour	Number of cases			Percentage incidence
	Male	Female	Total	
Osteosarcoma	62	27	89	60
Fibrosarcoma	16	12	28	19
Primary malignant unspecified	13	8	21	14
Giant-cell sarcoma	4	0	4	3
Chondrosarcoma	1	1	2	1·3
Reticulosarcoma	2	0	2	1·3
Malignant round cell tumour	0	2	2	1·3

HISTOLOGICAL TYPES OF SARCOMA (TABLE 6)

The commonest histological type of tumour was osteosarcoma of which there were 89. This was 60% of the series. The next most common tumour was fibrosarcoma; there were 28 cases—19% of the series. The next most frequent tumour was primary malignant bone tumour (sarcoma) unspecified, with 21 cases amounting to 14% of the series. There were then small numbers of cases of giant-cell sarcoma, chondrosarcoma, reticulosarcoma and malignant round cell tumour. All these tumours were more frequent in males than in females but Table 6 shows that the proportion of males affected was higher when the tumour was an osteosarcoma than when it was a fibrosarcoma or a primary malignant bone tumour (sarcoma) unspecified.

RADIOLOGICAL APPEARANCES

The radiological features of the sarcomata arising in Paget's disease are best described by presenting cases illustrating the various radiological signs in turn. Cases of osteosarcoma are used for this purpose as all the signs are in fact produced by these tumours. Examples of the other histological types are given later for comparison with those produced by the osteosarcomata.

OSTEOSARCOMA

DESTRUCTION OF MEDULLA AND CORTEX

CASE 1. OSTEOSARCOMA OF UPPER END OF LEFT FEMUR

The radiograph of the left hip showed the typical appearance of Paget's disease of the upper end of the femur (Fig. 1(a)). The head of the femur was sclerotic. The cortex was thickened and the trabeculation was coarse. The bone was expanded and bowed laterally. An important point was that the trabeculae were sharply defined. Twenty-one months later (Fig. 1(b)) the patient had developed an osteosarcoma in this femur and the presence of the tumour was shown by the considerable destruction of the bone which it had produced. The destruction was shown by obliteration of the architecture of the bone and dissolution of the trabecular pattern. However, at this time, the remaining trabeculae were poorly defined. There was also destruction of the cortex of the lesser and greater trochanters. The commonest sign produced by an osteosarcoma was destruction within the bone and this was present in 90% of the cases.

SOFT TISSUE TUMOUR

CASE 2. OSTEOSARCOMA OF LOWER END OF RIGHT FEMUR

The next most common radiological sign was a soft tissue tumour outside the bone (Fig. 2(a)). This was shown by a mass of soft tissue density which would be seen on the medial and lateral side of the lower end of the femur which was also affected by Paget's disease. The soft tissue tumour mass was sharply outlined by a thin translucent line representing a fat line between the tumour and the surrounding soft tissues. There was also some spiculated and amorphous periosteal new bone extending into the soft tissue mass. A large amount of destruction within the lower end of the femur was also shown. In the lateral view (Figs. 2(b) and (c)) the soft tissue tumour could be seen extending out from the back of the bone with fine irregular calcification within it. This view also showed another radiological sign; there may be displacement of surrounding structures by the tumour. The lower end of the femoral artery and the popliteal artery were shown by mural calcification and the popliteal artery was clearly displaced backwards by the tumour. The commonest structures to be displaced by a tumour mass were the surrounding radiolucent intermuscular planes. These became displaced and convex away from the affected bone but they tended to remain remarkably well-defined. Of course, when the tumour actually infiltrated across these planes then the radiolucent line was obliterated.

CASE 3. OSTEOSARCOMA OF THE LEFT ISCHIUM

The soft tissue tumour may not be so well-defined as it was in the last case. In Case 3 there was Paget's disease of the left pubic bone and rather sclerotic Paget's disease of the left ischium and ilium (Fig. 3). There was both cortical and medullary destruction of the ischium extending up round the region of the acetabulum. Below the neck of the femur there was irregular calcification in the soft tissues which inferred that there was tumour in the soft tissues though no soft tissue mass could be seen on the radiograph.

46

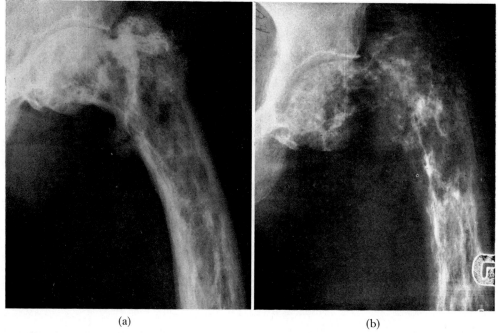

(a)   (b)

Fig. 1.   Bristol B.T.R. Case No. 705. Female aged 57 years. Osteosarcoma of the
upper end of the left femur. Radiograph of left hip. (a) Prior to the development of
the osteosarcoma showing Paget's disease of the femur. (b) Twenty-one months
later, considerable destruction of the neck and upper portion of the femoral shaft
due to the osteosarcoma which has developed within the Paget's disease.

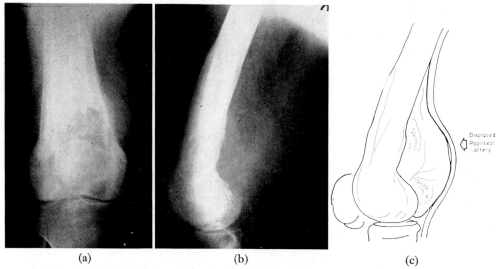

(a)   (b)   (c)

Fig. 2.   Bristol B.T.R. Case No. 406. Male aged 66 years. Osteosarcoma of the lower
end of the right femur. (a) Anteroposterior view. Paget's disease of lower end of the
femur with large central area of destruction and surrounding soft tissue tumour.
Amorphous and spiculated periosteal new bone on the medial side. (b) and (c) Lateral
view. Femoral and popliteal arteries outlined by medial calcification. Popliteal artery
displaced posteriorly by the soft tissue tumour mass.

New Bone Formation

CASE 4. OSTEOSARCOMA OF LOWER END OF LEFT FEMUR

The next two commonest signs were new bone formation and pathological fracture. The new bone formation took the form of sclerosis within the bone or ossification within the extra-osseous tumour mass. Both of these signs were shown in the radiograph of the lower end of the femur of Case 4 (Fig. 4). There was dense spiculated and amorphous new bone formation within the soft tissue tumour which surrounded the lower end of the femur, and some sclerosis within the bone itself. There was a pathological fracture across the upper part of the affected area. This radiograph also showed a radiolucency extending up the shaft from the site of the tumour and ending in a sharply-defined V directed up the shaft. This is a typical appearance of active Paget's disease.[3,4]

CASE 5. OSTEOSARCOMA OF RIGHT HUMERUS

This patient had an injury to the right arm and shortly after it the first radiograph (Fig. 5(a)) was taken. Sclerotic Paget's disease affecting the whole length of the humerus was shown. There was an area of dense sclerosis in the medulla of the middle third of the humerus with some irregular calcification in the soft tissues lateral to it. In a further radiograph (Fig. 5(b)) taken a fortnight later, a soft tissue tumour had developed at the same site and the calcification which was within the tumour, had increased in extent. A fortnight later still (Fig. 5(c)) the soft tissue tumour and the area of calcification were very much larger and the sclerosis within the bone had also increased in amount. Biopsy showed this tumour to be an osteosarcoma. In this case radiologically the tumour within the bone was shown by sclerosis only, and there has been no evidence of bone destruction whatsoever.

Pathological Fracture

CASE 6. OSTEOSARCOMA OF LOWER END OF LEFT FEMUR

Thirty-six per cent of the patients in this series showed pathological fracture at the site of the tumour in the bone affected by Paget's disease. Most of the pathological fractures were transverse or nearly transverse in direction. This patient presented with a fracture of the lower end of the femur (Fig. 6(a) and (b)) and the radiograph also revealed destruction of the cortex and medulla in the adjacent part of the distal fragment.

Metastases to Bone and Lungs

CASE 7. FRACTURE OF PELVIS. LATER DEVELOPMENT OF OSTEOSARCOMA OF LEFT FEMUR AND SUBSEQUENT BONE METASTASES

Not every patient having a fracture through bone which is the site of Paget's disease will develop a sarcoma at the site of the fracture.[5] This patient, who had extensive Paget's disease throughout the pelvis and the upper end of the left femur, was involved in a car accident. He sustained a fracture through the left ilium extending down to the region of the acetabulum. There was also a fracture of the left ischium (Fig. 7(a)). A radiograph nearly 2 years later (Fig. 7(b)) showed that these fractures had united and that some deformity of the ilio-pectineal line and ischium was all that remained to indicate their former site. Six weeks later the patient had pain in the left knee and a

48

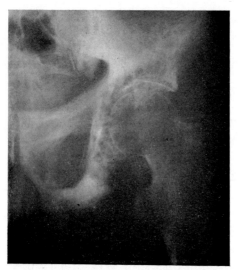

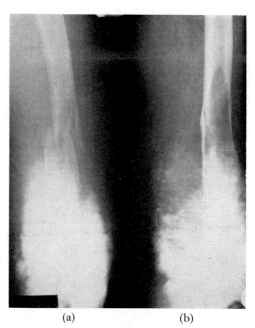

(a)　　　　　　　　　　(b)

Fig. 3. Leeds B.T.R. Case No. 8. Male aged 51 years. Osteosarcoma of the left ischium. Extensive Paget's disease of the pelvis, sclerotic in the left ischium. Destruction in the left ischium and region of the acetabulum with irregular calcification in the soft tissues below the neck of the femur.

Fig. 4. Bristol B.T.R. Case No. 2175. Female aged 62 years. Osteosarcoma of the lower end of the left femur, osteoblastic in type. (a) Lateral view. (b) Antero-posterior view. Pathological fracture. Well-defined V-shaped translucency extending up the shaft of the femur, characteristic of Paget's disease.

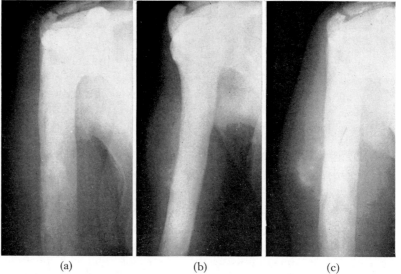

(a)　　　　　　　　　　(b)　　　　　　　　　　(c)

Fig 5. Leeds B.T.R. Case No. 161. Female aged 64 years. Osteosarcoma of the right humerus. Sclerotic Paget's disease of the whole length of the humerus. (a) 12.5.61. (b) 26.5.61. (c) 9.6.61. Rapid development of a soft tissue tumour containing calcification on the lateral aspect of the middle third of humerus with a sclerotic area within the underlying bone.

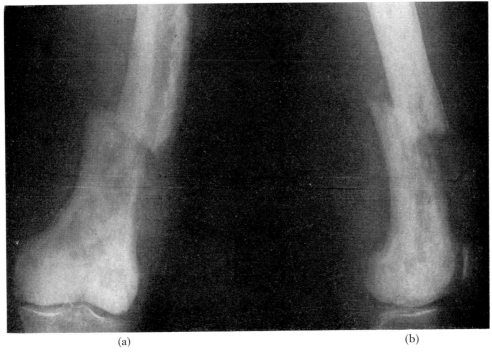

(a)   (b)

Fig. 6. Bristol B.T.R. Case No. 1332 (a) antero-posterior (b) lateral views. Female aged 72 years. Osteosarcoma of the lower end of the left femur. Sclerotic type of Paget's disease with pathological fracture, oblique in type. Medullary and cortical destruction in the lateral and anterior part of the distal fragment extending down from the fracture line. Soft tissue swelling.

radiograph (Fig. 7(c) and (d)) revealed that there was a large amount of destruction with some sclerosis in the lower end of the femur, which was also affected by Paget's disease. This therefore was a case of a Paget's sarcoma developing within a bone remote from the one which had previously been fractured. The patient subsequently had a disarticulation through the hip joint. Five months later (Fig. 7(e)) areas of destruction were shown in the region of the acetabulum, the left ischium and pubic bone and the right ilium due to metastases. At least 23 of the patients in the series showed metastases to other bones and this represents 16% of the series. The metastases were always to bones affected by Paget's disease.

CASE 8. OSTEOSARCOMA OF LEFT ISCHIUM WITH PULMONARY METASTASES

The radiograph of the hip of this patient with Paget's disease (Fig. 8(a)) showed destruction of the left ischium. Surrounding the area of destruction there was a soft tissue tumour containing fine calcification. The malignant nature of this tumour was confirmed by the presence of early metastases in the lungs (Fig. 8(b)). Metastases to the lungs were present in 55 patients in the series.

c*

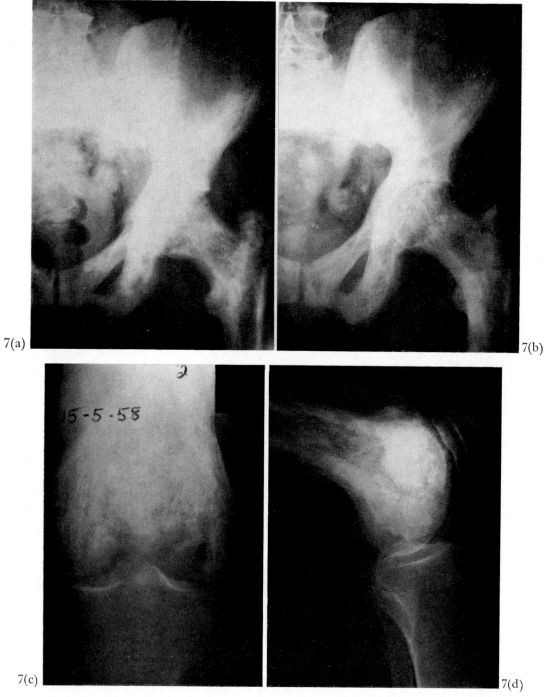

7(a)

7(b)

7(c)

7(d)

Fig. 7. Bristol B.T.R. Case No. 1309. Female aged 65 years. Osteosarcoma of the lower end of the femur. (a) Pelvis, 9.5.56. Traumatic fracture of left ilium and ischium. Extensive Paget's disease of the pelvis and left femur. (b) Pelvis, 25.2.58. The fractures have united. (c) and (d) Left knee, 15.5.58. Paget's disease of lower end of femur. Large area of destruction with some sclerosis in the intercondylar region of the femur due to the development of an osteosarcoma. (Fig. 7 continued on next page).

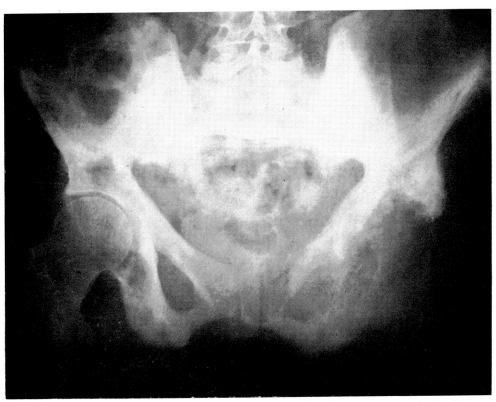

Fig. 7. (e)　　Pelvis, 13.10.58. Five months after disarticulation through the hip joint. Multiple osteolytic metastases in the Paget's disease of the left side of the pelvis and in the right ilium and sclerotic new bone above the left acetabulum.

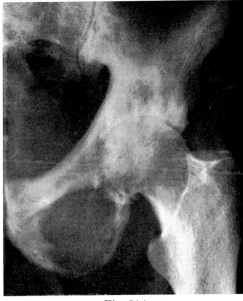

Fig. 8(a)

Fig. 8.　　Bristol B.T.R. Case No· 1885. Male aged 60 years. Osteo-sarcoma of the left ischium. (a) Left hip. Extensive Paget's disease of the left side of the pelvis with destruction of the left ischium and some calcification in a surrounding soft tissue mass. (Fig. 8 continued on next page).

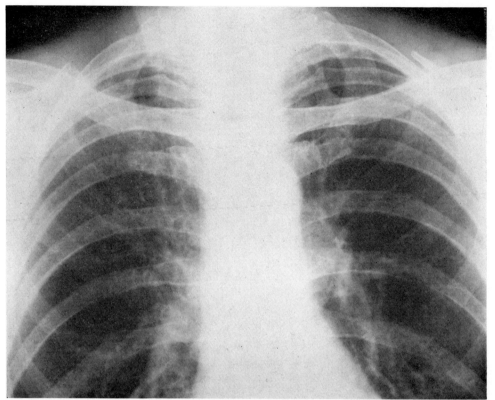

Fig. 8. (b) Chest radiograph taken at the same time showed multiple early metastases in the lungs.

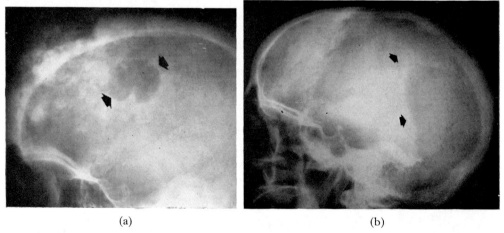

(a)   (b)

Fig. 9.   Bristol B.T.R. Case No. 212. Osteosarcoma of the left side of the calvarium. (a) Lateral view. Paget's disease of the frontal and parietal bone. Active stage of Paget's disease anteriorly in the frontal bone. A well-defined reniform area of destruction in the posterior frontal and anterior parietal region produced by an osteosarcoma (arrows). (b) Typical osteoporosis circumscripta of Paget's disease of the skull (arrows) in another patient.

Unusual Radiological Appearances

Case 9.   Osteosarcoma of the Vault of the Skull

In patients with Paget's disease of the skull, the area of destruction produced by a malignant tumour tends to be much more sharply defined radiologically than is usual in the long bones. In Case 9 the frontal and parietal bones were affected by Paget's disease, the active stage being evident in the frontal bone where there were ill-defined areas of translucency. However there was also a sharply defined reniform shaped area of destruction posteriorly in the frontal bone produced by an osteosarcoma.

This sharply defined destruction produced by a malignant tumour must be distinguished from the appearances of osteoporosis circumscripta which is the active stage of Paget's disease in the skull (Fig. 9(b)). In osteoporosis circumscripta the area of destruction is usually much larger than that produced by an osteosarcoma when first seen. Osteoporosis circumscripta is of course not a painful lesion and is not associated with an overlying tumour mass.

Case 10.   Osteosarcoma of right femur

In this patient there was Paget's disease of the lower end of the femur but there was also destruction of the cortex laterally with underlying destruction of the medulla Fig. 10(a). Within the area of destruction deep in the bone there was a small density and this was thought to be due to a sequestrum. Two months later (Fig. 10(b)) the tumour had burst out of the bone indicated by the presence of a large soft tissue tumour surrounding the lower end of the femur with irregular and spiculated bone within it. The destruction of the cortex and medulla had increased but the density previously seen within the bone was still present.

Further Radiological Investigations which may be Undertaken when Diagnosis is not Conclusive on the Original Examination

Doubt may arise as to the presence of a malignant tumour within the portion of a bone affected by Paget's disease when the trabecular pattern of a relatively small area is different from that of the surrounding Paget's disease but no certain localized area of destruction nor sclerosis can be identified. Four courses of action are possible in these circumstances from the radiological standpoint. Multiple oblique views with varying penetration can be taken or tomography can be performed in the hope of revealing an area of destruction. Alternatively a follow-up radiograph may be taken several weeks later and it is very likely to reveal progressive destruction or increased sclerosis if a tumour was present originally. Arteriography may be very helpful in giving a quick solution to this problem.

Case 11.   Osteosarcoma lower end of left femur

The destruction produced by the tumour within the bone may not be very convincing on the radiograph taken early after the onset of symptoms. In Case 11, the radiograph of the lower end of the femur (Fig. 11(a)) showed the typical spongy type of Paget's disease but in the intercondylar region there was an area where the pattern was very different from the rest of the affected bone. It was evident that there could well be

54

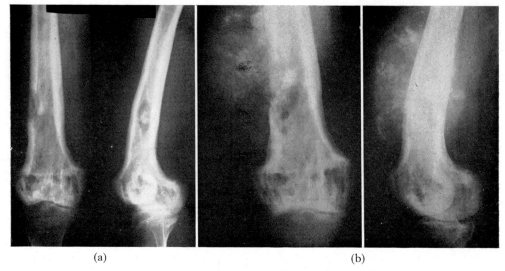

(a)   (b)

Fig. 10.   Bristol B.T.R. Case No. 2325. Female aged 73 years. Osteosarcoma of the lower end of the right femur. Antero-posterior and lateral views. (a) 27.2.67. Paget's disease of the lower end of the femur. Sequestrum within central area of destruction. (b) Two months later. Large soft tissue tumour with irregular calcification within it has developed. Displacement of soft tissue planes by tumour. Increased intramedullary destruction.

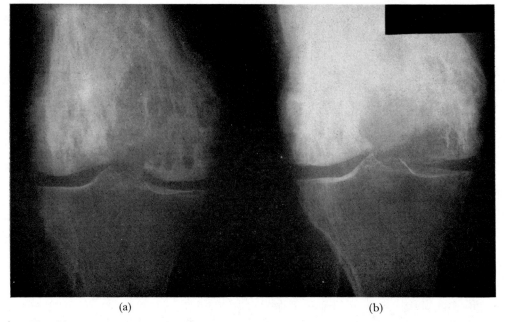

(a)   (b)

Fig. 11.   Bristol B.T.R. Case No. 440. Female aged 55 years. Osteosarcoma of lower end of right femur. Paget's disease clearly shown in the lower end of the femur. (a) 22.10.51. Early destruction in the intercondylar region. (b) 7.12.51. Area of destruction more evident.

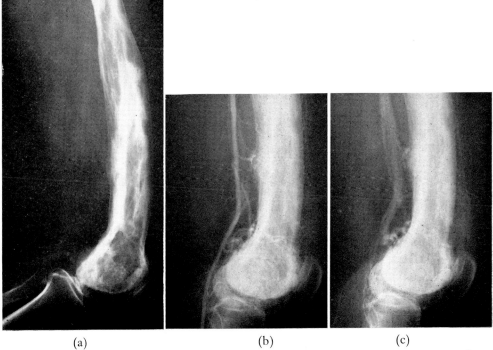

(a)   (b)   (c)

Fig. 12. Bristol B.T.R. Case No. 1599. Female aged 51 years. Osteosarcoma of lower end of left femur. Extensive Paget's disease of the lower two-thirds of the femur. (a) Lateral view of femur. Different trabecular pattern at lower end of bone from that above it. (b) Arterial phase of femoral arteriogram. Pathological circulation through the osteosarcoma at the lower end of the femur and its extension anteriorly outside the bone. Shunting of contrast medium superiorly through the bone affected by Paget's disease and inferiorly through the osteosarcoma. (c) Later venous phase of the arteriogram. Tumour "blush". Rapid shunting of contrast medium into the upper part of the femoral and popliteal veins. See text for full description.

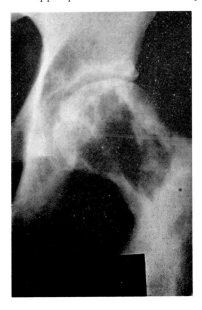

Fig. 13. Bristol B.T.R. Case No. 504. Male aged 49 years. Fibrosarcoma of the upper end of the left femur. Paget's disease of the left ischium and upper end of femur. Destruction in the head and neck of the femur.

destruction in this region. In fact a radiograph taken 6 weeks later (Fig. 11(b)) demonstrated that the destruction in the intercondylar region had increased to such an extent that it was easily visible. In this type of case, tomography applied early in the disease may enable destruction deep in the bone to be revealed without any discomfort to the patient and it is therefore well worth applying.

CASE 12. OSTEOSARCOMA OF THE LOWER END OF THE FEMUR, DEMONSTRATED BY ARTERIOGRAPHY

The lateral view of the lower half of the left femur in this patient (Fig. 12(a)) showed the coarse trabecular pattern of Paget's disease right down the shaft but at the lower end there was an area in which the trabecular pattern was different, giving an appearance as if it had been partially erased. There was doubt as to whether there was a tumour at the lower end of the femur and so arteriography was performed. Enlarged branches of the femoral artery (Fig. 12(b)) supplied the lower end of the bone and the vascular pattern within the bone was completely different from that higher up the shaft of the femur. Figure 12(c) showed a late stage of the examination in which there was a tumour blush within the bone where the tumour had taken up the contrast medium. The rapid shunting of the contrast medium by the tumour and also the bone which was the site of the

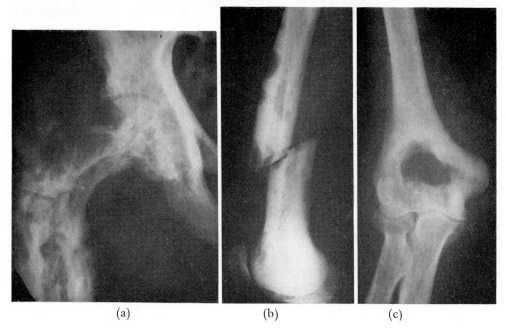

(a)   (b)   (c)

Fig. 14. Bristol B.T.R. Case No. 529. Female aged 59 years. Fibrosarcoma of the upper end of the right femur with metastases to the lower end of the right femur and the right humerus. (a) Right hip, 2.4.52. Destruction in the head and neck of the femur. Multiple cortical fractures. (b) 3.10.52, Lateral view of lower end of right femur. Paget's disease and oblique pathological fracture. Multiple well-defined areas of destruction due to metastases. (c) Same time. Antero-posterior view of right elbow. Paget's disease of the lower end of the humerus and a large area of destruction in the lower end due to metastasis.

Paget's disease into the popliteal and femoral veins was also well shown. This was the typical pathological circulation of a malignant tumour and the arteriogram therefore confirmed the presence of a malignant tumour in the lower end of the femur. It also revealed that the abnormal circulation extended anteriorly outside the bone (Fig. 12(b) and (c)) and therefore the tumour was not confined to the bone. Arteriography is very valuable when it shows a typical malignant circulation indicating the presence of a malignant tumour. There are, however, a small percentage of malignant tumours[6] which are avascular and do not show this pathological circulation. Therefore a negative result on arteriography does not exclude the presence of a malignant tumour.

RADIOLOGICAL APPEARANCES PRODUCED BY TUMOURS OF HISTOLOGICAL TYPES OTHER THAN OSTEOSARCOMA

Analysis showed that it was not possible to determine the histological type of tumour from the radiological appearances except for the tumour which produced dense sclerosis within the bone and a lot of new bone or calcification in the soft tissue mass, this tumour invariably being an osteosarcoma.

FIBROSARCOMA

Fibrosarcoma was the second commonest tumour and it occurred in 19% of the series.

CASE 13. FIBROSARCOMA OF THE NECK OF THE LEFT FEMUR

A radiograph of the left hip (Fig. 13) showed Paget's disease of the left ischium and upper end of the left femur with an area of fairly well-defined medullary destruction in the neck and head of the femur and some destruction of the superior cortex of the femoral neck.

CASE 14. FIBROSARCOMA OF THE UPPER END OF THE RIGHT FEMUR WITH METASTASES TO THE LOWER END OF THE SAME FEMUR AND THE HUMERUS

The radiograph of the pelvis (Fig. 14(a)) of this patient showed extensive Paget's disease of the pelvic bones and of the upper end of the right femur with cortical fractures in the upper end of the femur. There was also ill-defined destruction in the neck of the femur extending into the greater trochanter. The destruction in this case and in the previous case showed no distinguishing features that would lead to a diagnosis of fibrosarcoma. Six months later the patient had pain in the right thigh and a radiograph (Fig. 14(b)) showed that there was Paget's disease of the lower end of the femur through which area there was a pathological fracture and also multiple areas of sharply defined medullary and cortical destruction due to metastases. At the same time the patient had pain in the right elbow and on the radiograph (Fig. 14(c)) there was a destructive lesion, due to another metastasis, in the lower end of the humerus which was also affected by Paget's disease.

58

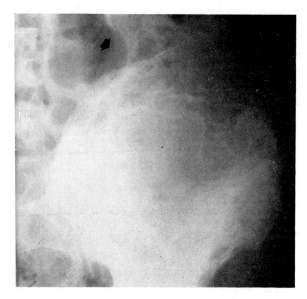

Fig. 15. Leeds B.T.R. Case No. 163. Male aged 49 years. Primary malignant bone tumour (sarcoma) unspecified of left ilium. Extensive Paget's disease of the left side of the pelvis with destruction in the region of the iliac crest and adjacent part of the blade of the ilium, soft tissue tumour (arrow) and displacement of fragment of the iliac crest into the soft tissue tumour.

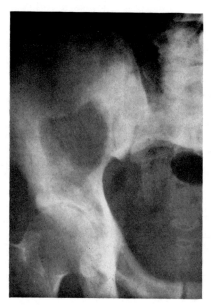

Fig. 16. Bristol B.T.R. Case No. 155. Male aged 71 years. Giant-cell sarcoma of the right ilium. Extensive Paget's disease of the right side of the pelvis. Large area of destruction in the right ilium.

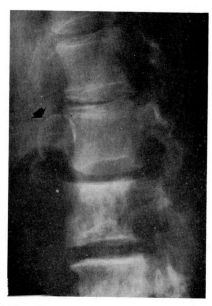

Fig. 17. C.R.C.B.T. Panel Case No. 601. Female aged 61 years. Chondrosarcoma of LV3. Paget's disease of LV3. Destruction of the posterior aspect of the body and pedicle. Calcified aneurysm of renal artery (arrow).

PRIMARY MALIGNANT BONE TUMOUR (SARCOMA) UNSPECIFIED

This tumour was the third commonest histological type and it accounted for 14% of the series.

CASE 15. PRIMARY MALIGNANT BONE TUMOUR (SARCOMA) UNSPECIFIED OF THE LEFT ILIUM

This patient had Paget's disease of the left ilium involving the crest (Fig. 15) and an area of destruction beneath it. There was a soft tissue tumour extending up from the iliac crest and a bit of the iliac crest medially had been elevated by the tumour. Again there was no feature in the radiological appearances which would help to indicate the histological type of this tumour.

GIANT CELL SARCOMA

There were four cases of giant cell sarcoma arising in Paget's disease in this series.

CASE 16. GIANT-CELL SARCOMA OF THE RIGHT ILIUM

In this case the radiograph showed extensive Paget's disease of the right side of the pelvis (Fig. 16) and the sacrum with an area of well-defined destruction in the blade of the right ilium which was affected by the Paget's disease. There were no features which would raise the suspicion that the histological type of tumour was anything other than an osteosarcoma.

CHONDROSARCOMA

In two patients chondrosarcoma developed within the Paget's disease.

CASE 17. CHONDROSARCOMA OF LV3

The lateral radiograph of this patient's spine (Fig. 17) showed Paget's disease of the body of LV3. There was well-defined destruction of the posterior aspect of the body with some destruction in the region of the pedicle. Again there were no distinguishing radiological features that would suggest the possibility that the tumour was a chondrosarcoma rather than an osteosarcoma.

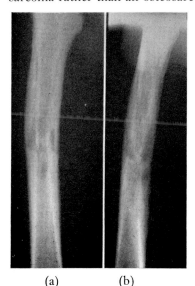

(a)   (b)

Fig. 18. Leeds B.T.R. Case No. 357. Male aged 59 years. Reticulosarcoma of the right femur. (a) Anteroposterior view. (b) Lateral view. Paget's disease. Several areas of destruction grouped together in the middle third of the shaft. In (a) a small periosteal reaction shown on the medial side of the femur.

RETICULOSARCOMA

There were two cases of reticulosarcoma developing within the Paget's disease in the series.

CASE 18. RETICULOSARCOMA OF THE RIGHT FEMUR

The radiograph of the right femur (Fig. 18) showed extensive Paget's disease of the shaft. There was a group of small areas of destruction in the middle of the shaft with some periosteal reaction on the medial side of the bone.

MALIGNANT ROUND CELL TUMOUR (UNSPECIFIED)

CASE 19. MALIGNANT ROUND CELL TUMOUR (UNSPECIFIED) OF THE RIGHT FEMUR

This patient had the sclerotic type of Paget's disease in the upper end of the right femur with a transverse pathological fracture through it. (Fig. 19(a)). Just distal to the lesser trochanter there was also a well-defined area of destruction involving the bone on each side of the fracture line. On the proximal side of the fracture the inner aspect of the lateral cortex of the femur was destroyed. The fracture was subsequently fixed by insertion of an intra-medullary nail and plating of the lateral aspect of the shaft. But 3 months later (Fig. 19(b)) there had been considerable increase in the amount of

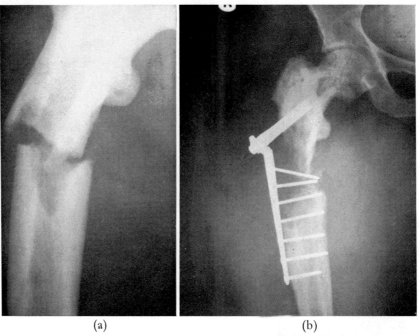

(a)   (b)

Fig. 19.   Bristol B.T.R. Case No. 2360. Female aged 77 years. Malignant round cell tumour (unspecified) upper end of right femur. Paget's disease of the upper half of the femur. (a) 3.4.67. Transverse pathological fracture through an area of well-defined medullary destruction. (b) 26.7.67. Fracture had been treated by insertion of an intramedullary nail and plate. Large soft tissue tumour now present around the upper end of the femur with considerable destruction of the bone around the fracture site.

destruction within the bone and there was now a huge soft tissue swelling around the bone with displacement of the inter-muscular planes.

SUMMARY OF RADIOLOGICAL FEATURES OF PAGET'S SARCOMA
(TABLE 7)

The radiological signs in 133 cases of Paget's sarcoma for whom there were analysable radiographs are given in Table 7. Soft tissue tumour occurred in 78 cases which is 57% of the series. Destruction, either cortical or medullary, occurred in nearly 90% of the cases. New bone formation, appearing as sclerosis in the bone, was seen in 15% of the cases and new bone formation, including calcification, outside the parent bone was seen in 32% of the patients. Fracture was present in 48 cases which is 36% of the series and sequestra were seen in two patients which is 1·5% of the series.

TABLE 7

PAGET'S SARCOMA. ANALYSIS OF RADIOLOGICAL SIGNS IN ADDITION TO THE PAGET'S DISEASE (133 CASES)

	Number of cases	Percentage incidence
Soft tissue tumour	78	57
Destruction		
Cortical	116	87
Medullary	119	89
New bone formation		
Sclerosis	20	15
Outside parent bone	42	32
Fracture	48	36
Sequestra	2	1·5

ACKNOWLEDGMENTS

The authors are indebted to many colleagues who have referred their cases to the Bristol and Leeds Bone Tumour Registries. The former is supported by generous grants from the Cancer Research Campaign. Thanks are also due to the members of the Cancer Research Campaign Bone Tumour Panel for permission to include the cases from the Bone Tumour Panel records in the present study.

REFERENCES

1. Barry, H. C. *Paget's Disease of Bone*, page 136. E. & S. Livingstone, Edinburgh & London, 1969.
2. Price, C. H. G. & Goldie, W. Paget's Sarcoma of Bone. *Journal of Bone and Joint Surgery*, **51-B**, 205–224, 1969.
3. Brailsford, J. F. *The Radiology of Bones and Joints*, 4th ed., page 613. J. & A. Churchill, London. 1948.
4. Murray, R. O. & Jacobson, H. G. *The Radiology of Skeletal Disorders*, page 698. Churchill Livingstone, Edinburgh & London, 1971.
5. Barry, H. C. *Paget's Disease of Bone*, page 120. E. & S. Livingstone, Edinburgh & London, 1969.
6. Strickland, B. The Value of Arteriography in the Diagnosis of Bone Tumours. *Brit. J. Radiol.*, **32**, 705, 1959.

Discussion

Professor Duthie I notice you showed one illustration of arteriography, but this has proved very unsatisfactory in any form of bone malignancy as regards showing the location of the lesion or the extent of the spread within it. I wonder if you have ever repeated your arteriography at intervals of say 24 hours and 96 hours in order to see if these pictures and patterns are reproducible for the same tumour? Have you ever used arteriography to show up occult lesions which have then gone on to become manifest tumour demonstrated either by histology or radiology?

Dr. Ross First of all in the cases on which we ourselves have performed arteriography I think we have found it to be a very reliable method of examination. Admittedly, in any one particular centre unfortunately one gets relatively few tumours to examine. It is interesting that in these 148 cases, only two of the patients had actually had arteriography performed on them, and equally interesting that none of them had had tomography, which in my opinion is a very useful method of examination. I think that when it is a positive case with abnormal circulation by arteriography then it is a very reliable sign, and we use it for identification of the malignancy if present. I think it is a very good indication to the surgeon as to where in the bone he should take his biopsy by showing the actual tumour site. In many cases arteriograms show the tumour is very much bigger than what one suspects. I must admit that sometimes it is difficult for us to do arteriograms on these patients because the orthopaedic surgeons are so anxious to get on with the biopsy and the treatment of the patient. When this situation arises, we tend to do arteriography on the operating table, just before the biopsy is done, and then of course there is no opportunity to repeat it, because the lesion has been interfered with by the surgeon afterwards. For demonstrating osseous metastases or other bone tumours I don't think we have done this; but on several occasions when one has done aortograms for other lesions or possible tumours such as in the kidneys, one has shown up metastases in surrounding bones.

Professor Bonfiglio My question concerns the 16% of your cases that had metastases in other bones—and they always go to "Pagetoid" bone. Are they in fact in your opinion metastases or are they primary tumours arising from mulitiple sites? This has always bothered me.

Dr. Ross A very good question, and this allows me to say something about the survival of these patients. We did analyse the survival and for osteosarcoma the survival was 11·3 months average survival, and in fibrosarcoma 22·5 months. Now at the end of one year only 32% of the patients were still alive: at the end of two years only 7% of the patients were still alive, and the prognosis is absolutely ghastly. As the tumour has such a very short natural history it seems to me very difficult to be able to differentiate as to what is a metastasis and what are primary tumours. I don't know how this can be done myself. I would like to know if anyone else has some idea, because many of these cases suggest that they are of multiple origin, but they could well be metastases and I am pretty certain they are.

Professor Campbell   I would like to ask a question along the same lines. Can the multi-focal bone tumours arising in Paget's disease be different types of sarcomas in the same patient? For example, can you have osteosarcoma on one side with chondrosarcoma on the other, or fibrosarcoma with giant-cell tumour in another bone.

Dr. Ross   No, not in the series that I have been able to look at. I haven't seen that.

Dr. Jacobs   I would like to congratulate you on the quality of your reproductions. I say this because of a sign we have found now on three occasions—that the malignancy wasn't evident at the initial examination when the patients sustained a fracture through the area of Paget's disease. I grant you that some of our films may not have been of the highest quality, being femoral X-rays in old people. But I notice that Barry, who you quote, has also made that point. I wonder if you have come across a case where the malignancy was missed on the initial examination, or where there was merely thought to be a pathological fracture through Paget's disease? The other question I would like to ask is about histological types. I have seen it quoted that giant-cell tumours can complicate Paget's disease, some of which may not be malignant. Is that a myth or is it true, Dr. Ross?

Dr. Ross   Taking the last question first. We definitely excluded all giant-cell tumours from this particular study and they certainly are reported as you know. Barry reports them, but we have excluded giant-cell tumours from this series. As not all these cases arose in Bristol and Leeds, I can say with confidence that in some of them in fact the primary tumour was missed on the first radiograph. With many of them I think you have got to look very carefully indeed and even with hindsight, knowing the tumour is there, actually to be able to see it. We have a very nice one where the biopsy was taken across the fracture, and sitting slap in the middle of it was this tiny sclerotic area where the radiograph showed the osteosarcoma. Months later you can see this bursting right out of the bone producing a huge sclerotic tumour. Certainly the answer is "Yes".

Mr. Wilson   Were any scans done in these cases?

Dr. Ross   Not recorded in these patients, "No".

Dr. Makley   I would like to say from a clinical standpoint that the increase in pain in a patient with a previously painless Paget's disease is usually a pretty good indication that the Paget's disease has become malignant. I would like to ask if you have been able to correlate the onset of Paget's disease with an increase in the blood alkaline phosphatase, particularly in those which are monostotic which ordinarily would be expected to have a rather low alkaline phosphatase level? Also how many patients with monostotic Paget's were in your series?

Dr. Ross   The last question first. I think virtually all the patients were polyostotic

Paget's disease; there wasn't one that I could really say was in fact monostotic. Of course the records tend to be a little bit difficult to follow, and you may not get all the information, but the implication of all the records was that there was polyostotic disease.

So far as pain is concerned, the history ranges from one patient who actually was putting on his trousers and felt a click in his thigh. He went to the hospital where they radiographed him, and there was a sarcoma in his Paget's disease. It wasn't until a fortnight after he had been in hospital that he started complaining of pain. There was another patient who had six years of pain, and he was so bad with the pain in his back and down his leg that actually for the last three years he was walking around on crutches. Then I think the pain got a little bit worse, and he was radiographed again, and this showed a sarcoma in what had been previously an ordinary common or garden Paget's disease. The sarcoma had developed then. It is a very variable thing.

Concerning the alkaline phosphatase—I regret only twenty patients had had an estimation done, and none of them showed a rise with certainty during the origin of the tumour. I don't think Barry subscribes to this—that the alkaline phosphatase level is of any value at all. Sometimes it is low and sometimes it is high. I don't think it is of value.

Extra-corporeal irradiation of bone tumours

by

H. J. BRENNER and E. SPIRA

SUMMARY

With no survivors amongst 40 patients with osteogenic sarcoma treated by surgery and/or radiotherapy, heavily irradiated autografts of tumourous bone have recently been employed. Technically, the sarcomatous bone is excised, irradiated with 250,000 rads from a radiocobalt source, then firmly replaced as an autograft. Of five patients treated thus (four osteosarcoma, one reticulosarcoma) four have died. One patient has survived four and a half years with a discharging sinus. Secondary infection is a problem and in two cases there were local recurrences of tumour.

In one tumour recovered at autopsy no viable sarcoma was found, the tumour cells showing no nuclear staining but having intact cell membranes. Although this regime does not provide any solution to the metastatic problem it is claimed:
1. The psychological trauma of amputation is avoided.
2. The bone tumour is destroyed, but reconstitution of the bone can slowly proceed.
3. Post-irradiation fibrosis of soft tissues is eliminated.
4. The intact dead tumour cells may stimulate antibody formation and perhaps provoke resistance of metastatic growth.

INTRODUCTION

THE PROBLEMS facing the clinician and research worker, when dealing with osteogenic sarcoma should be analysed from a dynamic and biological point of view.

A number of factors are involved in the spread of metastases (which are predominantly blood borne.)
1. The operation itself has been blamed for dissemination, and to this end the use of pre-operative X-ray therapy and either local or general use of chemotherapy has been tried with no really effective result.
2. Direct spread of the tumour into the bone marrow and tumour vessels has been suggested.
3. The absence of immunological resistance may be a further modifying factor.

However, all attempts at immunization have to our knowledge failed.

It can be safely said, that the treatment of osteogenic sarcoma presents an unsolved problem, and in our hands, using the accepted techniques of amputation or local irradiation we have had no survivals. Consent to the amputation is always only obtained by explaining that this is a life-saving procedure and in fact this is not true. All our juvenile

67

patients are lost within a few months, and they have all suffered the trauma of amputation to no avail.

The same disappointment is reflected in the varied clinical and experimental studies, such as those of Higinbotham and Coley (1950) who suggested that bone tumours should be resected and replaced by massive grafts, Merle D'Aubigné and Mazabraud (1962) who used autografts, while Scales *et al.* (1969) replaced tumours by a metallic device. Crile (1963), using the T241 tumour in the foot pads of mice, investigated the effect of heat with and without irradiation, and attempted to extrapolate the ideas to human patients in five cases. There were two survivors of 5 and $6\frac{1}{2}$ years, but there was severe limitation in the function and stability of the treated bone.

Gruca in 1937 introduced his idea of "Biological Resection" using open diathermy, and in 1964, among other tumours, he reported on 24 osteogenic sarcomata with 10 patients surviving 5 years. Knoch (1970) had similar results.

Chemotherapy has never been shown to be of much use; but in 1970 Fleming and Tooms gave a preliminary report on the use of Cytophosphan and Vincristine on a "prophylactic" basis with some promising results.

Bearing all this in mind, and especially the need to avoid the unnecessary trauma of amputation we adopted a technique which we call "Extra-corporeal Irradiation" of bone tumours. The tumour-containing bone as well as any soft tissues close by are resected, cleansed and the bone sent to a 20,000 ci. source ^{60}Co irradiator. There the bone is given a dose of 250,000 rads at 10,000 r/min. On its return the bone is immediately fixed into position using metal plates and screws. The bone is now an irradiated autograft.

Of the five cases so treated (four osteogenic sarcomata and one reticulum cell sarcoma) only one patient remains alive and well. There were two local recurrences, but death

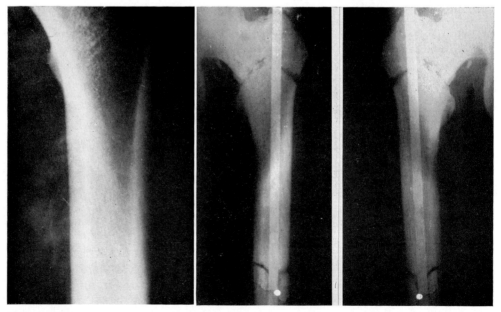

Fig. 1. X-Ray appearance before therapy in case 1

Fig. 2. Autograft replaced using intra-medullary pin (Case 1)

occurred in all four cases as a result of pulmonary metastases. The patient who still survives is at present free (4½ years later) of both local and distant metastases. There is however a locally draining sinus. It is possible that the tumour, although a proven osteogenic sarcoma by biopsy, could have been in fact a parosteal sarcoma having a natural history which is slow and relatively benign; nevertheless, this form of therapy was for this patient one which avoided amputation.

Secondary infection is to be feared, but was a major problem in one case only. This concurs with the experience as reported by Rubin and Casarett (1968).

CASE REPORTS

CASE 1. A young man aged 20 years complained of pain in the thigh for one month. At examination a protrusion could be felt in the anterior aspect of his thigh and there was limitation of movement at the hip joint. The X-ray showed a tumour protruding from the bone sclerosis of the endosteum (Fig. 1). Chest X-rays were negative. The tumour was resected and irradiated extra-corporeally. The bone was then replaced and fixed with an intramedullary pin (Fig. 2). Histology of the tumour confirmed that this

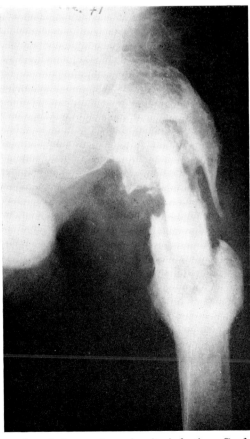

Fig. 3. Appearances of graft 4 years later despite infection. Graft is being resorbed. Pin has been removed (Case 1).

was an osteogenic sarcoma. The patient developed a draining sinus which persists to
this day, but he refuses any further surgical intervention. Recent chest X-rays are negative. The graft can now be shown to be partly resorbed with periosteal bone production
from both ends extending towards the centre (Fig. 3). In one of the cases we were
fortunate in being able to perform a post-mortem examination and then examine the
irradiated bone more closely some months after irradiation and replacement.

CASE 2. This was a 10-year-old boy who reportedly fell and hurt his knee one
month before admission. On admission the knee was swollen and painful. A biopsy was
performed at another hospital and then the patient sent to us. The tumour was bulging
into the scar which was adherent. The X-rays revealed irregular bone destruction in the
area of the previous biopsy (Fig. 4). The whole distal femur with the articular part was
resected, irradiated extra-corporeally and replaced, using a metal plate. Four months
later pulmonary metastases were evident and 2 months later the patient died. The
irradiated bone was recovered for histological examination. Macroscopically the bone
appeared to have united well, callus being formed, and the main body of the irradiated
bone had stood up well to a limited amount of weight bearing but the tumour area had
collapsed (Fig. 5). There was patchy necrosis of the articular cartilage.

On histological examination the most striking feature was the almost absolute lack of
nuclear material, but even after 6 months the bodies of the cells were clearly visible in
the lacunae. Even the bone marrow cavity in some areas showed cell envelope material
but no nuclear chromatin. It was easy to distinguish areas of malignant bone tissue,
and here again no nuclear material was visible although cell membranes were obviously
left *in situ*. The articular cartilage however showed islands of abnormal cells, the nuclear
material although clearly bizarre, nevertheless being visible. In the area close to non-
irradiated bone marrow there was early formation of new bone to replace the irradiated
bone marrow (Figs. 6 & 7).

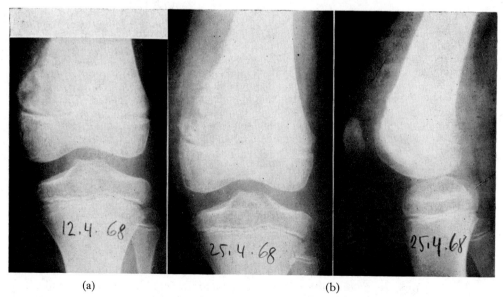

(a)   (b)

Fig. 4. X-Ray appearances (a) before biopsy and (b) 2 weeks later, showing scar
adherence (Case 2).

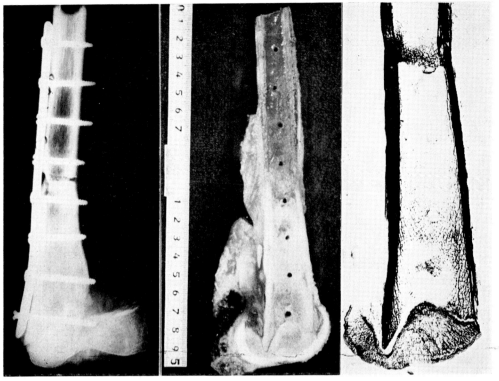

Fig. 5. Bone graft in place, but epiphysis collapsed.

Fig. 6. Post-mortem view of graft, showing good proximal union (Case 2).

Fig. 7. Slab radiograph of bone in Fig. 6 to show new bone formation at proximal junction.

DISCUSSION

In the first instance we would like to discuss briefly the effect of the massive dose of irradiation. The dose was decided upon because it was necessary to be sure that any tumour cells, that were either anoxic or inactive due to chilling procedures necessary for transporting the bone to the irradiator, would be destroyed. At the same time from the use of massively irradiated cadaveric bone grafts we were sure that the basic bone structure would not be changed. In fact when considering the body reaction to the graft we are able to say:

1. There was no immediate nausea or depression of the haemopoietic system.
2. The bone was invaded by granulation tissue, vessels and bone callus formed; that is, the body can cope with the graft, even if somewhat slowly.

The problem of local recurrence worried us, and in fact two of the five cases suffered from local recurrences. There are a number of ways in which this might be tackled—either by local irradiation, or by bathing the local area with a cytotoxic drug. We were afraid the damage might hamper or prevent the bone graft from taking, and in these cases no attempt at any local treatment of the bed was made.

The real and only major problem is the distant metastasis. Here we are still at a loss and have no adequate answer. In recent years, with investigation of the immunological defences of the body, and in view of the work of M. P. Finkel *et al.* (1969) who obtained a virus from human osteogenic sarcoma which produces osteogenic sarcoma in animals, we feel that this is the most exciting and profitable path to study. It is possible that the tumour cells and antigens from the primary that are reimplanted in our procedure may stimulate sufficient antibody production to prevent, or at least delay, the appearance of pulmonary metastases. This aspect of tumour therapy is being thoroughly investigated both by ourselves and others. Up to the present chemotherapy did not have any place in treatment as we had no drugs which effect osteogenic sarcoma; but a new drug, adriamycin may change this attitude.

Should a method be found to deal with distant metastases we feel that this procedure of "Extra-corporeal Bone Irradiation" might become the preferred method of therapy.

Its advantages:

1. It destroys the local tumour, but preserves skeletal stability.
2. It allows for a bone structure to be rebuilt by the body.
3. It avoids amputation.
4. It does not have the disadvantage of the massive fibrosis that accompanies conventional methods of external radiotherapy which must then be followed by amputation because of limitation in function.
5. The fact that the cell membrane remains intact may permit a certain stimulation of the body's own immunological system to respond to the tumour antigens. Immunotherapy may in fact help to deal with local residues of tumour tissue.

REFERENCES

Crile, G., Jr. The Effect of Heat and Radiation on Cancer implanted in the Feet of Mice. *Cancer Research*, **23**, 372, 1963.

Finkel, Miriam P., Biskis, Birute, O. & Farrell, Corinne. Non-malignant and Malignant Changes in Hamsters inoculated with Extracts of Human Osteosarcoma. *Radiology*, **92**, 1546–52, 1969.

Fleming, I. D. & Tooms, R. E. Chemotherapeutic Treatment of Osteogenic Sarcoma. *Interclinic Information Bulletin, Preliminary Report*, **9**, 7, 1, 1970.

Gruca, A. 1937. Cited by Gruca A. (1964).

Gruca, A. Biological Resection of Malignant Bone Tumours, 14*th. Bien. Int. Cong. Int. Coll. Surg. Vienna*, 715, 1964.

Hartman, J. T. & Crile, G., Jr. Heat Treatment of Osteogenic Sarcoma: Report of 5 cases. *Clinical Orthopaedics and Related Reasearch*, **61**, 269, 1968.

Higinbotham, N. L. & Coley, B. L. Treatment of Bone Tumours by Resection and Replacement with Massive Grafts. *The American Academy of Orthopaedic Surgeons, International Course Lectures*, **7**, 26, 1950.

Knoch, H.-G. Biological Resection of Bone Tumours, p. 71–72, in *Operative Treatment of Bone Tumours*. Edited by George Chapchal. Georg Thieme Verlag, Stuttgart, 1970.

Meile d'Aubigné, R. A. & Mazabraud, A. A propos de 22 observations de "vraies" tumeurs á cellules geantes, *Lyon chir*, **58**, 389, 1962.

Rubin, P. & Caserett, G. W. *Clinical Radiation Pathology*, Vol. 2, p. 557. 1968. W. B. Saunders, Philadelphia, 1968.

Scales, J. T., Duff-Barclay, I. & Burrows, H. J. Some Engineering and Medical Problems Associated with Massive Bone Replacement. *Biomechanics and Related Bioengineering Topics Symposium, Glasgow*, 205, 1964.

Discussion

Dr. Suit   I would like to ask the rationale for putting back a defective bone? I mean one that has been partially damaged by the tumour, particularly if one is going to go across the principle of removing the entire bone, that is if the entire affected bone has not either been irradiated or resected. Or what is the proposed advantage of putting back a bone partially destroyed by tumour even though one has presumably inactivated all the tumour cells which were taken to the irradiator? Secondly, I would like to ask for further documentation that this procedure controls the local disease when if I followed your comments correctly, there were two local recurrences out of five. I would judge that a local recurrence frequency of this magnitude might very well be equalled by radiation therapy alone in conventional doses.

Dr. Brenner   Where the bone structure is so completely destroyed that there is no hope of any structural advantage to be gained by putting the bone back, I agree with you that one must find other means of stabilising the limb. Our accent here was to avoid amputation because in all the cases studied to date in our Institute, we have no survivors of true osteogenic sarcoma, although there are some long survivors of the chondrosarcomas and so on. The question of the local recurrence is certainly a very worrying problem. The two cases where we did have local recurrences were in fact so gross in their local extent that we didn't really expect that there would be complete tumour control locally. We were just really studying the effect of the bone irradiation. I might add that in these cases, external radiation was tried and it made no effect at all on the tumour; in fact the tumour continued to grow. I have possibly not delivered such a big dose to the main bulk of tumour but in these two cases the tumour was involving the whole of the thigh where the bone had been excised and 6,000 rads just didn't touch it, and it was a huge volume. I really have no answer for the local recurrence, except that, as I mentioned, if at the time of the operation one could remove or irradiate the bed avoiding the massive doses one has to give normally to an osteogenic sarcoma to control it, this might help it or chemotherapy. Removing the bulk of the tumour and soft tissues might accept more chemotherapy into its milieu.

Prof. Campbell   I would like to ask about the patients during this period: How long do they hospitalize compared to those you amputated? To what extent were they real derelicts until they died or were they really rehabilitated?

Dr. Brenner   There is no doubt that there is a major problem in infection and the one case did in fact have a draining sinus for a long, long time. They really are vulnerable to infection but with adequate precautions we can overcome this. The four patients that I recall well didn't have an over-long stay in hospital. They were able to start walking immediately with partial weight bearing, at least at the beginning, far quicker than if they had had an amputation and having to start with the rehabilitation of the prosthesis and so on. I don't think that they were in any way harmed by the procedure in that

73

they were all advanced cases, except for the one fellow with this parosteal type osteogenic sarcoma and he refuses further surgical intervention. We in fact offered him further surgical intervention but he refuses, he says he can manage fine, thank you.

Mr. Eyre-Brook   Did you say you had no survivors?

Dr. Brenner   In the true osteogenic sarcoma among the children, yes: We had no survivors.

Mr. Eyre-Brook   But were these all children?

Dr. Brenner   These were all children.

Mr. Eyre-Brook   And the five that you did?

Dr. Brenner   They were young adults of the age of 21, I think.

Prof. Spira   That was the oldest.

Dr. Brenner   They were juveniles.

Prof. van Rijssel   How many osteosarcomas have you treated before with amputation? You said you had no survivors with amputation?

Dr. Brenner   Perhaps Prof. Spira could answer that better than I, he has been practising in Israel for many years, I am a relative newcomer.

Prof. Spira   I think we have lost more than forty cases during the last 15 years.

Prof. Barnes   Can Dr. Brenner tell us how he decided on what length of bone to resect?

Dr. Brenner   May I refer this question to Prof. Spira? I don't think this is a fair question for a radiotherapist.

Prof. Spira   Well, we went more or less some 10 cm above the levels of the tumours. We went down into the knee joint if it was in the epiphysis. This is an arbitrary decision I know, but you can do disarticulation in the hip joint for a tumour in the distal femur without having more success.

Dr. Byers   I was just wondering if the problem isn't the resection of the soft tissues. I am a morbid anatomist, and I haven't the practical experience of the surgeon, but one has an idea that the principle of local resection is to remove the tumour without actually seeing it. In the lower end of the femur this would suggest to me that possibly you have to remove a bulk of muscle with it. Is this the principle that you practice?

Prof. Spira   Yes it is.

Dr. Byers   How much of the muscle are you prepared to sacrifice with the limb?

Prof. Spira   How much you think you have to take out is another of these questionable points in the procedure. One has the feeling that if one could get these tumours earlier, and could get them without a biopsy a fortnight before and do the histological examination while the tumour is exposed one could have more chances.

Avoiding amputation might have some chances for a change of the immunological milieu; but this is all speculation.

Prof. van Ronnen   How many cases of osteosarcoma did you have?

Dr. Brenner   Well, I said just over forty.

Prof. von Ronnen   Just over forty in 15 years?

Dr. Brenner   In 15 years.

Prof. van Ronnen   And what was the mean survival time?

Dr. Brenner   Well, more or less a year.

Prof. van Rijssel   I don't understand that. We have about four hundred and fifty cases of osteosarcoma. We have a 5 years survival rate of 20%.

Dr. Price   The last time we investigated our osteosarcoma survival rate, which was I believe, 1966, on 130 cases including the Paget's sarcomas, the 5-year survival rate was 15%, the mean survival time was 18 months. Excluding the Paget sarcoma cases, the mean survival rate went up to 20%. The Paget cases usually die, their mean survival time being 13 months. That is the Bristol experience.

Prof. Bonfiglio   We have just recently completed a study of osteosarcomas in fifty patients followed over a 30-year period and we excluded anything that even smelled of any other histologic diagnosis other than bone-forming tumour. We excluded also the Paget's sarcomas. Our survival was 10% and in 20 years it was, 8%, and for those in the lower femur amputation or disarticulation made no difference. Just as good one way or another. I think really the question is one that begs the issue here about how one deals with it, because I am of the opinion that the survival rate is determined by the biologic behaviour of the tumour itself in the given patient and not by the treatment. We are really at a very primitive state in the management of the osteosarcoma, which is a true bone-forming tumour (not the fibro—nor the chondro—nor the small round cell nor the other groups that one might consider). So our luck is very, very poor in these patients. I still think that amputation is the treatment of choice, and an early immediate fitting gives as good function as the prolonged resection treatment for the osteosarcomas. Resection for other kinds, that is another matter.

Prof. Schajowicz There are two kinds of treatment generally used for osteosarcoma. Immediate amputation or amputation following radiotherapy. I would like to ask my English colleagues if they prefer pre-operative radiation, with these good results of 20% due to this type of treatment, because other schools like ours in Argentina prefer amputation. I would like to hear this argument because most people are asking it.

Mr. Lee Our figure was 20%, 21 to be exact, with the method of radiation and later amputation. It is the same figure near enough.

Mr. Eyre-Brook This is in 5 years?

Mr. Lee Five years. All cases including the Paget's.

Prof. Schajowicz What were the doses?

Mr. Lee Practically all had 6,000 to 6,500 rads of supervoltage therapy.

Dr. Brenner Could I in fact ask a question of Mr. Lee myself. Mr. Lee, we made the distinction of the juvenile osteogenic sarcoma with no addition of fibrosarcoma, or chondrosarcoma; the pure osteogenic sarcoma. You have just given us a figure of 20% including Paget's and so on; have you any information on the pure osteogenic sarcoma in the juvenile?

Mr. Lee Pure osteosarcoma is a very difficult expression, Sir. But if we exclude the Paget's sarcoma we have a very small number of patients who come in the intervening ages and then a vast number who are, as you say, up to the age of 21. If you take the juvenile ones up to the age of 21, the figure is about the same. It is about 20% 5 years survival, and I think this agrees pretty well with other figures.

Dr. Brenner We have the same treatment as that reported at the Westminster Hospital. We treat osteosarcomas with high voltage pre-operative treatment—6,000 rads with delayed amputation, arriving at about the same figure as everyone else with a 5-year survival of 10 to 15%. Our philosophy is that by treating these patients thus we let them wait some 2 to 3 months before we amputate. Some of these patients have already died having developed metastases and may be saved from amputation. On the other hand if we examine the operative specimen histologically we can see certain effects of irradiation in the tumour up to apparent sterilization.

Homologous bone and joint transplantation in bone tumour resections

by

ULF NILSONNE

SUMMARY

Experience is presented of six patients with bone tumours who received refrigerated cadaver homografts. In two patients with recurrent giant-cell tumours of the distal femur bony consolidation of the graft was radiographically demonstrated and the functional results were excellent. Of four patients with sarcoma, three have died with pulmonary metastases although two tumours were parosteal and one thought to be of low grade malignancy. In these cases bony union was mainly absent. In the other patient—a woman with chondrosarcoma of the proximal femur—graft union was obtained, but later a fatigue fracture ensued. Declining further surgery, she is now pain free and ambulant.

It is emphasized:

1. Massive homograft techniques should be reserved for patients under 40 years old in view of the long time needed for treatment.
2. Improved diagnostic criteria are essential for selecting tumours amenable to local surgery.

COMPLICATED PROBLEMS of reconstruction are often involved in major resections of all or a part of a joint. Many of those problems can be met with by specially designed endoprostheses. But since true union is ruled out with metallic implants the future mechanical stability will depend upon the extent to which the bone tissue tolerates the foreign material. This makes it desirable to look for a more biological solution. One possibility that presents itself is to carry out the substitution with big homografts.

It was the German surgeon Lexer who, in 1907, was the first to perform massive homografting of bone in man, mainly using material taken directly from amputated limbs. Lexer reviewed his cases in 1925 and was in some able to show good and long-lasting functional results. It is therefore surprising that only very few attempts at massive homografting of bone were published until the last decade. The largest series is reported from Russia where Volkow and collaborators developed a technique depending upon deep-freezing of the transplants. After studies in Moscow I have adopted this method in six cases.

The transplants are taken under sterile conditions from deceased persons within 6 hours from death. They are then put into a special refrigerator at a temperature of

−70°C for 48 hours and afterwards stored for one or more weeks at −20° before use. At the time of the operation the graft is thawed in a penicillin-containing physiological saline solution at body temperature and implanted after the tumour resection.

Case 1. A woman 20 years of age with a parosteal osteosarcoma of the distal part of the femur. In April 1966 16 cm of the distal part of the femur was resected including the tumour and the condyles with the joint surfaces. A homograft was fitted into the defect and fixed to the host femur by plates. The ligaments of the grafts were sutured side to side to the corresponding structures of the patient. Postoperatively infection developed and could not be controlled in spite of all kinds of treatment. A mid-thigh amputation was therefore performed 1 year after the first operation. In the specimen numerous areas of vital bone could be demonstrated within the graft. In 1970 the patient died from pulmonary metastases which is rather surprising in view of the relatively indolent nature of parosteal osteosarcomas.

Case 2. A woman 36 years of age with a chondrosarcoma in the region of the lesser trochanter of the femur. In January 1967 the femur, including the tumour, was resected at a distance of 21 cm from the acetabulum. The defect was filled by a homograft fixed with an intramedullary nail. Roentgenological consolidation of the osteosynthesis was observed after 10 months, and after 1 year there was a good range of active motion in the hip joint. The patient was able to walk with one cane. In 1969, $2\frac{1}{2}$ years after the operation the patient noticed pain in the hip. X-ray examination revealed a fatigue fracture of the femoral neck of the graft. A hip arthroplasty with endoprosthesis was proposed but the patient refused further surgery. The patient, who is a housewife, is still able to walk with only one cane and is pain-free. The condition seems to be comparable to the result of a Girdlestone operation. There are no metastases.

CASE 3. A woman 42 years of age with a recurrent giant-cell tumour of the lat eral condyle of the femur. In April 1967 a block resection was performed with a good mar gin to the tumoural region, the defect being filled with a homograft fixed with screws. There was roentgenological consolidation after 10 months and weight bearing was then allowed. Five years later the patient has a pain-free knee when walking, with a range of active mobility from 175°–130° and leads a normal life. There are no signs of osteoarthritis.

CASE 4. A woman 37 years of age with a fibrosarcoma of the condylar region of the femur, at the time thought to be of a very low-grade type. In September 1967 a resection was performed of the distal 16 cm of the femur and the defect filled by a homograft. Six months later there was a local recurrence of the tumour and pulmonary metastases were demonstrated. The disease took a very fulminant course and the patient died 2 months later. Evidently the true nature of the fibrosarcoma was originally under-estimated. At autopsy some areas of vital bone could be found in the graft.

CASE 5. A woman 18 years of age with a parosteal chondrosarcoma of the upper diaphysis of the femur. In June 1970 most of the diaphysis was resected with the tumour, the defect being filled by a homograft fixed with an intramedullary nail. Three months later a local recurrence necessitated a hip disarticulation. In the proximal region of the osteosynthesis there was already firm bony consolidation, the borderline between the host and the graft being almost invisible. The distal ostesynthesis was not healed. The patient died 11 months after the first operation of pulmonary metastases.

CASE 6. A man 28 years of age with a recurrent giant-cell tumour of the medial condyle of the femur. In July 1970 a block resection was performed of the condylar region and a homograft fitted into the defect fixed with screws. After 8 months consolidation could be demonstrated roentgenologically. The patient has now, 21 months after the operation, a range of mobility of the knee-joint of 180°–90° and walks without pain, unaided by a cane. He is re-employed as a road engineer.

Thus in my experience it has been possible to perform massive bone and joint homografting with revitalization of the graft by the host and with acceptable limb function. In some cases this procedure can be an alternative either to ablative surgery or to reconstructive surgery with artificial implants. As the time for the consolidation of the graft is long, I think however that the method should be reserved for the age group not above 40 years of age. Young adults can afford to lose the time caused by the treatment if the biological implant leads to true healing with lasting function. There still remains the question, however, of which tumours should be treated in this way. It is therefore necessary to arrive at a better understanding of the inherent nature of bone tumours, as within the same group appear indolent as well as fulminant types. Better diagnostic criteria are a prerequisite for the further development of local surgery in the treatment of bone tumours.

Discussion

Mr. Eyre-Brook I would like to ask a question about the parosteal sarcomas. I would very much doubt from the X-rays that I would have accepted either of those as parosteal.

Dr. Nilsonne I think the first case I demonstrated is a very typical picture of a parosteal osteosarcoma and also typical localization.

Mr. Eyre-Brook I would have said that if you had gone into the bone enough it would be an ordinary osteosarcoma. A very rare thing is a parosteal osteosarcoma. That is my opinion. I would like your general reaction.

Dr. Nilsonne Well, there were two cases here defined really as parosteal, the parosteal osteosarcoma and the parosteal chondrosarcoma. I agree that it is very difficult to make a very precise definition of this.

Professor Campbell The question comes up about the use of an homogenous graft in an articular surface, and what is the natural course of such an articular graft. We have done experimental work of this type in dogs, and usually a cartilaginous graft of homogenous type where there is a cancellous base will survive about 180 and sometimes 360 days looking almost normal. By about 500 or 600 days the dogs begin to deteriorate. So in this kind of case you are up against really the kind of tumour you are dealing with in the first place. You can possibly save the articular surface. If you cannot save it, then you have to accept that you are dealing with homogenous bone and homogenous cartilage. Now, if you are dealing with homogenous bone then you can expect those fractures occasionally, because that is a part of the natural replacement of an homogenous graft and you can expect cracks in it. The second thing is the osteoarthritic part: you are hardly getting in to it yet because of the pylon. A person can tolerate a lot of osteo-arthritis before pain. I think already in the cases which you have demonstrated you have articular changes, but they also are relatively early. Would you agree with this in principle?

Dr. Nilsonne Well, I must confess that I am myself a bit surprised at the good appearances of the joints still in the X-rays, because the cases I saw in Moscow had very bad X-rays but pain-free joints. But the two knee joints here, for example—the first one is 5 years and the other one almost 2 years, and I think there is a very slight osteoarthritic change in the X-rays but the cartilage is dead; I know that from the other specimens.

Prof. Campbell But that is a half joint really. So the other side of the joint contains a great deal of detritus.

Dr. Nilsonne That's true.

Prof. Bonfiglio I would like to suggest that there are two other factors involved in the repair of a half joint. Whether it is autogenous or homogenous the repair is quite similar except the delay in the homograft. Once the subchondral cortex is invaded by a vascular supply it destroys the cartilage in both instances. In the homograft I suggest that you are dealing with a half joint and a rheumatic joint, which may be one of the reasons why there is a delay in the pain mechanism that is involved in this. That is why the breakdown seems to be so dramatic in the late stages of the repair.

Prof. Dahlin I would like to second Mr. Eyre-Brook's comment and suggestion about the parosteal osteosarcomas. I think that unless we define exactly what we are talking about we get somewhat confused. I think that a tumour that should be called a parosteal or juxtacortical osteosarcoma must not only be on the surface of the bone radiographically and anatomically, but it also must be of a low order of malignancy. Because a periosteally located osteosarcoma that is highly undifferentiated will have the same biologic capacity as one that starts within bone.

Dr. Suit I would like to ask you to comment on the need for removal of all of the bone in patients with osteosarcoma. We have had an example here in a preceding paper where a portion of the bone was resected and then someone in the audience stated that it was equally as good to do an amputation as a disarticulation. If this is a valid concept I think it would be appropriate to have some comments regarding this.

Mr. Lee This is a thing that interests me very much because it depends on how you measure the results. If you measure the results in terms of survival, then I think there seems to be no difference between an amputation and a disarticulation, even perhaps a more local resection. But if you measure it in terms of local recurrence, then we have a few cases of stump recurrence after partial removal say of a femur. We feel that on the whole it is better to disarticulate just from that point of view.

Dr. Nilsonne I agree with that in those kinds of tumours, but in these more slowly developing tumours I feel now convinced that this is a possibility in young persons.

Mr. Wilson I am working with Dr. Scales on the resection of tumours and replacement by metal prostheses. I thought it might be wise to correct Dr. Nilsonne that we are not doing this for fast-growing tumours. In our opinion this is only applicable to slow-growing tumours. We have actually done parosteal sarcoma (which we have tried to diagnose), but that is the nearest thing to an osteosarcoma. The other tumours have all been locally malignant—such as chondrosarcoma and giant-cell tumour, that type of thing. The procedure has been done in error for osteosarcoma. They have all died, they all produced local recurrences. I don't think there is any place for local resection here in highly malignant tumours.

Dr. Lloyd I am interested in the repair process which you have going on here. There seems no doubt that new bone can latch on to dead bone, and make a perfectly good joint of it long before the dead bone comes anywhere near to being converted back into living bone again by the cell replacement. I think probably that this happened in some

D*

of your cases where you had new bone making what appeared to be good fusion with the graft; but what happens after that I am not quite clear. Do you not get a host versus graft reaction, and if so what form does it take? How much of the corruption that you showed us is due to that kind of reaction do you think?

Dr. Nilsonne   The Russians have tried to discuss this with me, which is not so easy, but apparently it is just an empirical technique. They have tried quite a lot of different modes of preparation and found that this worked clinically. Personally I think that maybe the deep freezing technique, where you very rapidly bring the transplant to this low temperature, creates a rupture of all the cells, and this might minimize the antigenicity of the transplant. We have done very little immunological work on this kind of transplant so I don't want to say anything more about that.

Prof. Bonfiglio   In discussing this very point, the question that you raise, most of my experimental work has been in just this area, about the immunological reactions to various types of bone. The autograft or homograft (which is the old term) does have a continuing immunological reaction to it as long as it is present. As long as there is cellular destruction of it there is an inflammatory reaction to it. In some of the lower animals we were able to produce titres of complement-fixing antibodies to that bone, to the bone there by doing certain tests with it. There is no question that this is one of the problems, and the only real experimental work that I have seen recently that might deal with the whole bone transplant has been done by a British surgeon, Brian Reeves in London. He did anastomoses of vessels for the whole bone—the geniculate artery for instance from the lower femur to the femoral artery and then used immuno-suppressive drugs as well and was therefore able to control the reaction just as they do with the kidney transplants—using it as a whole bone preparation, an organ preparation if you will. In instances where they have done this with autogenous grafts, Lance and others in England have done both kinds and you get total survival of an autogenous graft by using a vascular connection. You don't go through the phase of creeping substitution and replacement. If one could do this with the homograft and use drugs sufficiently long for new bone to form and make it living bone from the host, one might abort this phase that one is going through. I think that is the future for this kind of work and it is still in the experimental stage.

Progression in bone tumours

TH. G. VAN RIJSSEL

SUMMARY

Progression of malignancy may occur in several types of bone tumours (chordoma, giant-cell tumour, cartilaginous tumours).
On the whole cartilaginous tumours show the greatest tendency to progression.
Progression of chondrosarcoma often results in a more or less pleomorphic fibrosarcoma, rarely some areas may show features of osteosarcoma.[1]
Chondrosarcomas of the thoracic wall have the greatest tendency to progression.
Progression of chondrosarcoma occurs mostly in patients older than 50 years.

IN 1949, FOULDS[2] proposed the term "progression" to characterize the phenomenon of increasing malignancy shown by some tumours during their course. This irreversible qualitative alteration of the neoplastic tissue is expressed in an increased growth rate, rapid metastatic spread, loss of histological differentiation, anaplasia, and an increase in the mitotic index. Foulds stressed that it is not sufficient to divide tumours into benign and malignant types, and he pointed out that malignancy is not a well-defined property since it occurs in different grades. To characterize a neoplasm the grade of its malignancy must be indicated. Foulds' proposition was based on his observations in experimental cancer research, and he referred to similar observations made by Rous and Kidd and by Berenblum.

There are also many examples of progression in human pathology. It is not unusual to find that incompletely removed fibrosarcomas of the soft tissues contain more mitoses and show more pleomorphism in each successive recurrence.

In some well-differentiated mammary ductal carcinomas, areas can be found with infiltrating strands of anaplastic cancer cells, but large infiltrating undifferentiated carcinomas of the breast may contain a central part with much better differentiated cells proliferating mainly in the ducts. Both observations suggest that some cancers of the breast are well-differentiated in the early phases but may undergo a change in behaviour when cells with a higher growth rate and a lower tendency to differentiate develop locally, after which these cells rapidly overgrow the older parts of the tumour. We have observed a case in which this mechanism was very probably involved: an elderly woman who had had a solitary nodule in the left thyroid lobe for 30 years (she had refused surgical treatment) died one year after she had noticed rapid growth of the tumour. At autopsy a large aggressive anaplastic spindle-celled thyroid carcinoma was found, with metastases in the lungs. At the site of the left lobe of the thyroid there was a focus of well-differentiated papillary carcinoma in the anaplastic tumour tissue.

Clinically, this phenomenon is not so important in neoplasms with a high grade of malignancy from the beginning, but in tumours with a low or moderate grade of malignancy, progression may give rise to a dramatic change of the clinical course, Therefore it is of great importance, especially in the treatment of tumours of low or moderate malignancy, to prevent the occurrence of progression, where possible, by meticulous, complete removal of the neoplasm. This also holds for several types of bone tumours; and the cases in the series of the Netherlands Committee on Bone Tumours include several examples of progression.

This Committee consists of radiologists, orthopaedic and general surgeons, and pathologists, and is supported by the "Stichting Koningin Wilhelmina Fonds" (Queen Wilhelmina Fund) of the Netherlands Organization against Cancer. The Committee on Bone Tumours, which was founded in 1953, began by collecting sections of bone tumours and data concerning the patients from the archives of various departments of pathology. The clinicians who had treated the patients were asked to supply the radiographs and case histories. Files were established for all cases for which sufficient data were available, and in subsequent years follow-up information was obtained. This material was compared with the data in the literature. After some time, and with much hesitation, the Committee began to accede to requests for advice concerning diagnosis and treatment. These cases were also duly registered and followed. The number of requests for advice gradually increased, and at present the archives of the Committee contain data concerning more than 3,000 patients with a tumour or a tumour-like lesion.

Among the bone tumours that show progression, cartilaginous tumours predominate We have observed eight of these cases.

CASE 1.   *BA 1040*   woman   52 (born in 1900)
  Nov. 1952:   resection of a part of left 8th rib with large tumour (coconut). post-operative irradiation.
  path.:   chondrosarcoma, grade 1.
  May 1960:   local recurrence (20 × 16 × 14 cm).
  treatment: block resection of ribs and tumour.
  path.:   chondrosarcoma with fibrosarcomatous parts (Fig. 1).
  Dec. 1962:   died dyspnoeic. No autopsy.

CASE 2.   *BA 1864*   man   57 (born in 1907)
  Spring 1965:   rapidly growing tumour below right clavicle.
  X-ray: tumour of 3rd rib.
  July 1965:   resection of right ribs 2, 3, 4.
  path.:   chondrosarcoma grade II (8 cm) with local fibrosarcomatous progression.
  Feb. 1966:   local recurrence, juxta-sternal.
  April 1966:   another recurrence, in lateral border.
  July 1966:   methotrexate and irradiation.
  Dec. 1966:   died.

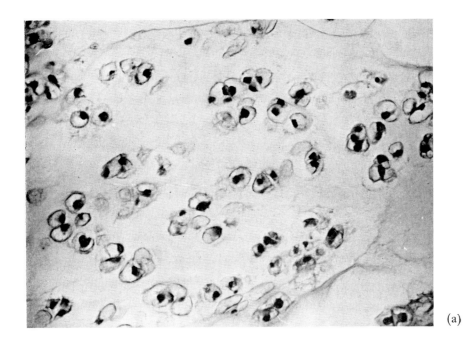

(a)

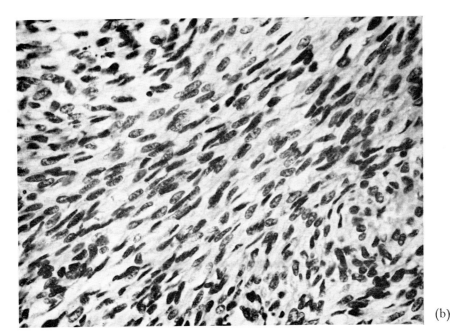

(b)

Fig. 1. Case 1: Chondrosarcoma (a) in which fibrosarcomatous areas (b) were found.

CASE 3.   *BA 2045* woman   54 (born in 1911)
  Oct. 1965:   patient noticed a slowly growing swelling on sternum.
  June 1966:   extirpation of corpus sterni.
      path.:   cartilaginous tumour (8 × 5 cm) in sternum.
         chondrosarcoma grade 1, containing a circumscribed focus (4 cm) which consisted of atypical chondrosarcomatous and fibrosarcomatous tissue.
  Jan. 1972:   patient in excellent condition.

In these three cases local fibrosarcomatous areas were found in tumours which elsewhere had the appearance of chondrosarcoma. In three other cases this relationship was reversed.

CASE 4.   *BA 2547* man   67 (born in 1901)
  Oct. 1968:   pain in left leg.
     X-ray: radiolucent focus in trochanteric region.
  treatment: curettage.
      path.:   pleomorphic fibrosarcoma with chondroid areas.
  Nov. 1968:   disarticulation.
      path.:   tumour mass (8 × 8 cm).
         chondrosarcoma (1·5 cm), surrounded by fibrosarcoma.
         removal incomplete.
  treatment: hemipelvectomy.
  April 1969:   recurrence, died with metastases in lungs, adrenals, thyroid and lymph nodes.

CASE 5.   *BA 2588* woman   71 (born in 1897)
  Dec. 1968:   fracture of left femur.
     X-ray: fracture in radiolucent area.
      path.:   fibrosarcoma.
  Jan. 1969:   disarticulation.
      path.:   tumour of 9 cm in the marrow space with fracture in the middle.
         the centre is chondrosarcomatous (well-differentiated);
         in the fracture area and the distal part the tumour is fibrosarcomatous (grade III).
  Feb. 1970:   died from metastases in the lungs.

CASE 6.   *BA 1178* man   57 (born in 1905)
  Jan. 1962:   complaints about right arm.
     X-ray: radiolucency in coracoid process.
  treatment: extirpation of cartilaginous tumour.
      path.:   chondrosarcoma (grade I).
  Nov. 1962:   recurrence (14 cm), rapidly growing.
  treatment: amputation.
      path.:   pleomorphic fibrosarcoma, with remnants of cartilaginous tumour.
      1964:   died (metastases).

In the cases 4 and 5 the tumour had the appearance of more or less pleomorphic fibrosarcoma, this diagnosis having been made on the biopsies. The examination of the resection specimen revealed that the tumour contained areas of well-differentiated chondrosarcoma (in both cases in the central part). In these cases the original cartilaginous tumour probably was overgrown by the faster growing fibrosarcomatous tissue when tumour cells had lost their ability to differentiate into cartilage and proliferated as fibroblastic sarcoma cells; this certainly happened in case 6 when the rapidly-growing recurrence developed.

In one case we have observed local progression in one recurrence, whereas other and later recurrences did not show progression:

CASE 7.   *BA 1393*   man   55 (born in 1905)
July 1960:   resection of part of a rib with tumour (5 cm).
     path.:   chondrosarcoma, grade I.
Oct. 1962:   recurrence (5 cm).
    treatment: more extensive resection.
     path.:   chondrosarcoma grade I, not completely removed.
March 1963:   two recurrences (3 and 6 cm).
    treatment: removal (not complete).
     path.:   a. pure chondrosarcoma grade I.
                 b. chondrosarcoma with fibrosarcomatous parts.
Aug. 1963:   recurrence.
    treatment: extensive resection.
     path.:   pure chondrosarcoma grade I (7 cm).
Jan. 1965:   X-ray: pulmonary metatasis.
May 1966:   sudden death (embolism?)

This case illustrates Foulds' first rule: progression occurs independently in different tumours in the same individual.[3] Fibrosarcomatous tissue has been found in one of the recurrences and apparently all the "progressed" tissue was removed surgically, as later recurrences had a chondrosarcomatous structure.

Our last case (no. 8) showed the development of fibrosarcomatous tissue between the lobules of a chondrosarcoma which had existed for many years. In the fibrosarcomatous tissue a focal bone formation resulted in the appearance of a fibroblastic osteosarcoma.

CASE 8.   *BA 2988*   woman   50 (born in 1920)
                 Complaints of back pain since 1960.
Oct. 1970:   paraesthesia in right leg.
    X-ray: large tumour of right iliac bone.
    biopsy: chondrosarcoma.
Jan. 1971:   resection of tumour and main part of iliac bone.
     path.:   lobulated tumour mass of 18 × 18 × 15 cm.
                 central part is cystic.
                 chondrosarcoma with fibrosarcomatous and osteosarcomatous parts.
March 1972:   patient in good condition.

It is remarkable that neither the localization of these progressing chondrosarcomas nor the age of the patients reflects the general distribution of chondrosarcomas over the skeleton nor their incidence among the different age groups.

TABLE 1

FREQUENCY OF PROGRESSION IN DIFFERENT SITES

Site	Total number of chondrosarcomas	Number with progression
Axial skeleton (skull, vertebr., sacr.)	25	0
Thorax Pelvis	80 { 46 / 34	6 { ribs 3 / scap. 1 / stern. 1 / pelvis 1
Limbs Long bones Small bones	150 / 22	2 / 0 } femur 2
Total	277	8

TABLE 2

NUMBER* OF CHONDROSARCOMAS IN DIFFERENT AGE GROUPS, AND PROGRESSION

Age	0	10	20	30	40	50	60	70	
Cases		2	51	41	34	42	46	38	17
Progression		—	—	—	—	—	6	1	1

| 170 cases under 50 no progression | 101 cases over 50 8 with progression |

* The total number in this table is a little lower than in Table 1 because we did not know exactly the age of 6 of the patients.

As to age, the development of progression in chondrosarcomas seems to have a marked preference for older age groups (Table 2). Chondrosarcomas localized in the bones of the thoracic wall seem to have more risk of progression than those in the more usual localizations, i.e. the long bones of the limbs (Table 1).

Chondrosarcomas are not the only bone tumours in which progression can occur. We have observed two patients suffering from sacral chordoma, in which pleomorphic sarcoma developed, rapidly overgrowing the chordomatous tissue.

CASE 9. | *BA 1215* man   46 (born in 1918)

May 1962:	complaints about micturition and defaecation.
	tumour in sacral bone; curettage.
path.:	*chordoma* (Fig. 2(a)).
April 1963:	recurrence, incomplete extirpation.
path.:	pleomorphic fibrosarcoma.
Dec. 1963:	died; huge tumour of sacrum, metastases in lungs.
path.:	*chordosarcoma* (Fig. 2(b)).

CASE 10. | *BA 2841* man   71 (born in 1898)

Jan. 1969:	low back pain.
Jan. 1970:	increasing complaints.
X-ray:	osteolytic destruction of right part of sacrum.
biopsy:	typical *chordoma* with pleomorphic *fibrosarcoma*.
March 1970:	operative treatment after irradiation (2,000 rad) complete removal not possible.
	patient died 3 weeks later from pneumonia.
Autopsy:	no metastases.
	tumour of circa 10 cm diameter in sacral region.
	tumour mainly typical *chordoma, partly pleomorphic fibrosarcoma*.

Sometimes a malignant growth develops in a benign lesion which had already existed for a long time. It is well known that this occurs in some tumour-like conditions arising from local disturbances of development, such as multiple exostosis, enchondromatosis and—rarely— fibrous dysplasia, and also from benign tumours sarcomatous growth may develop. This phenomenon which has been described as malignant degeneration or malignant transformation can be regarded as a manifestation of progression. In a few cases a malignant growth develops on the same site where many years earlier a benign lesion had been removed. We have observed this twice in giant-cell tumour. Our series comprises 161 cases of giant-cell tumour. Eight of these could be classified as malignant at the first histological examination. Three of these patients died of the tumour. Fifteen other tumours were histologically suspect but did not show conclusive evidence of malignancy. Of these patients, three died of the tumour which had progressed to clear histological malignancy and metastasized. The other 138 giant-cell tumours were considered benign. In the long run, however, two of these cases took a fatal course: in one of them a metastasizing malignant recurrence developed 25 years after curettage and irradiation of a seemingly non-malignant giant-cell tumour of the tibia, and in the other a pleomorphic fibrosarcoma developed in the femur, where a benign-looking giant-cell tumour had been curetted 19 years earlier.

We have observed a similar occurrence in a patient suffering from a benign chondroblastoma of the femur.

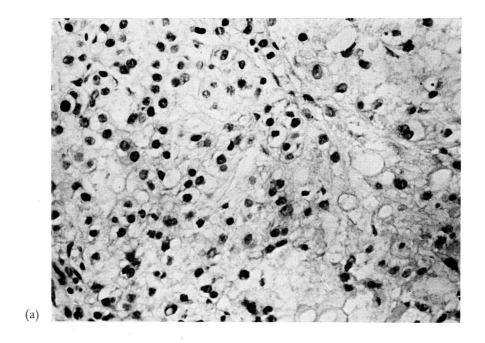

(a)

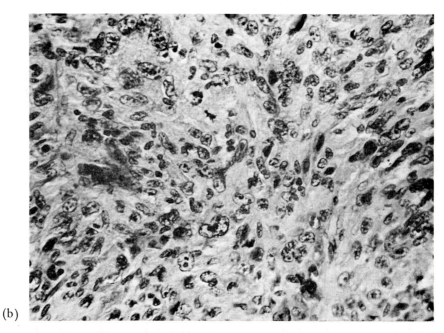

(b)

Fig. 2. Case 9: Chordoma (a), one year later transformed into a pleomorphic fibrosarcoma (b).

CASE 11.   *BA 207*   man   24 (born in 1930)
  1954:   trauma of left knee.
  1955:
    X-ray: large radiolucent area in lateral femoral condyle.
                curettage and chips.
    path.   *chondroblastoma benignum.*
  1956–1968:   excellent condition, good function.
  Sept. 1968:   pain and some swelling of left knee.
  Dec. 1968:   "spontaneous" fracture of lateral condyle.
                exploration, biopsy.
    path.:   pleomorphic *fibrosarcoma* (grade III).
  Jan. 1969:   amputation.
  Dec. 1969   died with metastases in the lungs.
  Summary: 14 years after treatment (*no irradiation*) for benign chondroblastoma:
                development of fibrosarcoma grade III in the lesional area.

An intriguing feature in this last case is that after the treatment of the original tumour the patient seemed to be free from tumour for so many years. It is not clear whether cells from the first tumour survived for all these years and progressed finally into undifferentiated neoplastic growth or whether a new tumour originated in the traumatized area.

If irradiation has been applied, it is usually held responsible for such late development of malignancy, but in our Case 11 (and in the last of our giant-cell tumours) no radiotherapy had been given.

There are sufficient examples of human bone tumours in which the transition to a more malignant type is well established for us to accept Foulds' concept of progression as being applicable to this field.

REFERENCES

1. Dahlin, D. C. & Beabout, J. W. Dedifferentiation of Low-grade Chondrosarcomas. *Cancer*, **28**, 461–467, 1971.
2. Foulds, L. Mammary Tumours in Hybrid Mice: Growth and Progression of Spontaneous Tumours. *Brit. J. Cancer*, **3**, 345–375, 1949.
3. Foulds, L. General principles of tumour progression. In: *Neoplastic development*, 69–75. Academic Press, London–New York, 1969.

Discussion

Prof. Lodwick Do you suppose the greater frequency of recurrence in the chondrosarcomatous lesions of the chest wall may be due to perhaps greater difficulty in getting a complete resection?

Prof. van Rijssel I do not think that the greater frequency of recurrence is the same as progression. We have seen recurrences of chondrosarcoma in the limbs too. So I cannot say that that explains anything.

Prof. Lodwick Is there any real biological difference in chondrosarcoma of the chest wall?

Prof. van Rijssel I thought that perhaps chondrosarcoma of the chest wall has been present for a longer time when it is discovered than similar tumours in the limbs, because weight bearing may give an earlier indication that there is a tumour—but that is a hypothesis.

Dr. Suit I wish you could document this point a little bit more carefully by supplying us with data as to the local recurrence frequency. For example, you gave six out of 80 progressions in the thoracic wall, I would like to know how many of the 80 patients showed recurrence and of those recurrences how many showed progression—was this the six? Out of so many recurrences which were progression, and how does this compare with the frequency of local recurrence in the long bones, of which there were 150 cases? This might be relevant to Prof. Lodwick's question as to whether or not there is any real biological difference between these tumours in these two sites.

Prof. van Rijssel Yes, I think this is a good point. But I have to study the number of recurrences in the long bones. I am not sure about that, but it can be found.

Prof. Duthie Foulds introduced his concept of progression of tumours based on mammary carcinoma in mice. Your adaption of his concept really is being influenced by the surgical intervention. In other words the change in the behaviour pattern of these has followed your diagnosis which is based upon the biopsy.

Prof. van Rijssel I tried to demonstrate eight cases in which the progression had taken place before surgery. Those were the cases where we diagnosed fibrosarcoma, but when we have had the whole tumour we found in the centre the remnants of the cartilaginous tumour. The surgery was not prior to the progression.

Prof. Duthie Eight cases were chondrosarcomas in which you had actually to get histological diagnosis to see them change their invasive properties, probably with metastases.

Prof. van Rijssel I demonstrated three cases in the beginning in which there was only partly fibrosarcoma, the bulk of the tumour was chondrosarcoma. Then I showed a few cases in which there was a large fibrosarcoma but within the centre there was a small area of chondrosarcoma. Of these cases two were diagnosed as mixed tumours at the first surgery.

Dr. Byers I think most pathologists with experience of bone tumours would agree with Professor van Rijssel that you do find tumours that have not been interfered with in any way where both these components are present—cartilaginous and spindle cell tissue. Whether you put these together in precisely the same way that he does is I think the point at issue.

Prof. Mackenzie I am a little bit unhappy as a pathologist by the use of this word "fibrosarcoma"; but I also know as a pathologist, how unfair one can be to judge something from a single or even a dozen photomicrographs. Some of the pictures seem to me just to indicate that a chondrosarcoma was becoming de-differentiated. I think the cells were anaplastic chondrocytes not collagen-producing fibroblasts. In some instances I would merely have said that this was a chondrosarcoma getting less differentiated, and not implied that there were two independent lines of mesenchymal differentiation. That would be one point I would like to make. The other thing is, in the last picture of all, and here I realize the risk of looking at a single photomicrograph, I am not one hundred per cent happy about that chordoma.

Prof. van Rijssel The last remark I cannot answer except by showing you sections. On the first I think the word de-differentiate is much worse than progression. Because the tissue, the cells do not de-differentiate; they do not differentiate any more. That's the difference. So I think the word de-differentiate is . . .

Prof. Mackenzie What I mean is that we are not dealing with two types of cells.

Prof. van Rijssel I think we just speak about the same as Foulds did. He thought that in a tumour with a uniform picture, after some time some cells may lose some of their possibilities to differentiate; and then you get a tumour with two cell clones. One differentiating, in our case, with the production of chondroid matrix and collagen fibres (because the chondrocytes also make collagen), and other cells which have lost the property of making cartilaginous matrix and grow more rapidly and look unlike fibroblasts and certainly producing some collagen too.

Dr. Price I am afraid I would rather back up Professor McKenzie about the rather loose usage of the term fibrosarcoma where in some instances this may be pure speculation. It is better to be factual and say this is a pleomorphic sarcoma, which may be fibrosarcoma. The point I would really like to make is that I personally think that progression may be observed in connective tissue tumours. Quite a number of these I would regard as of mixed structure *ab initio*— you can if you wish use the term "mesenchymoma". One has seen for example liposarcoma and osteosarcoma mixed *ab initio*.

Are you going to regard that as progression? Surely this really goes back to the concept that many sarcomas both of bone and soft tissue have a very mixed cell population.

Prof. van Rijssel   I think that the term progression has only sense when it is used for a change in the tumour morphology and the change in tumour morphology occurs when the new cell line overgrows the old line; then there is a change. That is the thing I wanted to demonstrate in these cases and I think they demonstrate it; and if you want to be convinced about the progression of chordomas, I can demonstrate another case.

But I do not think regarding the terminology whether you call a fibrosarcoma Grade III or pleomorphic sarcoma makes much difference in this case. The tumour cells produce some collagen that is certain.

SESSION II

Tumour Diagnosis

Chairman: PROFESSOR J. H. MIDDLEMISS

On the roentgenological diagnosis and differential diagnosis of bone sarcomas

J. R. VON RONNEN AND R. O. VAN DER HEUL

SUMMARY

McKenna *et al.* (1966) stated that precise radiological differential diagnosis of bone sarcomas is uncertain beyond indicating the presence of a tumour and that histological examination is required in all suspected cases. This was confirmed by examining the radiographs of a large series of tumours. With osteosarcoma and juxtacortical osteosarcoma about 50% of the radiographs could be considered typical: with other types rather fewer—even for the trained observer.

Conflicting diagnoses were repeatedly found between the radiologist and the pathologist. In some films a histologically proven sarcoma resembled a benign lesion, in others the type was incorrectly stated, and there was difficulty in recognizing early malignancy A "cystic" variant of osteosarcoma was distinguished with a better prognosis than the conventional form. It is emphasized that irrespective of radiographic appearances when diagnostic doubts still linger a prompt biopsy should be performed.

IN 1966 AN ARTICLE by McKenna and co-workers appeared in *The Journal of Bone and Joint Surgery* entitled: "Sarcomata of the Osteogenic Series (Osteosarcoma, Fibrosarcoma, Chondrosarcoma, Parosteal Osteogenic Sarcoma and Sarcomata arising in Abnormal Bone)." In this article the following statement drew our attention:

"The differential roentgendiagnosis of osteogenic sarcoma is only of academic interest since histological confirmation is required for definitive diagnosis. Maximum effort should be devoted toward deciding whether a bone tumour exists, and whether it is more likely benign or malignant."

This induced us to trace on the basis of material from the Netherlands Committee on Bone Tumours if this point of view is right and to investigate if a more exact formulation is desirable. For that purpose we tried to analyse the problems with regard to X-ray diagnosis of primary malignant lesions. Especially we were interested in those cases in which misjudgment causing harm to the patient, is liable to occur.

Although X-ray pictures of primary bone sarcomas show a marked variability it is possible to distinguish a characteristic picture for a number of tumour types. It is true that such a characteristic X-ray picture is not encountered in all cases, but, if present, it offers the possibility of making the correct diagnosis with a high degree of probability. In the following examples typical X-ray appearances are illustrated:

97

1. OSTEOSARCOMA

The radiographical appearance in typical cases is characterized by destruction of pre-existing bone by the tumour tissue, calcification in the tumour area often with recognizable bone structure and periosteal bone formation, often with formation of spicules and Codman's triangles. The tumour has an intra-osseous origin but may protrude beyond the bone after destruction of the cortex (Fig. 1). In our material we found amongst 252 osteosarcomas, located in the long bones, 139 typical cases.

2. CHONDROSARCOMA

(a) Typical cases of central chondrosarcoma show a centrally situated, more or less lobular radiolucency in a long bone. These radiolucencies often contain irregular densities, caused by calcification in the tumour tissue.

Cortex destruction occurs only in more advanced stages and periosteal bone formation is usually limited. The bone sometimes gives the impression of being "ballooned-out" (Fig. 2).

(b) Eccentric chondrosarcoma consists in typical cases of irregular appositions, containing irregular densities. Outgrowths in the surrounding soft tissue, sometimes of appreciable length, are present. The borderline between the tumour and the surrounding soft tissue, is indistinct (Fig. 3).

3. FIBROSARCOMA

We did not succeed in distinguishing a typical X-ray appearance, permitting diagnosis of this type of tumour with a high degree of probability.

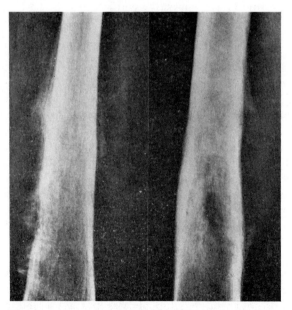

Fig. 1. Radiographically typical case of osteosarcoma.

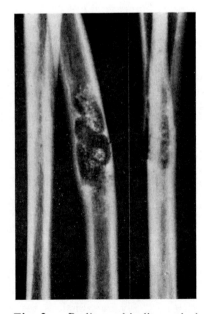

Fig. 2. Radiographically typical case of central chondrosarcoma.

4. EWING'S SARCOMA

Typical X-ray appearances are found in the long tubular bones. In these cases the tumour has involved a large part of the bone and penetrated the entire circumference, the structure of the bone has a mottled or dissociated appearance. There is distinct periosteal bone formation, consisting of spicules and/or lamellar appositions of bone. The layers are not continuous, although the interruptions are sometimes small (Fig. 4).

5. JUXTA-CORTICAL OSTEOSARCOMA

In typical cases the radiographic appearance shows a densely calcified tumour, adherent to the bone with a broad base and partially growing around the bone. Therefore, the cortex can often be traced for some distance underneath the tumour from which it is separated by a narrow radiolucent zone. The cortex under the tumour can be thickened by apposition of bone. Codman's triangles or spicules are not found (Fig. 5). In 10 out of 16 cases we found a typical X-ray appearance.

With regard to the above mentioned X-ray appearances the following can be observed:

1. Typical cases do not lead to difficulties if the radiologist has gained experience with the diagnosis of bone tumours. These roentgenologically typical pictures are found in osteosarcomas and in juxta-cortical osteosarcomas in about 50% of the cases; in the other types of bone sarcoma they occur considerably less frequently. Although these typical X-ray appearances indicate the correct diagnosis with a high degree of probability, one should never forget that certainty only can be obtained by means of histological examination of the tumour tissue.

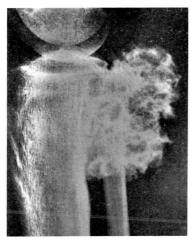

Fig. 3. Radiographically typical case of eccentric chondrosarcoma.

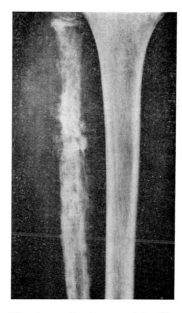

Fig. 4. Radiographically typical case of Ewing's sarcoma.

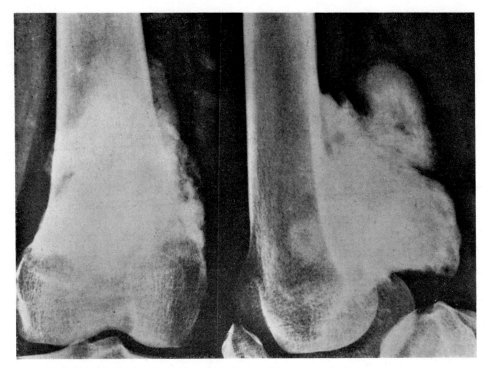

Fig. 5. Radiographiclly typical case of juxta-cortical osteosarcoma.

2. In the majority of the cases of primary bone sarcoma, however, the X-ray picture is atypical, and in these cases diagnostic difficulties arise.

It may be of interest to analyse *why one does not arrive at the correct diagnosis* and *to trace in which cases this is dangerous for the patient*. To make this easier, three groups can be distinguished:

(a) The malignant nature of the lesion is roentgenologically beyond doubt
but

a1 classification is difficult (Figs. 6 and 7).

a2 the radiological appearance closely resembles that of another type of bone sarcoma (Figs. 8 and 9).

a3 a benign lesion presents itself roentgenologically as a malignant tumour (Figs. 10 and 11).

In this group the necessity of biopsy is obvious and this procedure, if properly carried out, will provide in most cases the correct diagnosis. In other words, in this group there is no danger that the nature of the lesion remains unrecognized.

(b) A malignant lesion gives rise to a roentgen-picture of benign aspect.

Cases of bone sarcoma, manifesting themselves as roentgenologically benign lesions are, fortunately, rare but they do occur. Because of the sharp borders of the lesion, the intact cortex and the absence of periosteal bone formation, an osteoblastic osteosarcoma may sometimes resemble a benign process (e.g. chronic osteomyelitis of Garré (Fig. 12)).

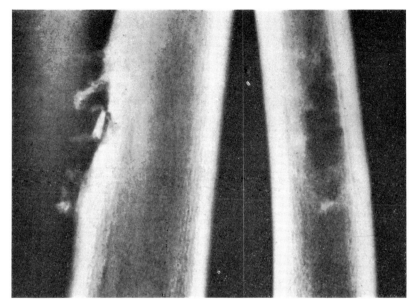

Fig. 6. Case BA 449, destruction of the cortex, some coarse spicule-like appositions. Clearly a malignant lesion. Classification? Histologically: Ewing's sarcoma!

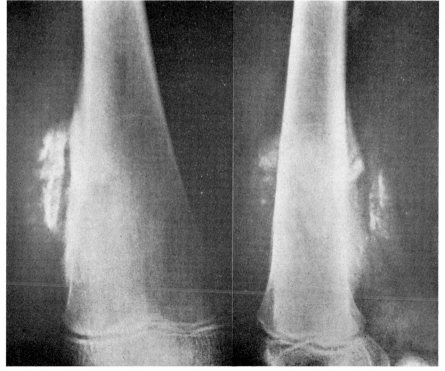

Fig. 7. Case BA 1067, slight destruction of the cortex in the lateral view, triangular periosteal appositions, some spicules, large loose calcified mass. Clearly a malignant lesion. Classification? Histologically: chondrosarcoma!

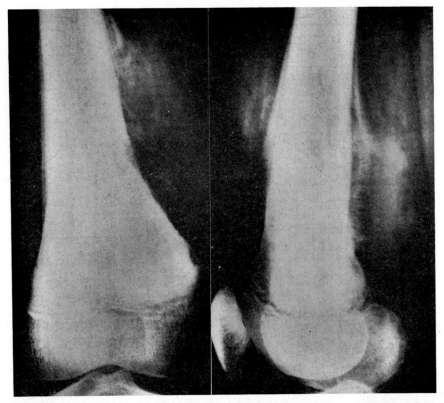

Fig. 8. Case BA 470, typical appearance of osteosarcoma. Histologically: Ewing's sarcoma!

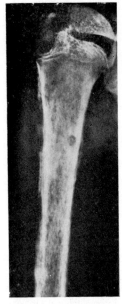

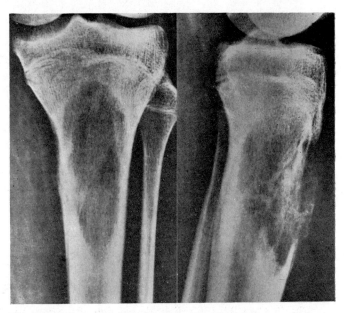

Fig. 9. Case BA 2067, we diagnosed this case as Ewing's sarcoma. Histologically: osteosarcoma!

Fig. 10. Case BA 787, the large cortical defect and the irregular periosteal bone formation suggest a malignant lesion. Histologically: aneurysmal bone-cyst!

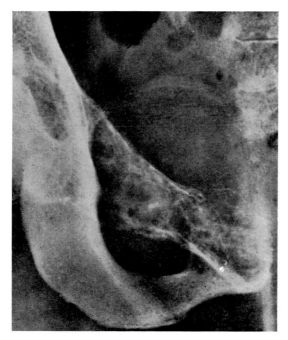

Fig. 11. Case BA 1833, cortex thinned and partially destroyed, vague periosteal apposition and structural changes suggest a malignant lesion. Histologically: fibrous dysplasia!

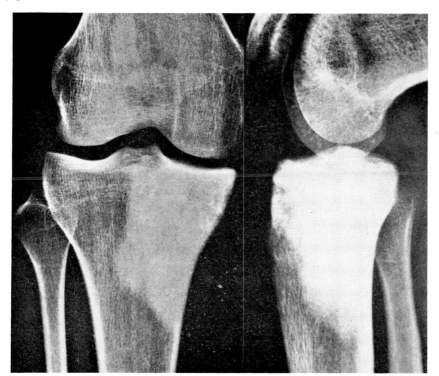

Fig. 12. Case 1321, well defined radiopacity, no cortex destruction, no periosteal bone formation. Benign appearance. Histologically: osteosarcoma!

Most of the cases with a benign roentgen picture we found however among osteosarcomas of a purely osteolytic form which we called "cystic" type because of the sharp
borders, the intact cortex and the slight regular periosteal bone formation (Figs. 13 and
14). Of this "cystic" type we found 12 cases amongst 252 cases of osteosarcoma located
in the long bones. It can be very difficult to differentiate these from an aneurysmal bone
cyst, a giant-cell tumour, or chondromyxoid fibroma. In one case a "cystic" lesion of
benign appearance proved to be a chondrosarcoma (Fig. 15).

These cases with a "cystic" radiographic appearance are insidious in onset, so there is
a great chance that because a benign lesion is diagnosed, the taking of a biopsy is post-
poned. Thus the real nature of the lesion remains for some time undiscovered and treatment, if given, in all probability will be inadequate.

(c) Early cases of bone sarcoma

Early cases of all bone sarcomas mostly show only a periosteal bone formation of limited extent, sometimes of a lamellar appearance, sometimes irregular and ill-defined
(Fig. 16). In some cases small subcortical radiopacities are present. Sometimes small
cortical or subcortical destruction is visible.
On the basis of the X-ray picture alone differentiation from innocent lesions as e.g. a
stress fracture, a local osteomyelitis, or a small osteoid osteoma, proves in most cases to
be difficult or even impossible (Fig. 17). In these cases repeated roentgen examinations
with short intervals are necessary, and biopsy is imperative as soon as suspicion about
the nature of the lesion arises (Fig. 18).

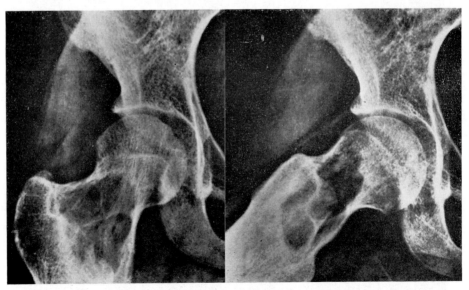

Fig. 13. Case BA 1298, well-defined "cystic" lesion, slight bulging of the cortex,
some septa or ridges. The patient was 15 years of age, our diagnosis therefore was
aneurysmal bone cyst. Histologically: osteosarcoma!

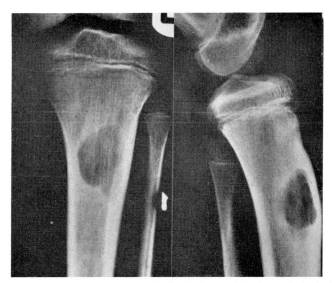

Fig. 14. Case BA 2524, lobulated well-defined "cystic" lesion, slight bulging of the cortex, no signs of malignancy. Our diagnosis was non ossifying fibroma? aneurysmal bone cyst? Histologically: osteosarcoma!

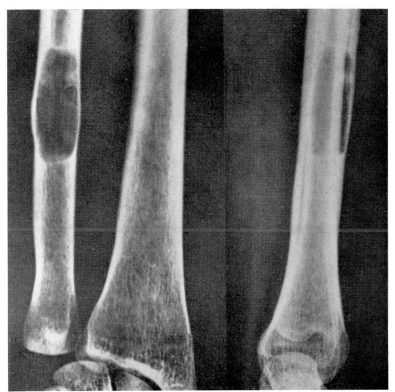

Fig. 15. Case BA 1441, well-defined radiolucent area, bulging and thinning of the cortex, some fine septa or ridges are visible. Our diagnosis was bone cyst or chondroma. Histologically: chondrosarcoma!

E

106

Figure 16. (a) Early case of osteosarcoma.
(b) Early case of Ewing's sarcoma.
(c) Early case of juxtacortical osteosarcoma.

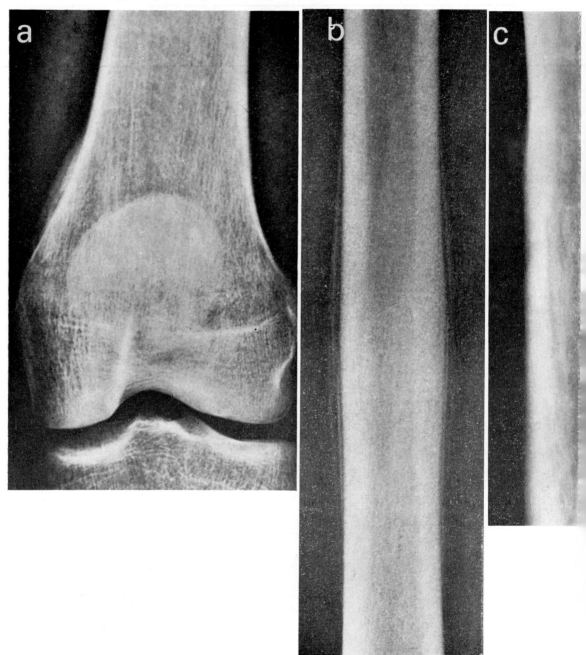

An interesting question is whether or not osteosarcomas producing a roentgenologically benign picture, differ from the others in histological features or behaviour. Comparing the 12 cases, showing radiographically a "cystic" type, with the other osteosarcomas located in long tubular bones (252 cases) the following remarks can be made:

(a) Of the 12 cases five have already a survival of more than 5 years: this is statistically significant ($P < 0.01$).

(b) Concerning the distribution of age, sex and location in the skeleton no difference is evident.

(c) As to the therapy applied, no difference was found compared with the whole series, nor with the group of patients, having a survival of more than 5 years (that is 37 out of 252).

(d) Histologically, two cases belong to the osteosarcomas having a basic pattern of interlacing bundles of fibroblast-like cells and fibres: this type of osteosarcoma has a better prognosis than osteosarcomas in general.

(e) Three cases have a low mitotic activity (one, five and two mitoses per 1,000 tumour cell nuclei), a histological feature favouring a better prognosis.

(f) Two cases belong to the telangiectatic type of osteosarcoma (cystic appearance throughout the whole tumour); one had large telangiectatic areas; three cases contained large cysts, due to secondary changes in the tumour tissue.

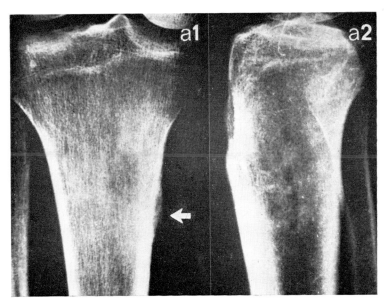

Fig. 17. (a) Case 2891, periosteal apposition of irregular density medially, ill-defined borders; on the lateral view small radiolucencies bordered by vague osteosclerosis. Malignant aspect. Biopsy: osteoid osteoma!

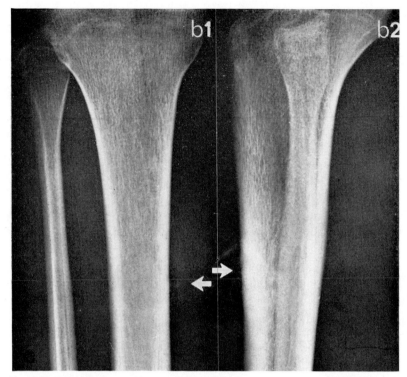

Fig. 17. (b) Case 1136, small irregular periosteal apposition anteriorly ill-defined borders, vague sclerosis in and underneath the cortex. Biopsy: osteosarcoma!

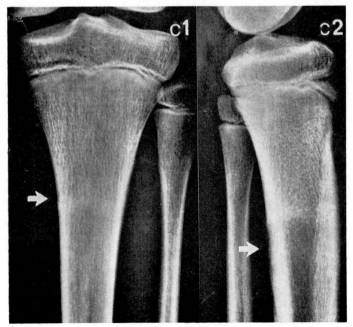

Fig. 17. (c) Case 1068, slight hazy periosteal apposition posteriorly horizontal sclerotic zone extending through the shaft at the same height. Our diagnosis stress-fracture was confirmed by biopsy: only formation of reactive bone.

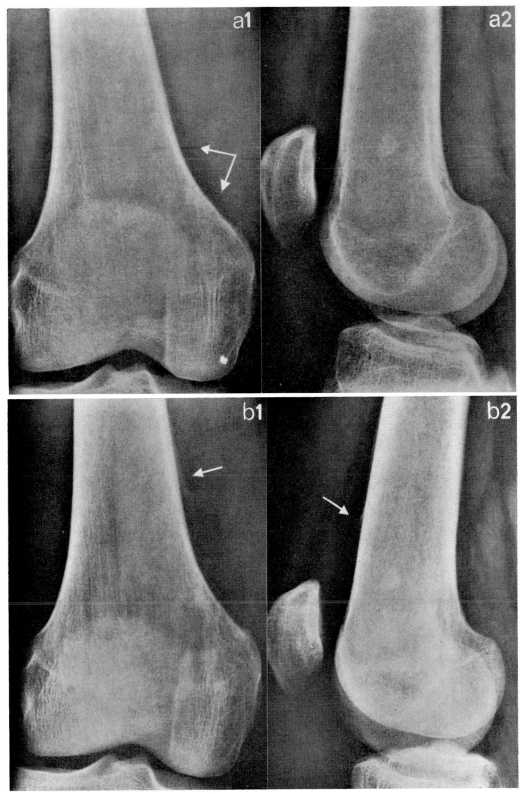

Fig. 18. Case 1541, 20 year old patient complaining for a few weeks of pain in the right knee. (a) Cortex medially poorly defined, distally slight hazy periosteal apposition. (b) 3 weeks later: marked progression of periosteal reaction now showing a malignant character. Biopsy: chondrosarcoma grade III.

In other words, osteosarcomas, showing radiographically a "cystic" appearance have a better prognosis than the other osteosarcomas. In most cases this better prognosis might be due to the presence of histological features favouring a longer survival time. In many cases the "cystic" appearance of the tumour in the radiogram can be explained by the presence of large cystic cavities filled with blood or other fluid.

From the foregoing it will be clear that we not only agree with the opinion of McKenna and co-workers, that the "differential roentgen diagnosis of osteogenic sarcoma is only of academic interest since histological confirmation is required for definitive diagnosis", but that in our opinion this statement holds for all cases in which the X-ray picture suggests a malignant lesion. *But one should not forget that these cases are not the treacherous ones*—which are the bone sarcomas producing a benign X-ray picture (early cases, "cystic" lesions, sclerotic lesions). Therefore, in cases of a benign X-ray appearance it is of the highest importance to analyse not only the X-ray appearance of the lesion itself but also to take into account other data, such as site of the lesion, age of the patient, clinical symptoms, etc. If these are not in accordance with the roentgenologically presumed lesion, one should keep in mind the possibllty of a bone sarcoma and perform a biopsy.

CONCLUSION

We agree with McKenna *et al.* that: "The differential roentgendiagnosis of osteogenic sarcoma is only of academic interest since histological confirmation is required for definitive diagnosis. Maximum effort should be devoted toward deciding whether a bone tumour exists, and whether it is more likely benign or malignant." We would however extend their statement in the following way:

(1) To avoid diagnostic errors one should perform a biopsy in all cases of primary lesions showing a malignant X-ray picture, because roentgendiagnosis never can be certain about the nature of the lesion.

(2) In all cases showing a benign X-ray picture one should keep the possibility in mind that one is dealing with a bone sarcoma when the site, the size, the age or the clinical symptoms are not in accordance with the presumed lesion. In these cases a biopsy should be performed.

(3) Especially, for a small lesion of uncertain nature, X-ray examination should be repeated at short intervals, and if suspicion of malignancy lingers, a biopsy is imperative.

REFERENCE

McKenna, R. J., Schwinn, C. P., Soong, K. Y. & Higinbotham, N. L.   Sarcomata of the Osteogenic Series (Osteosarcoma, Fibrosarcoma, Chondrosarcoma, Parosteal Osteogenic Sarcoma, and Sarcoma arising in Abnormal Bone). *J. Bone Jt. Surg.*, **48-A**, 1, 1966.

Discussion

Prof. Ackerman   Do you feel that arteriography has any value in making a differential diagnosis between a benign and malignant bone tumour?

Prof. von Ronnen   We are not so sure about that. If it is clearly positive—yes. But there are tumours that show an arteriogram that has a benign aspect, but the tumour is a malignant one. We don't believe so much in arteriography as a differential method. As soon as doubt arises we perform a biopsy, as we think it is the most reliable method to see what type of tumour you have.

Dr. Ross   May I ask Professor von Ronnen whether arteriography was in fact performed on these patients or not?

Prof. von Ronnen   Not on the demonstrated cases.

Prof. Lodwick   I noticed with interest that some of your cases which appeared to lie largely outside the bone occupied circumferentially only a small segment on the surface. I did a study of a large number of tumours some years ago in which I looked at this factor of the number of quadrants of cortex which were involved, and it was quite clear that the lesions which were involving only one quarter of the quadrant of circumference of one bone for example had a very high rate of survival as compared with others which extended around the bone periphery.

Prof. von Ronnen   This is a very interesting point, but we didn't investigate it.

Prof. Middlemiss   There is one other point which I would like to bring up. I wonder if we are all using the same terms. Do our Dutch colleagues and their pathologist colleagues recognize different types of osteosarcoma? One which you showed us which looked like an osteosarcoma, and you told us in fact that it was a chondrosarcoma at the lower end of the femur with sclerosis in the shaft in an individual whose epiphysis had not united, I would have expected to be an chondroblastic osteosarcoma. Is this an entity which other people recognize? How do we diagnose osteosarcoma and chondrosarcoma histologically?

Prof. von Ronnen   I think I can now ask my colleague, the pathologist, to answer this question.

Prof. van der Heul   We can diagnose osteosarcoma immediately by the sarcomatous tumour cells. It is not dependent on the amount of cartilage or fibrous tissues. It is I think the criterion most pathologists use to diagnose osteosarcoma.

Prof. Ackerman I think that pathologists are improving over the years and we are getting a little bit better in this area. I think in the past that this was mixed up; but I think at the present moment when we have a chondrosarcoma it is a chondrosarcoma throughout. One of the areas of confusion in the past is that in association with chondrosarcoma there may at times be metaplastic normal bone and this is not an indication to throw that case into the osteosarcoma group. So in our meeting with the WHO group, I think we have thoroughly defined this as a specific entity.

Dr. Cortes Do you have any correlation between the elevation of alkaline phosphatase in your benign and malignant tissues?

Prof. von Ronnen No. We couldn't find it.

Dr. Roylance In Bristol we make a diagnosis, I think it is fair to say, from correlation between all the parameters, radiological, histological, clinical, and behaviour. I understand from your talk the final diagnosis was a histological one, and one in which you use radiology to predict histology. I would like to ask the question whether this was done; because I feel that the importance of radiology is to assist in interpretation of the histology which I believe is as difficult as the radiology you have shown us?

Prof. von Ronnen This is right: but the presence of a bone lesion is shown by the X-ray examination. In our opinion when you find in the X-ray a lesion of a malignant aspect then we think biopsy is imperative; but as I told you before, these lesions are not the treacherous ones. When on the X-ray you find a malignant lesion roentgenologically then I think what we say is—a biopsy should be done and you will find the real nature of the lesion. The difficulty is with benign lesions, and in benign lesions we use all sorts of various parameters to decide—e.g. the age of the patient, the size of the lesion, the blood chemical changes, etc.

The periosteal reaction in bone tumours

by

J. VERMEIJ

SUMMARY

Many osseous lesions cause the formation of reactive new periosteal bone which, on account of the structure of periosteum, the nature of the stimulus and type of bone, characteristically appears in four patterns:

1. Single boneshell.
2. Lamellar boneshells.
3. Spicules.
4. Codman's triangle.

There may often be a combination of these. The single boneshell, often more slowly formed, resembles the cortical structure. Lamellar boneshells indicate a more rapid and intense reaction. The spicular pattern is associated with cortical destruction and periosteal displacement. With cortical perforation and rapid extraosseous spread of a tumour, any new subperiosteal bone is destroyed and a Codman's triangle is produced. These changes may be demonstrated histologically and radiographically and are related to the type of bone involved—long bone, vertebra, skull, etc.

An analysis is presented of periosteal reactions seen in 213 benign tumours, 168 tumour-like lesions and for 234 bone sarcomas, and reflect the histological grading of the malignant tumours.

WHEN A PATHOLOGICAL process develops in the marrow cavity of a bone and reaches or even destroys the cortex, a periosteal reaction is likely to occur.

It is well known that a periosteal reaction, which is visible on the radiograph, may be the first sign of a process taking place inside the bone, for example in cases of osteomyelitis and malignant bone tumours.

What is the anatomical relationship between the periosteum and cortical bone? The periosteum contains osteoblasts, scattered as isolated cells over the cortical surface, and to the outside there is fibrous tissue, several layers thick, in which the periosteal blood vessels are situated. These blood vessels communicate with the circulatory system within the Haversian canals of the cortex, via ramifications passing through the deeper layers of the periosteum and through the Volkmann canals. In addition, collagenous fibres anchor the periosteum to the cortex.

The stimulus to which the periosteum reacts is formed by a complex of physical and chemical changes originating from the underlying process. There are changes in tissue tension or pressure, disturbances in chemical equilibrium affecting the circulation of intercellular fluid, and differences in electric potential. This causes tissue reactions and changes in the blood circulation in the vicinity of the process. Such stimulation of the periosteum results in proliferation of osteoblasts as well as of fibroblasts.

113

The osteoblasts will form new bone, and since within one or two weeks calcium salts are deposited in this bone, the resulting periosteal reaction will be visible on the radiograph.

The periosteal reaction can take four forms (Fig. 1):

      1. A single boneshell.
      2. Lamellar boneshells.
      3. Spicules.
      4. Codman's triangle.

These four forms often occur in various combinations, but a periosteal reaction may also be absent, with or without the occurrence of destruction of the cortex.

The changes taking place in the four periosteal reactions can be described as follows:

The Single Boneshell

The stimulus leading to the formation of a single boneshell may be present for a period ranging from months to several years. The phenomenon differs from the normal bone formation and remodelling by the domination of osteoblastic activity over osteoclastic bone absorption. The single boneshell has the same structure as the normal cortex except that its thickness may be smaller in cases in which the primary process causes increased bone absorption from the inside of the cortex (Fig. 1).

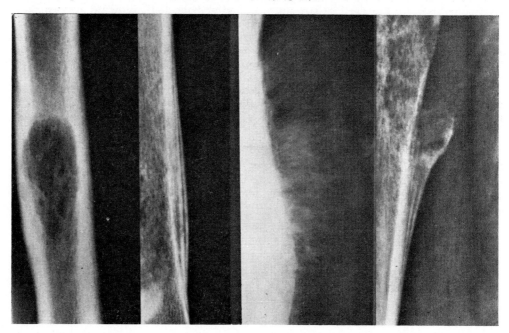

Fig. 1. The four forms of periosteal reaction; from left to right: single bone shell, lamellar boneshells, spicules and Codman's triangle.

Lamellar Boneshells　　　(Fig. 2).

Here, the stimulus is more intense than in the case of the single boneshell. The periosteum becomes many cell layers thicker than in the case of a single boneshell.

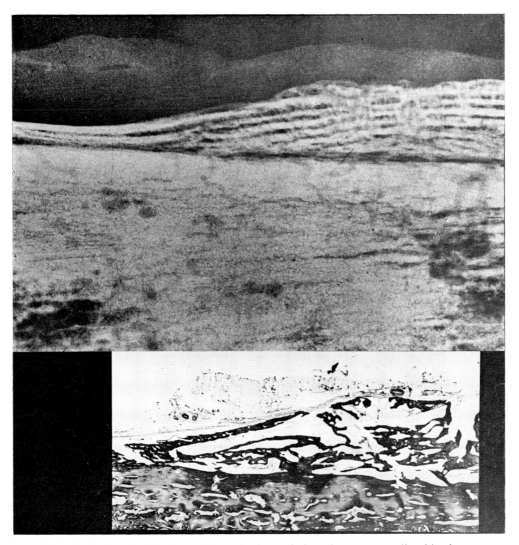

Fig. 2. Codman's triangle: radiograph above; below the corresponding histology.

The new boneshell is formed by multiple layers of osteoblasts on its cortical and outer sides. Still the bone layer thus formed has perforations permitting blood vessels to reach the cortex as well to make communication possible between the deeper and superficial layers of osteoblasts. When stimulation persists, the superficial layers of the periosteum proliferate still further, outside the newly formed boneshell, while the osteoblasts on the cortical side of the boneshell become inactive and disappear, to be replaced by loose fibrous tissue. In this way, separate, parallel boneshells are formed. The radiological picture does not show the perforations, due to superimposition of the bony struc·tures.

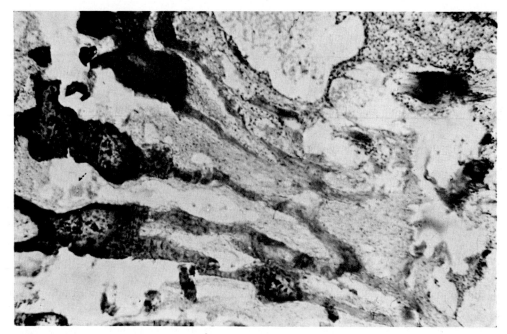

Fig. 3. Histological appearance of bone spicules.

SPICULES   (Figs. 1 and 3.)

The primary process causes destruction of the cortex with dissociation of the cortical bone. Besides the proliferation of the periosteum, the tumour pushes the periosteum outward. In some cases this lifting up of the periosteum is caused by the accumulation of exudate or by haemorrhage. The osteoblasts are then situated along the stretched blood vessels, and anchoring fibres. The reactive bone shows a radiating pattern or the spicules lie perpendicular to the cortex. On the outer side, the process is bordered by the fibrous layer of the periosteum, and when its development is arrested, for example after irradiation, a boneshell is formed on the periphery of the process, resting on the previously formed spicules.

CODMAN'S TRIANGLE   (Figs. 1 and 2.)

The tumour breaks through the cortex, destroying the structure of the periosteal reaction. The periosteum will be pushed forward, the fibrous layer holding out as long as possible. There is no time for spicules to be formed, and reactive bone is only formed at the proximal and distal ends of the tilted periosteum. This new bone takes the form of a triangle, its base turned toward the tumour tissue and being excavated thereby.

The anatomical structures of the various periosteal reactions are identical in the radiological and histologic pictures (Figs. 4 and 6).

As is generally known, the periosteal reaction is non-specific. Nevertheless, the occurrence of the four forms alone or in combination differs in certain diseases. The

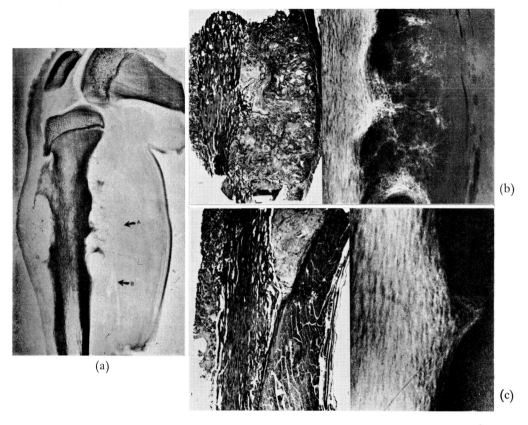

Fig. 4. Osteosarcoma of tibia. (a) Survey radiograph. (b) and (c) are enlarged details indicated by the corresponding arrows in the survey radiograph. In (b) and (c) on the left side are the histologic pictures and on the right side the corresponding radiographs.

formation of a periosteal reaction is different in different parts of the skeleton. The four mentioned forms of reaction are most clearly visible in limb bones. In bone lesions of the vertebral column a periosteal reaction usually will be visible in the vertebral arch. (Aneurysmal bone cyst, benign osteoblastoma.)

Of the malignant bone tumours, Ewing's sarcoma often causes the formation of spicules when localized in pelvis and ribs. The formation of a periosteal reaction, other than a single boneshell, in tumours of the skull is rare. Well known is the formation of spicules in cases of metastases of medulloblastoma and in haematoma.

The tables show the incidence of periosteal reaction for 213 benign primary bone tumours (Table 1) and also for 168 tumour-like lesions (Table 2). All the material comes from the archives of the Dutch Committee on Bone Tumours.

In 110 cases of benign tumours and 64 cases of tumour-like lesions, single boneshells were found; in 85 and 71 cases, respectively, there was no periosteal reaction.

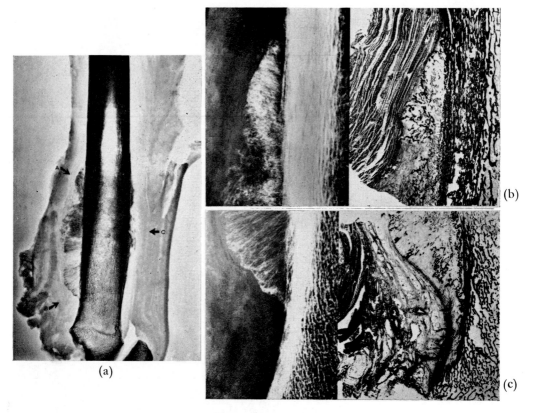

(a)

(b)

(c)

Fig. 5. Osteosarcoma of femur. (a) Survey radiograph. (b) and (c) are enlarged details indicated by the corresponding arrows in the survey radiograph. In (b) and (c), the histologic pictures are on the right side and the corresponding radiographs on the left side.

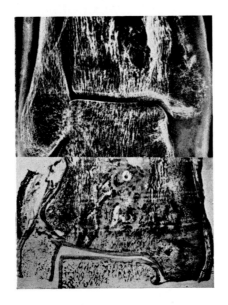

Fig. 6. Ewing's sarcoma of tibia. The radiograph above shows the same details of bone structure as the histologic slide underneath. Note the structure of the spicules on the right.

TABLE 1. NUMBER OF BENIGN TUMOURS IN THE SKELETON

Tumour	Periosteal Reaction						
	No reaction	Single sh.	Lamell. sh.	Single-lamell.	Codm. tri.	Lam. -Codm. -spic.	
Osteoblastoma	5	6					11
Osteoid-osteoma	7	7		3			17
Chondroblastoma	15	6					21
Chondroma	11	13					24
Condro-myx. fibroma		8					8
Exostosis, osteochondroma	16						16
Non-ossif. fibroma		21					21
Giant-cell tumour groups I, II	15	27	3	2	1		48
Haematoma	9						9
Aneurysmal cyst	7	22		7			36
	85	110	3	12	1		211

Abbreviations: sh. = shell. lamell. = lamella. Codm. = Codman's triangle. spic. = spicules.

TABLE 2. NUMBER OF BENIGN TUMOUR-LIKE LESIONS IN THE SKELETON

Lesion	Periosteal Reaction						
	No reaction	Single sh.	Lamell. sh.	Single-lamell.	Codm. tri.	Lam. -Codm. -spic.	
Fibrous dysplasia	15	26		1			42
Paget's disease	10						10
Fibrous cortical defect	1						1
Solitary cyst	8	20					28
Eosinophil granuloma	6	7	5	1			19
Hyperparathyroidism	4	1					5
Myositis ossificans	11						11
Reactive bone formation	8	8	12	1		1	30
Osteomyelitis	8	2	11		1		22
	71	64	28	3	1	1	168

Abbreviations: sh. = shell. lamell. = lamella. Codm. = Codman's triangle. spic. = spicules.

In malignant bone tumours the variety of periosteal reactions is greater. For localizations in extremities, the histograms show the frequency in 127 osteosarcomas, 54 chondrosarcomas, 29 fibrosarcomas, and 24 Ewing's sarcomas. (Figs. 7, 8, 9 and 10.)

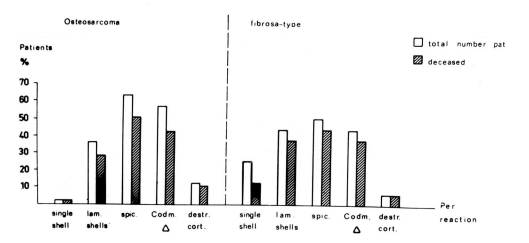

Fig. 7.

Abbreviations: Lam.—lamellar. Spic.—spicules. Codm.—Codman's. destr. cort.— destruction of cortex. Per.—periosteal.

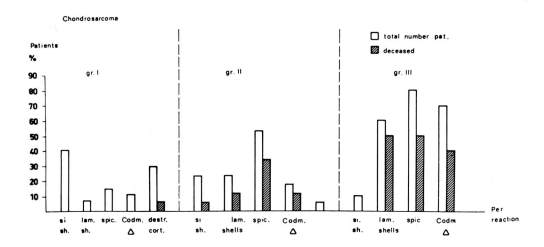

Fig. 8.

Abbreviations: Lam.—lamellar. Spic.—spicules. Codm.—Codman's. destr. cort.— destruction of cortex. Per.—periosteal.

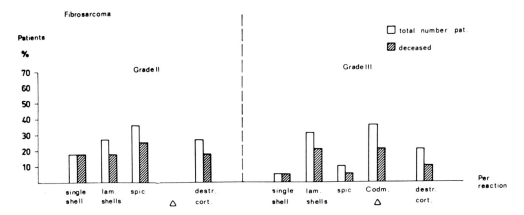

Fig. 9.

Abbreviations: Lam.—lamellar. Spic.—spicules. Codm.—Codman's. destr. cort.—destruction of cortex. Per.—periosteal.

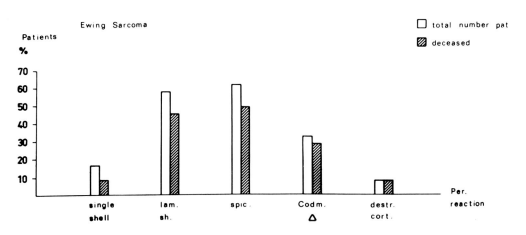

Fig. 10.

Abbreviations: Lam.—lamellar. Spic.—spicules. Codm.—Codman's. destr. cort.—destruction of cortex. Per.—periosteal.

In osteosarcoma the spicules and Codman's triangles are predominant. In chondrosarcoma grade I the single boneshell occurs most frequently, in grade II the spicules, and in grade III spicules and Codman's triangles. In fibrosarcoma grade II spicules predominate and in grade III the Codman's triangles. In Ewing's sarcoma lamellar boneshells and spicules, often in combination, are the most frequent periosteal reactions.

There is a positive correlation between histological grading and the sequence single boneshell, lamellar boneshells, spicules, and Codman's triangles.

BIBLIOGRAPHY

Atlas of Tumor Pathology, Section II, Fascicle 4.

Ackermann, L. V. & Spjut, H. J. *Tumors of Bone and Cartilage.* Armed Forces Institute of Pathology, Washington, D.C. 1962.

Bassett, C., *et al.* Biologic Significance of Piezoelectricity, *Calc. Tiss. Res.*, **1**, No. 4, 252–272, 1968.

Bloom, W. & Fawcett, D. W. *A Textbook of Histology*, W. B. Saunders Comp., Philadelphia, 1968.

Bourne, G. H. *The Biochemistry and Physiology of Bone.* Academic Press Inc., New York, 1956.

Codman, E. A. *The Shoulder.* Boston, 1934.

Committee on Bone Tumours, Dutch, Radiological Atlas of Bone Tumours. Mouton, The Hague, 1966.

Day, S. B. Ossified Subperiosteal Hematoma. *J. Amer. Med. Ass.*, **173**, 986–990, 1960.

Edeiken, J. & Hodes, Ph. J. *Roentgen Diagnosis of Diseases of Bone.* Williams and Williams, Baltimore, 1968.

Garber, C. Z. Reactive Bone Formation in Ewing's Sarcoma. *Cancer*, **4**, 839, 1951.

Ham, A. W. A Histological Study of the Early Phases of Bone Repair. *J. Bone Jt. Surg.*, **12**, 827–844, 1939.

van der Heul, R. O. *Het periostale Ossificerende fibrosarcom en de Gradering van Osteosarcomen.* Thesis, Leiden, 1962.

Jaffe, H. L. *Tumors and Tumorous Conditions of the Bones and Joints.* Lea and Febiger, Philadelphia, 1964.

Lodwick, G. S. Solitary Malignant Tumours of Bone. *Seminars of Roentgenol.*, **1**, No. 3, 1966.

von Ronnen, J. R. *Frühdiagnostik von Bösartigen Knochentumoren.* Referat Deutscher Röntgen Kongres, 1964.

Vermeij, J., *The Periosteal Reaction in Malignant Bone Tumours, Proceedings Symposium Ossium*, ed. by A. M. Jelliffe & B. Strickland, p. 310. Livingstone, London, 1968.

Discussion

Dr. Lloyd Before anybody starts tearing the speaker to pieces, may I congratulate him please on his lovely pictures, particularly where you are putting the radiological and histological appearances next to one another in such a way that each one tells you what the other one means. I think it was very nice.

Dr. Vermeij I have to say that I didn't make the pictures myself completely but with our photographer of course; but I selected them.

Prof. Sissons I would like to go along with that comment. I would like to follow by asking Dr. Vermeij if, in his experience, he has ever found the spicular appearance that he commented on and illustrated to us as a result of tumour ossification as opposed to a process of periosteal reaction?

Dr. Vermeij As a process of periosteal reaction yes, but I must admit that there is a kind of very porous spicules which are formed by tumour tissue in osteosarcoma. But what I have shown you is periosteal reaction.

Dr. Friedman Perhaps you could tell us what causes the absence of periosteal reaction say in multiple myeloma which is quite aggressive and in metastatic carcinoma?

Dr. Vermeij I cannot answer the question completely, but we know that in slow-growing processes you don't see a reaction perhaps at a given moment. It is only a momentary picture you get. In other cases the process is growing so fast that there is no time for a periosteal reaction to take place, but then you usually see destruction of the cortex. Apart from that there are factors we don't know about—chemical factors, physical factors—I would say specific for the process perhaps. In the case of myeloma they are the reason that you do not see the periosteal reaction. In many cases of metastases you don't find it, but I must say in myeloma it is usual. I cannot answer that completely but you always have to look at the cortex itself. If it is dissociated there will probably be a rapidly growing process.

Mr. Fitton I would like to ask Dr. Vermeij if you ever find the single shell and the lamellae at the same time in the same patient. It seems to me that it may represent a natural history that the lamellar formation of the periosteum precedes what is later the single shell?

Dr. Vermeij Yes, and that is what we don't find. We find combinations of the other periosteal reactions, but not of the single shell and lamellar shells. That is the reason why I say, in the cases of lamellar bone shells, you have a more actively growing process.

123

Prof. Campbell   Have you analyzed the endosteal reaction and reaction of the cancellous bone on the inner side of the bone and compared it with your periosteal reaction in any of these cases?

Dr. Vermeij   In most cases of the tumours I have looked after, there was destruction of the cortex and then you don't see the endosteal reaction, you usually don't see it in the radiographs. Endosteal reaction you find in the femur neck often and perhaps in vertebral bodies, but in the limb bones you see expansion of the cortex and no endosteal reaction but on the outside the periosteal reaction; so I don't see this.

Prof. Middlemiss   Professor von Ronnen emphasized how difficult diagnosis is in his presentation this morning. In this very careful analysis of periosteal changes, are you able to tell us, how to differentiate between a malignant periosteal reaction and a non-malignant periosteal reaction? Is there anything emerging on this?

Dr. Vermeij   Well, here you come to the difficult field of perhaps the benign lesion such as osteomyelitis and reactive bone formation, callus formation and so on and the malignant tumours. I must say that the periosteal reaction is unspecific and you cannot depend on that, you see. There are of course other criteria in the radiograph too which enable you to decide between a malignant or benign lesion, but again you heard from Professor von Ronnen how difficult it can be. You cannot judge on the periosteal reaction itself; you can judge probably on the combinations.

A syntactical approach to analysis of bone neoplasia

by

GWILYM S. LODWICK

SUMMARY

In radiodiagnosis methodical image analysis followed by logical synthesis leads to interpretive accuracy—whether by the eye alone or with computer assistance. Some observed features are certain—e.g. lesional site; others require probabilistic assessment. In every example a sequence of data is sought and studied—site and size, growth rate, edge peculiarities, bone reaction, matrix formation and the pattern of intrinsic mineralization.

Either visually or by computer analysis this information is recorded, classified, evaluated and summed. With computer assisted diagnosis the chance of the first diagnosis being correct is about 75%; if extended to include the first three alternatives about 95% correct. The process may be developed to computer data collection and analysis of radiant image techniques, but may require recognition of arrays not normally used for visual inspection. Future progress in automated pattern recognition is anticipated.

WHEN I CHOSE "Syntactical Approach" as the title of this paper, I was thinking of a rather specific kind of logic which we employ in the completely automated computer analysis of radiant images, where we start with the largest identifiable object, then proceed to identify smaller and yet smaller objects in fields until we have found the object which we have been looking for. In thinking it through however, it is apparent that in the sense of the definition of syntax "an orderly progression of words or elements", the syntactical approach has equal application to what follows.

First a few generalizations about the logic of diagnosis.

1. Diagnosis is a process of data reduction. Here the application "syntactical" comes into full bloom, because we start with the large and through a logical string of events, wind up with the small. In diagnosis we often begin the process with an almost unlimited number of possibilities, and hopefully at the end have one correct diagnosis, or perhaps several good possibilities.

2. Data treatment is either Boolean or probabilistic. In considering the data which are being reduced, in number, there are two kinds (a) those which represent powerful predictors, and which ordinarily are Boolean in nature in that they are either present or absent. (b) Those where the probability of presence varies dependent upon the particular kind of disease. An example of the former might be location, where a lesion either is or is not centered within the epiphysis. Of the latter, we can consider flocculent calcification, where the probability of presence in chondroblastoma is about 35%.

3. The sequence of data use is important. In decision making, the best logic is to use the most positive evidence, or the most powerful predictors, in the first order of priority reserving the less powerful predictors for lower orders of priorities. Where there is a significant doubt about the presence of absence of a certain symptom or finding, it is best not to use that information rather than to guess.

Passing on to some generalizations about lesions within bone we can accept the following:

4. In lesions of bone there are certain natural rules of behavior relative to site and size. Because of this fact, location and size are excellent variables with which to accomplish data reduction. For example, a lesion arising within the medullary canal certainly cannot be myositis ossificans which always is in the soft tissues or on the surface of bone. Further, a lesion out in the soft tissues cannot be non-ossifying fibroma, which always is in the cortex or medullary canal. As an example of size, primary malignant bone tumors are rarely less than 6 cm in diameter.

5. Some kinds of lesions grow slowly, others may be highly variable in their rate of growth. For example, chondroblastoma can be depended upon to be a slowly progressing lesion. On the other hand, chondrosarcoma or fibrosarcoma may be found throughout the entire spectrum of rate of growth, sometimes slowly growing, sometimes rapidly growing, and sometimes intermediate. For this reason, the histologic diagnosis of certain lesions such as fibrosarcoma often does not always provide a clear image of the character of the disease process.

6. Slowly growing (benign) tumors obey the natural rules relative to site and size. Rapidly growing tumors (malignant) do not. For example, the giant-cell tumor of a long bone is always found in the end or in a metaphysis analogue. One never finds giant-cell tumor in the middle of a long bone. However, osteosarcoma, while having sites of predilection, may arise almost anywhere in the skeletal system.

7. Slowly growing lesions remain circumscribed; rapidly growing lesions do not. Radiologists and others from the beginning have recognized intuitively the character of circumscription or encapsulation for certain lesions.

8. Degree of circumscription is reflected by one or both of two types of reactive phenomena; destruction or proliferation of bone. By way of illustration, geographic bone destruction with its sharp edge reflects circumscription, the permeated destruction blending into intact cortex reflects a diffuse spread. Also, the sclerotic rim of expanded shell around a lesion reflects circumscription, whereas Codman's triangles and mottled proliferative response reflects disorganized defense patterns. Circumscription seems to be a function of slow or moderate growth rate.

In the radiant image of a soft tissue tumor, circumscription, if present, cannot ordinarily be detected. For this reason, it is extremely difficult to assess rate of growth of soft tissue tumors from X-rays.

9. Specific kinds of lesions can induce peculiarities in edge patterns or in reactive response which indirectly identify the cell type of such lesions. It is perfectly clear that one cannot see tumor cells in the X-rays. However, each kind of tumor has its own peculiarities of behavior, and these perculiarities, if looked for, can be valuable predictive clues as to diagnosis. For example, chondrosarcoma in its well-differentiated form destroys bone with an edge pattern unlike that of other kinds of tumors. Osteosarcoma produces the sunburst pattern of spiculation. Ewing's sarcoma produces the hair-on-end pattern.

10. Certain kinds of neoplasms are capable of forming matrices (cartilage, bone) which mineralize. Patterns of mineralization can reflect (a) the kind of matrix, and (b) the degree of differentiation of the tumor. For example, the parosteal sarcoma forms an unusually mature bone matrix. Tumor bone may be so perfect that it may be mistaken by radiologists and pathologists alike for a non-neoplastic process.

Osteosarcoma, ordinarily much more poorly differentiated, produces a calcifiable matrix which appears highly disorganized. Parenthetically, it is important to point out that actively growing neoplasms with calcifiable matrix tend to calcify centrally; osteosarcoma for the reason that more mature matrix is likely to be in the center of the tumor; and chondrosarcoma for the reason that calcification often occurs in the central degenerated portion of the tumor. By contrast, most injury and repair reactions such as myositis ossificans or bone marrow infarct calcify around the periphery at the interface between normal and damaged tissue.

11. The variables of size, shape, location, bone destruction, edge characteristics, proliferative response and matrix mineralization can be identified and classified through radiant imaging techniques. Through such constellations of patterns which reflect gross morphology, the growth characteristics of disease in bone can be clearly identified, and cellular types often inferred.

In practice, the application of these principles can apply to human diagnosis, computer-assisted diagnosis, or completely automated diagnosis of radiant images. The recently published atlas, *The Bones and Joints*, defines a language of communication about bone disease, and shows how to apply the language and these principles in human diagnosis. The book was prepared with computer assistance, and the differential diagnoses shown on each plate are arrived at by the computer after receiving information which the radiologist has extracted from the radiant image. If one accepts the 99% probability as the classic image, it is possible to see how images vary within the same diagnostic category and overlap with other categories. Such overlap is a fact of life, and is the most obvious source of error in medical diagnosis.

The logic applied to obtain data reduction in this particular application is based on the principles enumerated above. These principles are embodied in a decision tree which employs a Boolean treatment of data to accomplish preliminary reduction. This is followed by a Bayesian application of decision theory to narrow the diagnostic range to the ultimate degree. For this particular computer-assisted system, the probability of the first diagnosis being correct is about three out of four. The probability of one of the first three choices being corrected is about 95 out of 100. I am not completely certain how this ranks with my own diagnostic ability, but in a sense this is a kind of a game, because from the radiologist's point of view, to arrive at the right cell type is impressive but not as valuable as his estimation of rate of growth. Where a lesion is aggressive enough to endanger the future health of the patient, evaluation of histologic cell type is better left in the hands of the pathologist.

For the past several years, we have been moving into a new phase of this effort where the computer not only calculates probabilities but accomplishes the initial acquisition of image information. This is an exciting field, because we can see that there are many approaches to the problem of making a diagnosis other than those which are most effectively managed in human hands. In our initial effort to diagnose acquired heart disease through direct computer scanning and evaluation, the rate of diagnosis substantially exceeds that of a team of radiologists. Of special interest, however, is the fact that this was accomplished through data arrays quite different from those ordinarily used by humans. Our efforts to date lie in the area of analyzing chest films, where our goals are the diagnosis of heart disease, lung cancer, and coal miners' black lung disease. These are health problems of great interest in the United States. We have moreover been working on the problem of direct computer diagnosis of bone disease, focusing on the knee. It is necessary in this kind of application to use an image system which has certain standard characteristics which permit the computer to "find itself", so to speak.

The problem of automated diagnosis from images is now one of world-wide interest. We know that the Japanese are now planning to spend nearly 100 million dollars (40 million pounds) in the next several years on the problem of automated pattern recognition. The pay-off is great, not only in the medical field of where the computer may relieve the radiologist of a substantial element of his burden, but also in industry for quality control and automated inspection, and in communication for recognition and simulation of the human voice. It appears that we are living in an era of technology where progress in automated pattern recognition can be expected to be extremely rapid.

BIBLIOGRAPHY

Lodwick, G. S., Haun, C. L., Smith, W. D., Keller, R. F., & Robertson, E. D. Computer Diagnosis of Primary Bone Tumors: A Preliminary Report. *Radiology*, 80, 273–275, February 1963.

Lodwick, G. S., Keats, R. E. & Dorst, J. P. The Coding of Roentgen Images for Computer Analysis as Applied to Lung Cancer. *Radiology*, 81, No. 2, pp. 185–200, August 1963.

Lodwick, G. S. Reactive Response to Local Injury in Bone. *Radiologic Clinics of North America*, Vol. II, No. 2, pp. 209–219, August 1964.

Lodwick, G. S. Radiographic Diagnosis and Grading of Bone Tumors, with Comments on Computer Evaluation. *Proceedings of Fifth National Cancer Conference, Philadelphia, September 1964*, pp. 369–380. J. B. Lippincott Company.

Lodwick, G. S. A Probabilistic Approach to the Diagnosis of Bone Tumors. *Radiological Clinics of North America*, Vol. III, No. 3, pp. 487–497, December 1965.

Lodwick, G. S. Solitary Malignant Tumors of Bone: The Application of Predictor Variables in Diagnosis. *Seminars in Roentgenology*, Vol. 1, No. 3, pp. 293–313, July 1966.

Lodwick, G. S. & Reichertz, P. Computer Assisted Diagnosis of Tumors and Tumor-Like Lesions of Bone. The Limited Bayes' Concept. *Proceedings of Symposium Osseum, London*, 1970. 305. Ed. by A. M. Jelliffe & B. Strickland. Livingstone, Edinburgh & London.

Lehr, J. L., Parkey, R. W., Garrotto, L. J., Harlow, C. A. & Lodwick, G. S. Computer Algorithms for Detection of Brain Scintigram Abnormalities. *Radiology*, 97, 269, 1970.

Sutton, R. N., Hall, E. L. & Lodwick, G. S. Texture Measurement of Pulmonary Pathology, *24th ACEMB*, 1971.

Lodwick, G. S. *The Bones and Joints*. Year Book Medical Publishers, Inc. *Chicago* 1971.

Ausherman, D. A., Dwyer, S. J. & Lodwick, G. S. Feature Extraction for Computer Diagnosis of Primary Bone Tumors. *Proceedings, Two Dimentional Digital Signal Processing Conference Columbia, Missouri*. October 1971.

Henderson, S. E., Harlow, C. A. & Lodwick, G. S. Feature Extraction of Knee X-Rays. Technical, Report. Published in the Special Issue of *IEEE Computer Transactions on Feature Extraction and Selection in Pattern Recognition*, September 1971.

Hall, D. L., Lodwick, G. S., Kruger, R. P., Townes, J. R. & Dwyer, S. J. Direct Computer Diagnosis of Rheumatic Heart Disease. *Radiology*, **101**, 497, December 1971.

DeGroot, J. M., Hall, E. L., Sutton, R. N., Dwyer, S. J. & Lodwick, G. S. Perception of Computer Simulated Lesions in Chest Radiographs, ACM 1972 Conference, Submitted.

Discussion

Dr. Vermeij   In the first place I want to compliment Professor Lodwick on his excellent paper. I want to ask you about the size of the tumour. I think in my experience this is not a reliable, and sometimes even a dangerous, criterion where we are making a diagnosis of a bone tumour. We know that many benign tumours grow very rapidly—e.g. aneurysmal bone cyst—and may be quite large. On the other hand we know that malignant tumours are often small lesions if seen early in the course of the disease. So I want to know what are the results of your investigations. Is it better to leave this criterion out when you use a computer?

Prof. Lodwick   In considering size, it is only one of a number of signs that you are going to use, you will use many other things. In the grading situation I have a special rhythm which the computer traces down through a whole series of steps; the size I regard as one of the least powerful of the predicted variables. I was thinking more in terms of human interpretation. When I see a lesion size is one of the things that I always look at. Then I see a small lesion and then I start fitting the other components of the image together which are important, such as its location, its exact location in bone, whether it is in the epiphysis, the metaphysis, the shaft, whether it is in the cortex and so forth, whether it is circumscribed, and all these things. Now if I see a lesion which is larger than 6 cm, I know that there are many slowly growing lesions—chondrosarcomas, for example—which do get beyond 6 cm, they grow to a huge size and they are still slowly growing, but they take many years to get there. So you have to consider size, you can't reject size, it is a useful tool. You can only put it in as well in the constellation of symptoms that you have. Each of these symptoms together may comprise a pattern, and all of them will focus in, so to speak, on a certain diagnosis. So you just can't isolate size and point out and say yes or no, but you have to use it as part of the whole.

Dr. Jacobs   You must excuse my complete ignorance about this if I ask this question. When you say the computer is seventy odd per cent correct, or ninety odd per cent in its first differential diagnosis of three, what are you comparing it with, and what is its base line; what do you think it ought to say on the histologist's final report?

Prof. Lodwick   I think this is a very important point. I think it brings up the point that is illustrated here today. We have a group from Holland, they have their pathologist. If I were to try to focus on every pathologist that was in this group, I would be hung up completely because pathologists are not in agreement in the classifications. So far as I am concerned, I take a pathologist that I trust and I stick to him. I had my training with pathology of bone by Lent Johnson at the Armed Forces Institute of Pathology, and from my point of view, his diagnosis is the last diagnosis and that is what I am comparing computer diagnosis or my diagnosis with. Now, this gets me into trouble from time to time because each pathologist may have his peculiarities and if I accept that pathologist, I can't just take what I like and reject the rest but I have to go along

130

with his peculiarities. So sometimes I could look a little screwey because the particular pathologist that I am working with doesn't necessarily agree with every other pathologist in the country in the particular element. I looked screwey for example in the consideration of cysts because Lent Johnson rejects the concept of aneurysmal bone cyst. Personally I don't, but in my atlas that I published recently I don't really make a diagnosis of aneurysmal bone cyst because I have to depend on my pathologist's point of view.

Dr. Ball   Do you have any information about changes in growth rate with time?

Prof. Lodwick   I have not made a special study of it, but I think it is perfectly clear that there are a number of lesions which do have changes of growth rate in time and I think that certainly one of these is aneurysmal bone cyst; and I will speak as Lodwick this time—not Johnson. Aneurysmal bone cyst, you know starts out with a tremendous burst of growth and during the period of time when it is growing most rapidly you see extremely thin or no cortex over it and the edges may be moth-eaten. There is usually this geographic pattern of bone destruction which is predominant. Then over a period of time, even without radiation, or treatment, this lesion may slow down, and indeed it seems almost to be self limited. That is one example where a lesion grows rapidly to begin with and then slows down as it goes along. We commented on myeloma a while ago as being a very rapidly growing disease and true enough myeloma does kill a patient very rapidly. I think this is not so much because it focally is a rapidly growing lesion; focally it has all the characteristics of slow growth.

   Those of you who have had experience with numbers of cases of myeloma will certainly remember cases where a single lesion has been present in the skeletal system over a very long period of time. Even those multiple lesions around the skeleton are very characteristic of slow growth, and it is rather unusual to see myeloma which has a permeated pattern of bone response or evidence of really rapid growth. It kills because it is so widely disseminated that it destroys all blood forming elements or for other reasons.

Dr. Murray   I would like you to support your figures, Dr. Lodwick, regarding the accuracy of diagnosis by emphasizing that you have been, I think I am correct in saying, including a large number of difficult lesions. You see most of us would get, I think 99 out of 100 metaphyseal fibrous defects right; and we probably get 99 out of 100 exostoses right. Can you give us some indication out of the cases you analysed by the computer, of how many were malignant or difficult benign tumours from the ordinary radiological diagnostic point of view?

Prof. Lodwick   Well, to me the diagnosis of osteosarcoma with my pathologist is a fairly easy diagnosis. I think that the diagnostic probability would be very high—in the low nineties. There is a feeling you know, you can't get much higher than 93, 94, 95%. The same thing is true with chondroblastoma. The principle cause for misdiagnosis in the X-ray, as far as I am concerned, is overlapping patterns and there is nothing unique about circumscription or an expanded shell. One of the really unique things about slowly growing lesions is their specific location in bone. It would seem to me that the principle source of error is in overlapping patterns—that you really don't have a good clue to the cell type. I think it is very impressive when we can come up with a high diagnostic rate in the terms of the pathologists. But we are not working in our own dimension, we are working in their dimension. I think our dimension is assessment of rate of growth and the estimation of rate of growth morphology, and the decision-making process as to whether this patient should go on and be biopsied, or whether this is something that we don't need to worry about. I feel so assured about this that I would certainly not send up my non-ossifying fibromas of bone to be biopsied; I just don't send the fibroxanthomas. I don't feel that this is a requirement. I feel quite certain about most of these lesions and feel that the possibility of error is very small. If I feel that there is any question that the lesion is going to progress and handicap or destroy the patient then I feel that biopsy is an obvious next step.

Some roentgenological features of bone tumours

by

N. P. G. EDLING

SUMMARY

The marked vascularity and cellular activity of the physis provides the commonest site of origin for tumours and tumour-like lesions. With continued length growth of a bone, these will gradually recede from the physis with time, and, if benign, may undergo remodelling, sometimes without actual increase in size. Following the cessation of growth, this migration stops. Malignant tumours also arise mainly in this region—often on young people. Rarely, benign and malignant tumours may co-exist in analogous situations in paired bones, their migration from the physis being assumed. Sarcoma may very rarely invade and destroy both physis and epiphysis. Dysfibroplastic defects may be simulated by cartilage rests, only recognized by subsequent mineralization.

The precise osseous location of 191 sarcomas is presented and shows different patterns for juveniles and mature adults, also between girdle bones and long bones. This is due to their peculiarities of growth and anatomical structure. In juveniles the osteosarcomas dominate in the long tubular bones and occur near the physes; in adults osteosarcomas and fibrosarcomas are found in the long tubular bones while chondrosarcomas display a distribution in the pelvis, scapulae, ribs and femora.

IN DIAGNOSTIC radiology of bone lesions at every occasion we are reminded of the different structures of cancellous and compact bone. This should also remind us of the various environments that may be offered a bone process, thus explaining that it may appear different. The cancellous bone with its rich vascularity has a higher metabolic activity than the compact bone. There is a variation of the cancellous structure from individual to individual and with age—the process of bone formation in the physes of the growing long bones presenting the most intense activity (Fig. 1). This difference in vascularization is roentgenologically demonstrable also in old patients (Fig. 2). This ankle belongs to a female patient 57 years of age inactivated for 2 months after a fracture. An osteopenia is present with the greatest loss of bone within the fused physes of the tibia and fibula. It seems clear that an osteogenic process, in an area where the intensity is reflected by extensive vascularization, might be exposed to disorders both of benign and malignant nature, especially in growing individuals. We also know that the great majority of bone tumours start in these areas and then will be localized according to the growth in length and modelling of the bone and the duration of the process itself.

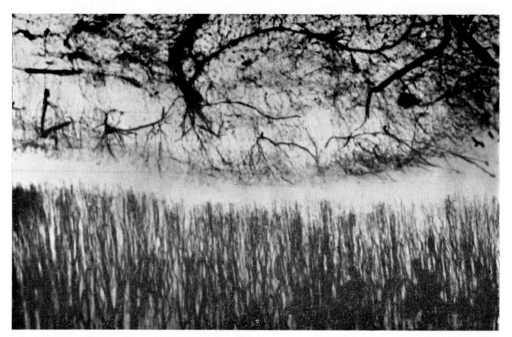

Fig. 1. Microradiograph of the physis in a specimen of a growing long bone after contrast filling of the nutrient artery. The intense vascularization of the metaphyseal side is visualized. (Epiphysis above, metaphysis below.)

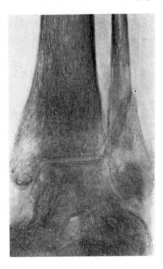

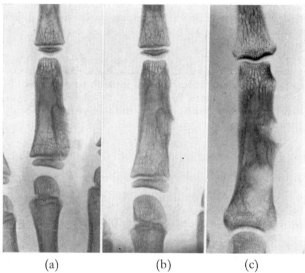

(a)   (b)   (c)

Fig. 2. Osteopenia in the ankle of a 57-year-old female patient, immobilized for two months after a fracture. The most marked loss of bone is found in the fused physes of tibia and fibula.

Fig. 3. Dysfibrochondroplasia. Female born 1945. (a) 1949. In the proximal part of the proximal phalanx of right ring finger there is a translucent area up to the physis. Biopsy (curettage): Contents of soft consistence with highly differentiated chondromatous islands in collagenous tissue. No malignancy. (b) 1952. Postoperatively decrease in size, and "migration" of the lesion in distal direction due to growth of the phalanx proximally. Close to the physics a second lesion has appeared. (c) 1962. The first lesion has grown and "migrated" further in correlation to the growth of the phalanx. The second lesion has expanded until fusion of the physis.

From these biological points of view the radiologist must study his cases. At every occasion the question should be: Is this a process starting long ago during bone formation in the physis, or by appositional growth, or is it a more recent lesion? A good knowledge of these conditions is offered by a study of the course of the lesions over an interval of years.

A disorder in the bone formation in the right ring finger of a girl at the ages of 4, 7 and 17 years is the first example (Fig. 3). At the first occasion (Fig. 3(a)) the radial part of the phalanx was occupied by a slightly protruding lesion extending from the middle to close to the physis. The ulnar border was marked by a cortex, the structure was more loose than normal and irregular at the surface. It seems reasonable to propose that the disorder in bone formation occurred soon after birth, and then continued. Curettage revealed rather smooth contents in which were found small areas of highly differentiated cartilage in collagenous tissue without signs of malignancy. The lesion had the character of dysfibrochondroplasia. Three years later (Fig. 3(b)) the lesion remained as a slightly protruding postoperative deformity and a small area in the middle of the phalanx. In addition, again a disorder in the bone formation radially in the physis was revealed. When the patient was 17 years of age (Fig. 3(c)) the deformity was more marked from the appositional growth in volume of the phalanx and during the growth in length the second lesion developed to a long and broad smoothly bordered translucency up to the fused physis. There it stopped as the growth in length had ceased. Nine years later, when the patient was 26 years of age, the protrusion was more bony but the rest of the area relatively unchanged. In such a series the nature of a lesion in a bone may be better understood than when examined at a single occasion.

The developmental fate of dysfibroplastic changes when present in the long tubular bones is still more striking and interesting. Two such courses will be shown, both starting fairly similarly.

The first picture (Fig. 4(a)) from a boy, 3 years of age, shows a big, expanding lesion situated in the distal metaphyseal part of left femur extending down to the physis. The most lateral part of the metaphysis, the width of the physis and the epiphysis appear intact. From curettage, the histological examination revealed dysfibroplastic tissue and the diagnosis was aneurysmal bone cyst. At the intervention, the distal border of the lesion grossly touched the physis. At an examination two years later (Fig. 4(b)) the lesion had changed appearance due to growth in length and remodelling of the femur. Medially the cortex seems to be resorbed. Without knowing the further course one should propose a biopsy from this area; however, when the boy was 10 years of age there was still no signs of malignancy (Fig. 4(c)). The whole area was still more modelled and had a diaphyseal character. The lateral views also tell us that the expanding character had decreased as the anterior and posterior surfaces were no longer bulging. Distally the bone had grown normally in the physis. At an examination when the boy was 16 years of age (Fig. 4(d)) there was further modelling. The difference in appearance was not large, as the boy is short in stature.

The second case, a boy one year of age had at the start a lesion similar in appearance as the first one (Fig. 5(a)). Again we see a lesion of cystic character expanding anteriorly and to the sides distally in the left femur down to the physis, which seems to form the distal wall. There was a periostal callus due to a fracture 3 weeks previously. At curettage the distal bordering at the physis was confirmed and microscopic examination revealed

136

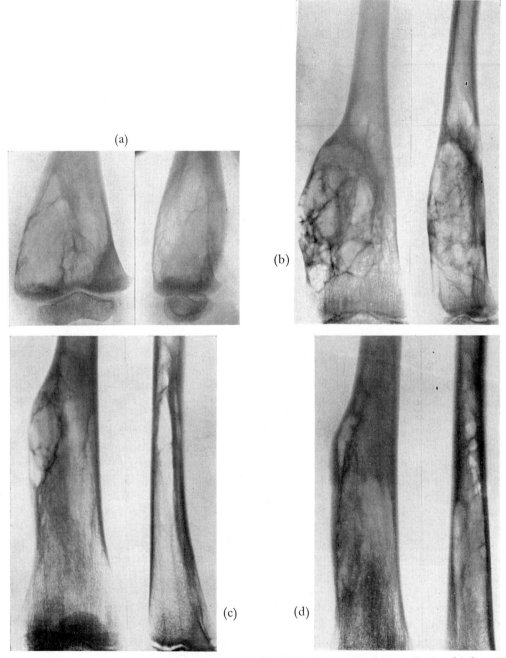

(a)

(b)

(c)   (d)

Fig. 4.   Dysfibroplasia. Male born 1954. (a) 1957. In the distal metaphysis of left femur an expanding translucent lesion. Biopsy (curettage + bone chips): Aneurysmal bone cyst, distal wall formed by the physis. (b) 1959. Length and deformity of the lesion increased. Normal bone formed between the lesion and the physis. (c) 1964. Length of the lesion unchanged, deformity decreased. Further ordinary bone formation. (d) 1971. Further diaphyseal modelling.

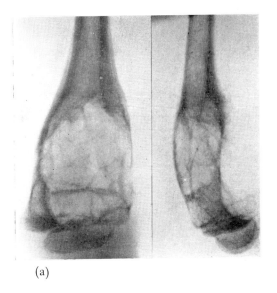

(a)

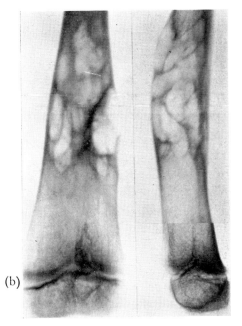

(b)

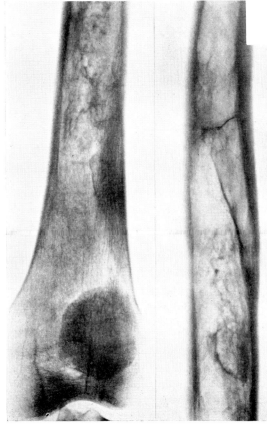

(c)

Fig. 5. Dysfibroplasia. Male born 1942. (a) 1943. In the distal metaphysis of the left femur an expanding translucent lesion; fracture 3 weeks previously and periosteal callus. Biopsy (curettage + bone chips): fibrous dysplasia with giant cells revised to aneurysmal bone cyst; distal wall formed by the physis. In addition, a rounded lesion laterally in the epiphysis. (b) 1947. Length of the lesion increased, deformity decreased. Additional metaphyseal lesion opposite to the epiphyseal one that remains unchanged. (c) 1964. The lesion now extending in the distal half of the femur shaft except for the area close to the physis; the epiphyseal lesion remaining. The frontal view shows the lower part of the diaphyseal and the epiphyseal lesions, the lateral view most part of the diaphyseal one.

F

fibrous dysplasia with giant cells, revised to aneurysmal bone cyst. In addition the
epiphysis also had a small cystic change laterally. In the next picture (Fig. 5(b)) the
boy was 5 years of age and the lesion had already a diaphyseal site. Again we find a
different structure and the shape is modified. Distally to the lesion there seems to be
some years of normal bone formation, but close to the physis a new disorder was present
opposite to the lesion in the epiphysis. The epiphysis had increased in size by appositional growth but the lesion had remained about the same size and site. Next, Fig. 5(c)
shows the situation when the patient was 22 years of age. He is a tall man. The modelling
of the diaphysis was almost normal, however, there is a long part of the shaft that has
an irregular structure. It seems to have the character of fibrous dysplasia; in fact, it is
the same dysfibroplastic process as before. The bone formation seemed to have been
fairly normal during the last years of the growth in length. The lesion in the epiphysis
is still recognizable and had not expanded in spite of its site in spongiosa.

The last two cases demonstrate the fate of dysfibroplastic lesions in long bones
occurring early in life. During the growth in length of the bones they had to adapt
themselves to the modelling in shape, but the disorder in rebuilding remained.

The situation is different when dysfibroplastic changes occur late in life and remain
localized to an epiphysis or metaphysis (Fig. 6). The female patient was 41 years of age
and had a big cystic change in the epiphysis and metaphysis proximally in the right
tibia. There was no chance for this lesion to "migrate" or to be modelled due to growth
in length of the tibia. The microscopic diagnosis was a benign giant-cell tumour, however, 20 years later there developed a fibrosarcomatous degeneration. There has been
and is still a discussion of the nature of giant-cell tumours. Jaffe[2] claims that the aneurysmal bone cyst and the giant-cell tumour are two different entities. However, he admits
that it may be impossible to differentiate them without the help of roentgen pictures to
indicate whether the lesion is located in an epiphyseal or metaphyseal area. Both may
contain giant cells. These are present in dysfibroplastic and fibrosarcomatous lesions in
the spongious bone tissue where the expanding process causes destruction and haemorrhages. However, this is not typical for epiphyseal processes. Giant cells may also
occur in abundance following on a previous exploratory operation upon bone, and in
soft tissue conditions with necrosis and haemorrhage, such as highly malignant tumours
and destructive inflammatory conditions [2,1]. In these cases their presence is not claimed
to be indicative of a pathologic entity. I think, therefore, that it is reasonable to consider
the giant cells as a secondary feature also in bone lesions. In the case of malignant giant-
cell tumours all authorities in pathology agree that the tumour has a fibrosarcomatous
ground substance according to which the degree of malignancy is assessed; nevertheless
the giant cells are given first place in the classification of the process.

The malignant bone tumours with fibrosarcomatous character have the same tendency
as the benign dysfibroplastic lesions to develop in the area of intensive bone formation
in the physes of the long tubular bones. Therefore they may also attack children and
teenagers.

In rare cases it is possible to demonstrate a corresponding development of benign
and malignant processes (Fig. 7). In this female patient (20 years of age) there was a
benign lesion of the type, that is usually called a non-ossifying fibroma, postero-medially
in the sub-metaphyseal area in the left femur. Laterally in the same area in the right
femur the structure was irregular due to destruction and bone formation, the latter also

found in the soft tissues. The microscopic examination after amputation revealed osteogenic sarcoma including osteoid tissue and calcification centrally and mainly fibrosarcomatous tissues peripherically. Unfortunately, there were no previous examinations in this case; however, it is interesting that two processes of quite different differentiation occurred in the same individual so similarly situated and suggestive of disorders in the bone formation in the physis some years ago. Also the malignant change had had time to "migrate" during the growth of the femur before it was clinically manifest and roentgenologically diagnosed.

The primary bone sarcomas have eventually a destructive character but are able for periods to stimulate new bone formation (Fig. 8). Proximally in the left tibia in a boy 7 years of age there was an irregular structure with marked new bone formation—and also areas of destruction. Microscopic examination after amputation revealed a fibrosarcomatous tumour, more specifically osteoblastic osteogenic sarcoma. The physis formed a distinct upper border of the tumour. In my youth it was said that the cartilaginous physis was a barrier to the expansion of any tumourous growth, however, due to the growth in length of the bone in the physis it might be suggested that the tumour growth all the time is receding from the physis.

A second tumour in similar situation in the right tibia in a patient 15 years of age is shown in Fig. 9. This tumour had a destructive character and not only the metaphysis but also the anterior and medial part of the epiphysis were attacked. The modelling was disturbed by moderate expansion of the tumour. The close relation to the physis is again found. Microscopic examination after amputation revealed a marked polymorphism, including spindle cell groups, several multinucleated giant cells, and also areas with bone formation.

Thus, the above three malignant tumours had in common a fibrosarcomatous ground substance with different degrees of remaining osteogenic capacity. As known, there are not only dysfibroplastic and fibrosarcomatous lesions that disrupt ordinary bone formation but also disorders where the bone formation is impaired at a later stage, and cartilaginous tissue laid down. If these changes are situated in the bone and not calcified they cannot be differentiated from the dysfibroplastic processes (Fig. 10). In this case a translucent area with poor cortex was situated in the metaphysis of the femur in a female 45 years of age. At a new examination 14 years later the area was calcified, revealing the true nature of the lesion.

The majority of the malignant cartilaginous lesions are also localized to physical areas, however, in parts of the skeleton with less intensive growth than in the long tubular bones. The tri-radiate cartilage and the trochanteric physes are the most usual areas. The case illustrated in Fig. 11 is an exception. In the proximal part of right humerous in a male patient 30 years of age, there were circumscribed radiolucent areas with faint calcifications (Fig. 11 (a)). Microscopic examination after curettage revealed osteitis fibrosa. Two years later (Fig. 11(b)) the changes were more marked and after further curettage the diagnosis was fibro-myxo-chondroma without malignancy. After a further two years (Fig. 11(c)) there was marked progression of the process with very irregular bone structure, calcification and bone formation in the soft tissues. The microscopic diagnosis after amputation was now osteo-chondro-myxosarcoma. Seven years later the patient was still alive. It seems reasonable to suggest this lesion to be a prototype of a disorder in bone formation, including all developmental stages in abnormal relations.

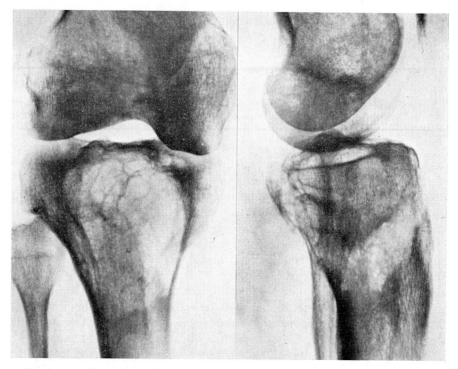

Fig. 6. Dysfibroplasia. Female 41 years. Proximally in the right tibia a big radiolucent lesion. Biopsy: Benign giant-cell tumour.

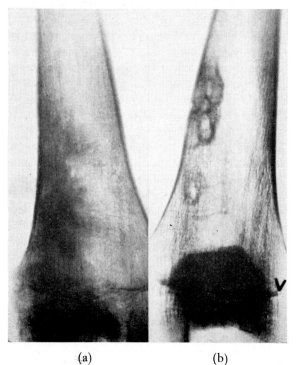

(a)   (b)

Fig. 7. Osteosarcoma and dysfibroplasia. Female 20 years. (a) Laterally in the distal part of the diaphysis and in the metaphysis of the right femur, irregular structure and new bone formation in bone and soft tissues. Biopsy (amputation): Osteogenic sarcoma including osteoid tissue and calcification centrally and mainly fibrosarcomatous tissue peripherally. (b) Superficially in corresponding portion of left femur radiolucent areas of dysfibroplastic type.

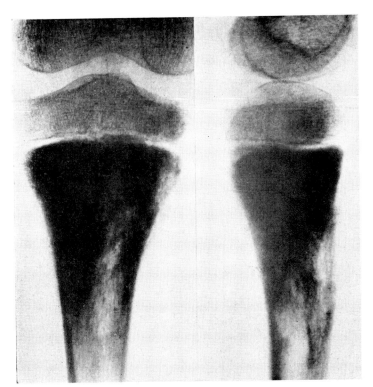

Fig. 8. Osteosarcoma. Male 7 years. In the proximal metaphysis of right tibia irregular structure, marked new bone formation, and also areas of bone resorption. Biopsy (amputation): Sarcomatous tumour, rather osteoblastic osteogenic sarcoma (appearances similar to fibrosarcoma).

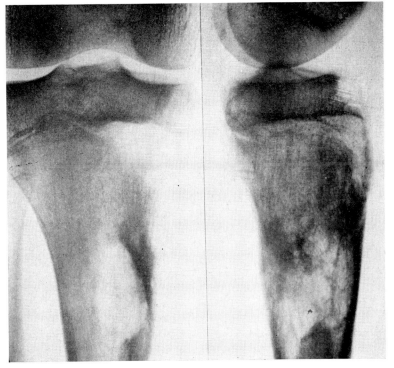

Fig. 9. Osteosarcoma. Male 15 years. Medially in the proximal metaphyseal and diaphyseal portions of right tibia resorption of bone and irregular structure. Biopsy (amputation): Spindle cell groups, marked polymorphism and areas with new bone formation. Several multinucleated giant cells. Osteogenic sarcoma.

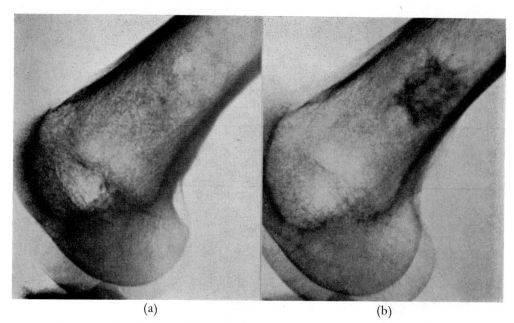

(a)   (b)

Fig. 10. Dyschondroplasia. Female born 1909. (a) 1954. In the distal metaphysis of right femur a radiolucent lesion with poor cortex. (b) 1968. Calcification of the lesion.

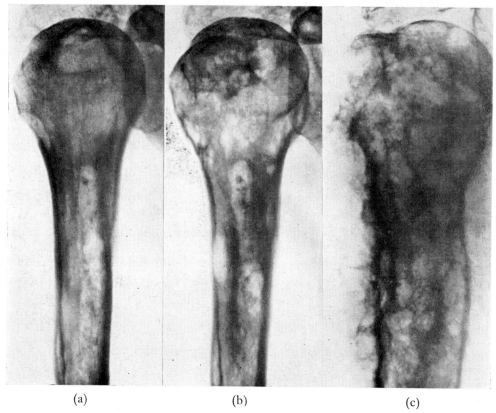

(a)   (b)   (c)

Fig. 11. Chondrosarcoma. Male born 1922. (a) 1952. In the proximal portion of right humerus circumscribed radiolucent areas with faint calcification. Biopsy (curettage): Osteitis fibrosa. (b) 1954. Progression. Biopsy (curettage): Fibro-myxo-chondroma, no malignancy. (c) 1956. Marked progression indicating malignancy. Biopsy (amputation): Osteo-chondro-myxo-sarcoma.

The cases discussed have been examples of disorders in bone formation suggested to be localized to the physes of the long tubular bones. However, a disorder in bone formation may also occur in mature bone. An interesting example is the so called osteitis deformans, or Paget's disease where the vascularization and the osteogenic activity of the diseased bone are very high. In about 10% of the cases malignant degeneration also develops suggested to be due to the intense rebuilding of the bone tissue. This is in agreement with the occurrence of the vast majority of benign and malignant lesions in the rapid growing long bones of young people.

Finally, I will show the distribution of 191 bone sarcomas that are included in our bone tumour file at Karolinska Sjukhuset in Stockholm. At the microscopic examination 28 were diagnosed as fibrosarcomas, 110 as osteosarcomas or osteogenic sarcomas and 53 as chondrosarcomas. Figure 12 shows the number of the cases that were found in

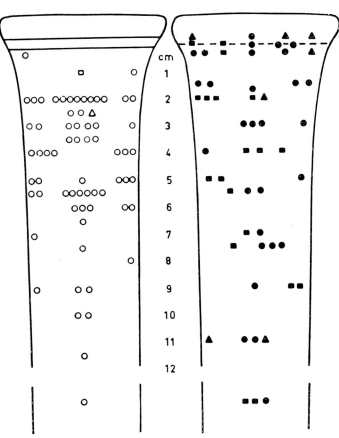

Fig. 12. Distribution of 191 sarcomas of bone, microscopically diagnosed as fibrosarcomas (□ or ■), chondrosarcomas (△ or ▲) and osteosarcomas (○ or ◉). Blank figures indicate patients under 21 years of age, black figures those 21 years or older. (a) In growing and matured long bones. (b) In pelvis, trochanteric areas and remaining sites.

long tubular bones, in the schematic drawing of them the open and fused physes are indicated. The fibrosarcomas are plotted as squares, the osteosarcomas as circles and the chondrosarcomas as triangles. The unshaded figures indicate patients under 21 years of age, black figures indicative those 21 years or older. The osteosarcomas dominate in the young tubular bones—there we only find one fibrosarcoma and one chondrosarcoma. In the older tubular bones the distribution is different, another, however, with dominance for fibro- and osteo-sarcomas. We also see that the tumours are more distally localized in the young bones than in the adult ones. This must depend upon the tumour "migrating" with the growth in length of the bone. When the physes are fused the tumour growth must stay where it has started.

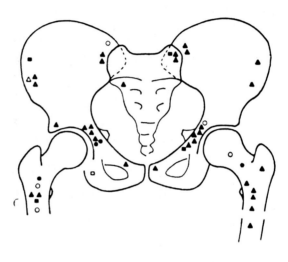

Anterior part of the squamous occipital bone					▲	
Maxilla				■	•	
Scapula		▲	▲	▲	•	•
Sternum				▲	•	
Ribs		■	△	△	▲	▲
Proximal ulna				■	○	
Metacarpal bones				▲	▲	
Phalanges				▲		
Calcaneum				•		
Metatarsal bones				○		

Fig. 13.

The distribution of the sarcomas was different in other parts of the skeleton (Fig. 13). In the schematic drawing of the pelvis the tumours are localized to the peripherial parts of ilia, the fused triradiate cartilages or the trochanteric areas. These areas have not the high degree of osteogenic capacity as the physes of the long tubular bones. In the ilia the lesions are situated in the peripheral parts that have been formed by appositional bone formation—the tumours must therefore have started relatively late. The chondrosarcomas now play a dominant role. These patients also had a higher average age (46 years) than the patients with osteosarcomas. It might be reasonable to suggest that the tumours have started as chondromas, then grew slowly and progressed to malignant degeneration late in life.

The tumours that remain occurred in other parts of the skeleton. The chondrosarcomas were more than half, and most of them found in the ribs, scapulae and hands. One chondrosarcoma was found in the skull, where most of the bones are developed in membrane. However, it was localized to the ventral part of the occipital bone which part is developed in cartilage.

About two-thirds of the osteosarcomas occurred in children and adolescents. The remaining third of the osteosarcomas and the great majority of the fibrosarcomas and the chondrosarcomas were found in adults. However, among the adults the average age of those with osteosarcomas was 10 years lower than the average age of those with fibrosarcomas or chondrosarcomas.

With all respect for my colleagues of pathology I should like to ask if it is reasonable that instead of fibrosarcomas and osteosarcomas or osteogenic sarcomas to talk of fibrosarcomas with different degrees of residual osteogenic capacity as the ground substance is fibrosarcomatous in all these cases. With this classification the fibrosarcomas will be the less differentiated and more malignant, the chondrosarcomas the higher differentiated and less malignant of the bone sarcomas, and there should be a good correlation between microscopy and clinical findings.

REFERENCES

1. Boyd, W. *A Textbook of Pathology*, 7th ed. Lea & Febiger, Philadelphia, 1961.
2. Jaffe, H. L. *Tumors and Tumorous Conditions of the Bones and Joints*. Lea & Febiger, Philadelphia, 1958.

F*

The radiological appearance of lesions resembling malignant bone tumours

by

R. O. MURRAY

SUMMARY

For the radiologist the differential diagnosis of a primary bone sarcoma includes a wide variety of diseases extending through the whole field of bone and joint pathology. Discordant features may be noted in radiographs and note should be taken of anomalous details of history and site of the lesion and age of the patient. Such points should arouse caution in definitive diagnosis. Particular confusion may occur with traumatic conditions and the rarer types of infective diseases. Likewise a typical benign primary tumours and unusual metastases may cause diagnostic difficulty. Examples of these various problems are illustrated.

THIS SYMPOSIUM clearly represents the way we all behave in our own little groups when we strive to make the accurate diagnosis of a bone tumour. The three disciplines, clinician, radiologist and the pathologist all work together. We all do our best, and if one of us falls down we rely upon the others to help us out. The tragedies occur when all three of us fall down together. Looking back over the years it has been possible to extract some examples of controversial cases which cover very largely the major groups of pathology. When faced with a problem film, we think of congenital, traumatic, infective and neoplastic lesions and then go on to the metabolic and endocrine group, the collagen diseases, the reticuloses, and we finish up with that miscellaneous collection of disorders of unknown origin, such as Paget's disease and infantile cortical hyperostosis.

CONGENITAL

Confusion may arise with osteopoikylosis in a pelvis. I recall a woman who had had carcinoma of the breast two years before, and because of this she was regarded as having metastases—I don't think that most of us would have agreed with the diagnosis—but I report it to you. However, in the congenital group, we are much more likely to be confused by the pseudo-tumours and the massive callus formation that can occur in osteogenesis imperfecta. A woman was known to have had osteogenesis imperfecta all her life, but she developed a particularly large painful swelling of the distal end of the femur, and it was in fact a manifestation of that disease. We did tomograms and we did a biopsy, because we were not happy about it.

Figure 1 illustrates another case of a young man with known osteogenesis imperfecta, who had a tooth extracted. Six weeks later he presented with this huge bulge growing

147

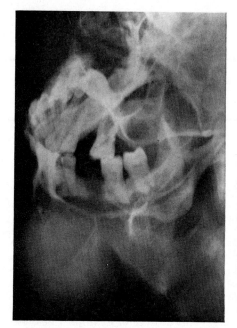

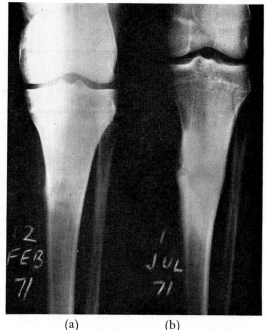

Fig. 1.   Osteogenesis imperfecta of
mandible.

(a)   (b)

Fig. 2.   Stress fracture of tibia: (a) 12.2.71;
(b) 1.7.71.

from his mandible. Here again the worry existed, but it was, in fact, not a true tumour.
In osteogenesis imperfecta we frequently see solitary lesions like this which have massive
new bone formation and closely simulate the pattern of an ostengenic sarcoma.

TRAUMA

When we turn to the lesions due to trauma I think confusion is even more liable to
occur. In this group I remember the case of a professional footballer who complained of
pain in the leg. A film taken was at that time passed as normal, although with hindsight
we could see a tiny crack in the fibula. But it was missed and he subsequently developed
a huge bony mass two months later which was queried as an osteosarcoma. Later, of
course, we realised that the lesion was a stress fracture with reactive callus formation
and the man is now well and active for the next football season. But the following case
was more of a problem. A boy of 20 presented with pain below the knee of 6 weeks duration and this lesion in the tibia was also seriously questioned as being an osteosarcoma
(Fig. 2). I think at this particular site the first diagnosis should always be a stress fracture.
I get at least one a year referred to me with the same question. But this case was a stress
fracture—then it went on to produce a good deal of bone formation, and a biopsy was
performed. This was shown to my colleague, Professor Sissons, and there was no doubt
that it was indeed a stress fracture, but people were worried.

A 16-year-old girl presented with a painful swelling in the right thigh and an effusion
in the right knee joint which limited movement. Three weeks earlier she had suffered a
kick in this area while playing with her sister. On the following morning the pain was

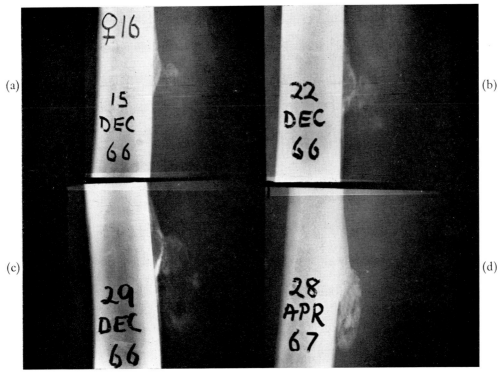

Fig. 3. Traumatic subperiosteal ossification arising from right femur: (a) 15.12.66; (b) 22.12.66; (c) 29.12.66; (d) 28.4.67.

sufficiently severe to prevent her walking. Clinically an extreme tender diffuse mass was found in the front of the middle of the thigh, appearing to be firmly attached to the bone with some localized increase of warmth. Radiological examination revealed a periosteal reaction (Fig. 3(a)) and further examinations one (Fig. 3(b)) and two weeks later (Fig. 3(c)) showed increased localized calcification, although the symptoms tended to diminish. During the course of this illness the patient ran a low-grade fever. Although the radio-logical findings were considered to be post-traumatic in origin, the films were submitted for an opinion concerning possible malignancy. This was confidently refuted, the appearances being characteristic of traumatic subperiosteal ossification. Further examination 5 months later (Fig. 3(d)) when the patient was totally asymptomatic, revealed an ossified mass at the site of calcification. This had well-defined and smooth margins and was also associated with an organized periosteal reaction on the anterior aspect of the femoral shaft.

Then we see some lesions which occur in the absence of pain sense. This child was a known bilateral congenital dislocation of hip with a meningocoele and on attending for follow-up some years after the hip had been reduced her mother remarked, as she was leaving the clinic, that there was a swelling below the knee. There was this pattern of destruction around the metaphysis of the tibia with irregular lumps of bone (Fig. 4). This at once raised the question—could it be sarcoma? Well, in the absence of pain sense, we all know this is a neuropathic lesion and this in fact remodelled perfectly well

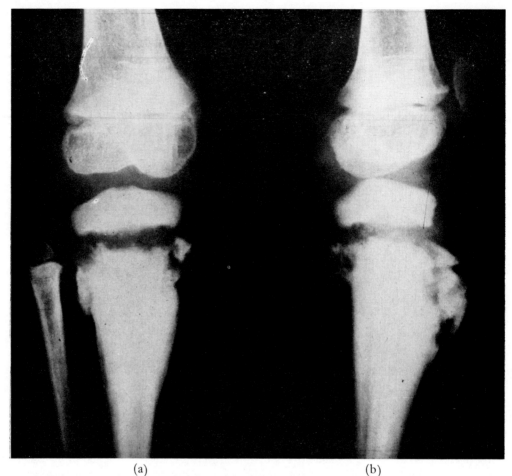

(a)   (b)

Fig. 4. Neuropathic fracture of tibia associated with loss of pain sense due to spina bifida. (a) Antero-posterior. (b) Lateral.

with no treatment other than protection. We see this again with the paraplegic child, from injuries which are totally unappreciated in routine nursing and without any brutality. Occasionally, such lesions are quite overlooked until they are organized, and then suddenly may be felt clinically as a bony hard mass in relation to the shaft of a long bone.

This case, a patient of Mr. J. N. Wilson, created a little difficulty for us. A man of 47 presented with pain in the knee and had a destructive lesion in the lateral femoral condyle which was suspected of being a tumour. Plain X-ray films were not diagnostic (Fig. 5(a)) but a tomogram showed an articuler defect (Fig. 5(b)). The diagnosis of a post-traumatic subchondral bone cyst was confirmed at operation.

I remember another patient also familiar to Professor Sissons. Six weeks after an injection of gamma globulin a girl presented with a tender swelling at the injection site in her arm. Histologically this was myositis ossificans, but this may be confused with a soft tissue sarcoma by an unsophisticated pathologist, for whom it is a diagnostic problem rather than for the radiologist.

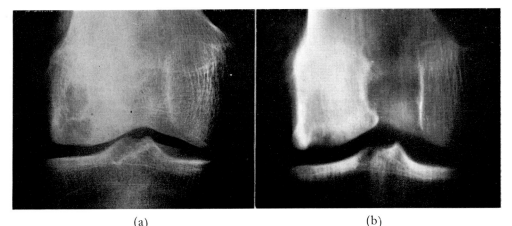

(a)   (b)

Fig. 5. Traumatic subchondral bone cyst of femur. Antero-posterior view: (a) plain film; (b) tomograph.

INFECTION

When we come to infection, even greater problems arise. A young soldier who had had pain in the forearm for a month was sent back to this country with this film (Fig. 6(a)). He had a periosteal reaction around the distal end of the radius. When we saw him it was pretty well organized; there was some medullary destruction—but my this time the diagnosis was pretty clear—it was osteomyelitis (Fig. 6(b)). But at each stage I think it should have been clear, and the radiological point which I would emphasize is that the soft tissue swelling which was originally manifest was not clearly defined—it was diffuse. Had that lesion been explored at that time no pus would have been present. The tissues

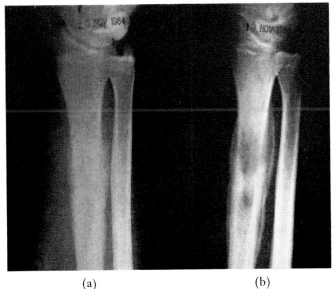

(a)   (b)
Fig. 6. Acute osteomyelitis of right radius: (a) 5.11.64; (b) 14 days later.

would have been boggy and oedematous as any surgeon will know. A genuine osteo-sarcoma of course shows clear delineation of the soft tissue tumour extension with displacement of the other soft tissue planes. To the radiologist I believe this differentiating feature to be of enormous value. It doesn't work always; you get clearly defined para-vertebral abscesses, and in some infections you may occasionally get a mass which bears resemblance to a tumour.

The osseous lesions of some other infections may resemble malignant tumours, for example, a syphilitic gumma (Fig. 7). And another patient had this very large destructive lesion which in the lateral view had a rather clearly defined soft tissue shadow (Fig. 8). This was hydatid disease. Hydatid disease can simulate a bone tumour, and it can be wrongly interpreted. Dr. R. I. Lewis of Halifax recently sent me this interesting film (Fig. 9). In 1916 a woman aged 20 presented with a swelling of the left shoulder for which amputation was advised but declined. Figure 9 shows the condition at the age of 76 years and in the meanwhile she has had a useful limb. Although no histology was carried out, the appearances resemble those seen in the pelvis of another patient which were proven to be due to hydatid disease and the films of which were given to the Museum of the Institute of Orthopaedics by Dr. Weston of New Zealand.

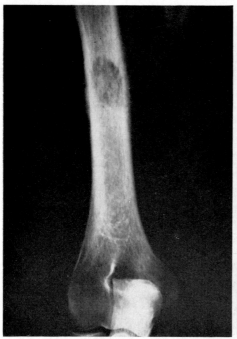

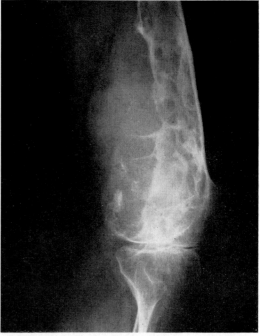

Fig. 7.   Syphilis of right humerus. In this middle-aged adult a lesion of acquired tertiary syphilis shows as a well-defined lytic area which has stimulated the production of organized periosteal new bone.

Fig. 8.   Hydatid disease of left femur. Numerous loculated areas of destruction of the posterior cortex with sclerotic margins and a large, well-defined soft tissue extension.

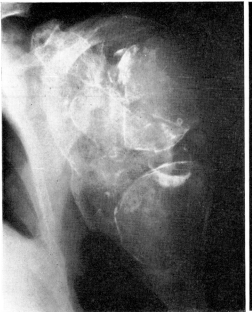

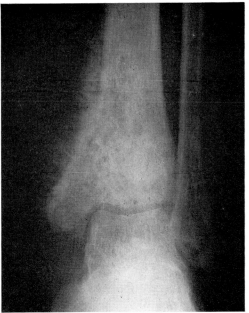

Fig. 9. Presumed hydatid disease of left humerus. See text. At the age of 76 years, the radiological pattern of an extensive, loculated and expanding lesion of the proximal end of the humerus is quite bizarre in its appearance.

Fig. 10. Mycetoma of right tibia.

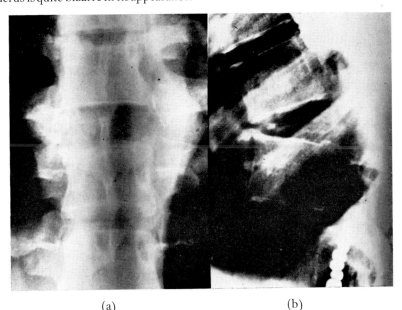

(a)   (b)

Fig. 11. Benign osteoblastoma of vertebral body. A young female, presenting with paraplegic symptoms. There is a grossly destructive lesion of the body of D8 with collapse and bilateral paravertebral masses. (a) Antero-posterior. (b) Lateral.

154

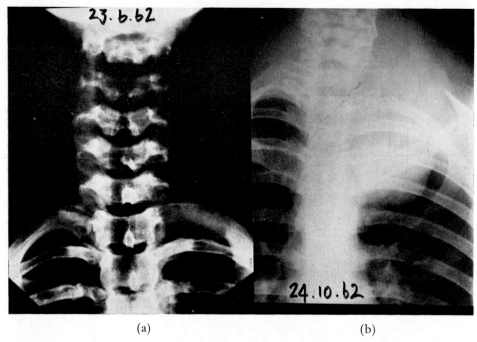

(a)   (b)

Fig. 12.   Rapidly growing aneurysmal bone cyst of first left rib. Eighteen-year-old
female complained of pain and swelling in the left side of the neck since May 1962:
(a) 23.6.62. destruction in the first rib; (b) 4 months later considerable further destruction of the rib and a large soft tissue tumour has developed.

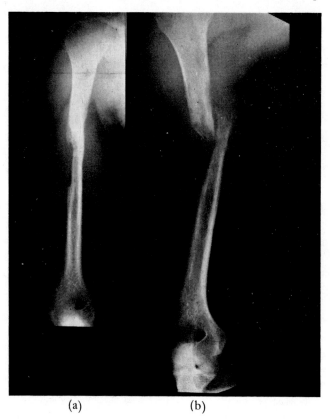

(a)   (b)

Fig. 13. Haemangiomatosis of right humerus. Young
male negro had suffered
mild pain in the right shoulder for 2 years. Swelling
and increased pain had followed a fall 2 weeks before
presentation: (a) Destructive lesion on the lateral
aspect of the humeral
shaft with a healing in-
fraction. Abnormal trans-
lucency of the medial cortex
of the proximal portion of
the humerus; (b) Three
months later. Gross and
rapid absorption of the fracture surfaces, with severe
displacement, has taken
place, which is a characteristic feature of haemangiomatosis.

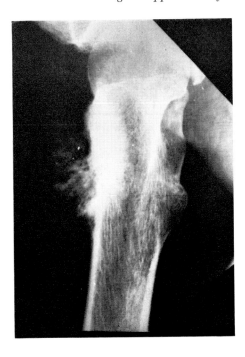

Fig. 14. Metastasis in femur from carcinoma of rectum. Spiculated new bone projecting from the femur of this elderly male, with cortical and intramedullary new bone formation, resembles a primary malignant tumour.

But what about this—the spiculation which is not uncommon with mycetoma infections may simulate sarcoma. A Sudanese patient presented with a brawny swelling above the ankle, due to this fungus infection of the tibia and producing bony spiculation similar to an osteosarcoma (Fig. 10). Such changes occur not infrequently with bizarre infections of fungal origin. Observe extension of the infection into the medulla. This diffuse type of infiltration was due to the non-encapsulated yellow-spore type of fungus. Destructive lesions in bone due to a black thorn lodged in the adjacent soft tissues may also simulate a tumour.

NEOPLASMS

(*a*) PRIMARY

I put this case in to remind us of the rate of growth of the aneurysmal bone cyst. I have encountered this with atypical examples of osteoblastoma (Fig. 11), occasionally with chondroblastoma and chondromyxoid fibroma. In all these the radiological pattern may suggest malignancy.

I put this case in to remind us of the rate of growth of the aneurysmal bone cyst. I think that this can be almost the most confusing entity of all of the benign tumours in simulating malignancy. I saw this film of a girl of 18 years, 2 months after it had been taken at another hospital, showing destructive changes in the first rib and this large mass (Fig. 12(a)). Well, I got it wrong in a big way, because I thought nothing could grow so fast as this except a very highly aggressive malignant tumour (Fig. 12(b)) and I made a diagnosis of haemangiosarcoma. I was wrong, it was indeed an aneurysmal bone cyst. But we learn from the case and we have seen similar episodes occur. You don't always get with an aneurysmal bone cyst a clearly defined endosteal margin. They can be very aggressive in their appearance. Such lesions if misinterpreted can lead to the tragic error of amputation which I have known to be needlessly performed both for aneurysmal bone cyst and giant-cell tumour.

Similar problems may be encountered in lesions of joints where pigmented villo-nodular synovitis may be confused with malignant synovioma. This in fact occurred in a man of 40 who complained of pain and swelling of the first metatarso-phalangeal joint. In this case para-articular lesions on both sides of the intact articular surface were taken to indicate synovial sarcoma, but the precise margins of the bone destruction should have indicated the benign nature of the condition which was not recognized until the specimen was re-examined 35 years later.

A young male negro had suffered pain in the right shoulder for 2 years. Swelling and increased pain followed a fall 2 weeks before he was examined (Fig. 13(a)). The films showed a destructive lesion of the lateral aspect of the humerus shaft with a healing infraction. A fibrosarcoma was orginally suspected but gross and rapid absorption of the fracture surfaces took place which is a characteristic feature of haemangiomatosis or "Vanishing bone" Disease (Fig. 13(b)). This diagnosis was histologically confirmed and prosthetic replacement carried out. Five years later he is alive and well with a useful arm.

(b) SECONDARY

Then there are the secondary malignant neoplasms. When we meet the "maverick" metastasis, turning up at the wrong age and in the wrong place, anyone is liable to make the wrong interpretation. For example, a young woman of 30 had a destructive lesion of the fibula with a soft tissue mass; this was a secondary from a carcinoma of breast. Unusual of course, but such things happen. I saw a man of 60, with pain in the hip, with bone spiculation and reactive sclerosis (Fig. 14)—although this resembled a primary osteogenic sarcoma it was in fact a secondary form carcinoma of rectum. Another which mimicked a sarcoma of pelvis, with widespread bone density, irregular spiculated new bone formation and a soft tissue mass displacing the bladder, was due to metastatic prostatic carcinoma. In the absence of Paget's disease the patient's advanced age was strongly against a primary malignant tumour of bone. Other anomalous metastatic lesions are perhaps more familiar—destruction of a terminal phalanx from a metastasis of bronchial carcinoma. There are also of course the occasional very late metastatic lesions. I remember an elderly woman who presented with pain and an unexplained area of bone destruction in the pelvis. This was later proven to be a late metastatis of a salivary gland tumour of the parotid, the primary having been removed 28 years before.

METABOLIC AND ENDOCRINE DISORDERS

Now briefly, the metabolic and endocrine disorders; the only one I need mention is the "brown tumour" of hyperparathyroidism which may be confused with a geniune giant-cell tumour. In the former however we are helped by evidence elsewhere of abnormal bone texture and sub-periosteal resorption of the phalanges. Moreover, there are biochemical changes which usually indicate the correct diagnosis.

MISCELLANEOUS CONDITIONS OF UNKNOWN ORIGIN

I had to hunt through the collagen diseases to find one which would interest you. This film shows irregular periosteal reaction on the tibia which is organizing and due to peri-arteritis nodosa (Fig. 15). This is a typical place for it to occur—in the proximal end of the tibia and fibula—unusual, but rather characteristic.

Amongst the reticuloses the one that matters is the solitary eosinophil granuloma. A young child of 6 was suspected of having a malignant tumour of the femoral shaft owing to the presence of an area of destruction. It showed an organized cortical reaction and we felt it was benign, but a biopsy report was equivocal. A year later it was densely sclerosed and the presence of eosinophil granuloma was confirmed when the biopsy was reviewed by an experienced bone pathologist.

Amongst the haemopoietic disorders should be mentioned the haemophiliac pseudo-tumour (Fig. 16). The site of this lesion in the ilium is characteristic and usually one knows the patient to be a haemophiliac; moreover the characteristic joint changes may be found as in this man. I must also mention the occasional flattened lumbar vertebral body in which Paget's disease may be indicated by coarse striation of the neutral arch. By the unwary this may be misinterpreted as a malignant tumour.

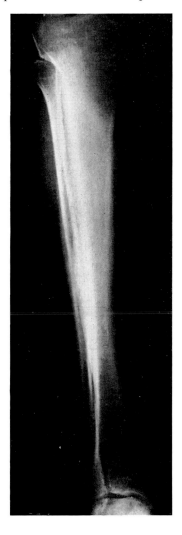

Fig. 15. Polyarteritis nodosa involving right tibia and fibula. Middle-aged patient. An irregular pattern of new bone formation on the tibia — a common site of involvement in polyarteritis nodosa.

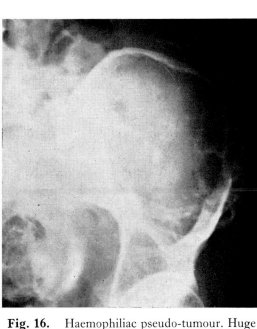

Fig. 16. Haemophiliac pseudo-tumour. Huge destructive lesion in the left ilium occurred in a known haemophiliac. The major joints in this patient showed the characteristic changes of haemophilia.

158

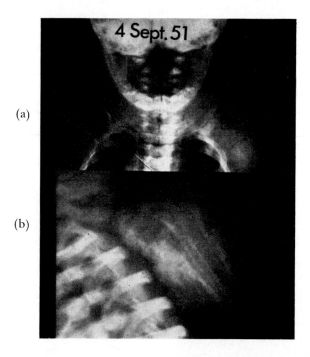

(a)

(b)

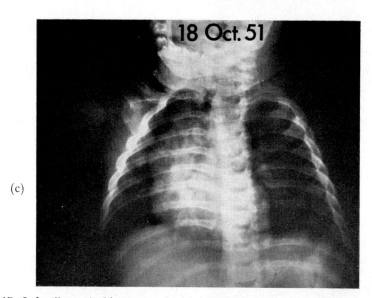

(c)

Fig. 17. Infantile cortical hyperostosis: (a) 4.9.51. Periosteal reaction can be discerned around the mandible and the original film did show involvement also of the clavicle and ribs; (b) 4.9.51. Extensive new bone on all surfaces of the left scapula; (c) 18.10.51. Shows the appearances after an unnecessary forequarter amputation had been performed. Periosteal reactions are still evident on some of the left ribs and on right clavicle, but those on the mandible have resolved.

And then finally this case which occurred back in 1951. An infant presented with a hard swelling of the scapula over which a mass of new bone had formed. There was also periosteal reaction around the mandible (Fig. 17(a) and (b)). This was not appreciated, but in fairness this is Caffey's infantile cortical hyperostosis. This was missed and a horrible thing happened—a forequarter amputation was carried out. The diagnostic radiological feature was there, but Caffey had only described this a few years before in 1945. It was at this time a new disease. This condition is accompanied by a low grade fever and large tender bony swellings. Originally involvement of the mandible was considered mandatory for his diagnosis, but in fact this is no longer believed to be essential. I think today we would not have considered a sarcoma simply because of the age. I personally have never seen a bone sarcoma under 4 years, and I would be very dubious about making such a diagnosis at this age. At any rate, here it was just 6 weeks later after the forequarter amputation (Fig. 17(c)). Further periosteal reactions had developed on the clavicle and on the ribs, and the diagnosis of this completely benign condition was radiologically clear.

And so, ladies and gentlemen, we have looked at all the various groups of pathology. I feel there is always hope when we have that ghastly sensation of taking a film as it comes from being developed and saying, "Oh God—it is a malignant tumour." It might conceivably be one of the less typical benign lesions of the several types I have tried to describe. We can never completely rectify, to the patient or to the parents, an erroneous diagnosis of malignancy. My own reaction is that, personally, I am only happy when my opinion regarding malignancy is supported by a colleague in whom I have every confidence.

Discussion

Prof. Campbell I would like to ask Dr. Murray if a biopsy was done in the case of Caffey's disease.

Dr. Murray Really, I think that biopsy was completely unnecessary. But it was regarded as a sarcoma. I won't tell you where it came from because it wouldn't be fair.

Prof. Lodwick I would like to ask Dr. Murray if he would generalize a little bit on how he makes a distinction between infection of bone and neoplasm of bone.

Dr. Murray I think this is the thing I have probably got wrong most of all—the differentiation between inflammatory lesions and neoplasms. I think most of us have got it wrong both ways at least once in our lives. I am getting more and more impressed, as I have tried to show you, with those films, by really close examination of the soft tissues If you can delineate clearly a soft tissue tumour extension in relation to an area of bone alteration in texture then I think the weight should go for tumour. I had a beautiful example I couldn't get ready in time to bring to you that someone gave me just the other day, of a girl of 19 who presented with pain below the knee, just with about three or four minute spicules of bone in the lateral view. It was an over-penetrated film and I was able to get a solarization of it with underpenetration. This solarization showed so clearly the well-delineated mass. The girl refused biopsy. A year later it was a gross fungating sarcoma. I believe the diagnosis was there on the original film, and indeed the radiologist who sent it to me had made this diagnosis. On the other hand, with the inflammatory lesions the soft tissue thickening is diffuse; it is not clearly defined and the lesions may smoulder on and go very slowly, in low-grade staphylococcal infection particularly, and these are the ones that are liable to be confused with tumours. But they will never, in a limb especially, as far as I know, produce a localized clearly defined mass. I think that is the fundamental differentiating feature I would use and I would emphasize the value of close examination of the soft tissues.

Dr. Burwood Dr. Murray has reviewed some of the interpretive observer errors in radiology; I would just like to ask his opinion whether he thinks the same errors exist to a comparable extent in histology.

Dr. Murray Well they do sometimes, you know. There are times when a radiologist beats the pathologist, but we don't do it very often. Just occasionally we win. There is the chap with the highly malignant aggressive sarcoma who is alive 15 years later looking just the same! But this is exceptional. I think we owe a tremendous debt to our pathologists. I know there have been a number of cracks about them disagreeing, but I couldn't support Lodwick more than by saying, hang your hat on a good bunch of pathologists, and believe them. I do, I have done so all my professional life. I have benefited from it

160

enormously. I suspect regretfully that their margin of error is very considerably less than mine.

Prof. Bonfiglio I think we are back to point zero. I am a clinician with an amateur interest in pathology and an amateur interest in radiology as a part of orthopaedic surgery. I think this last demonstration by Dr. Murray is a very clear exposition of the errors and difficulties that we can get into as clinicians and it brings us back to the thing we teach so often to medical students, the business about the history, the physical examination being correlated with the roentgenographic and the gross post-amputation and histologic aspects of the disease before we can really make a definitive diagnosis so we can hang our hats up quite clearly, and determine how the biological behaviour of the process we are dealing with is going to go. I think this is really a very important illustration of the problem that we all face when we are addressing ourselves to this Symposium.

Dr. Jacobs So may I make a plea that we talk about limitations of radiology and limitations of pathology rather than radiologists and pathologists. It is the method that is limited rather than the practitioners. I would cite two cases I have seen relatively recently where very distinguished pathologists both regarded lesions in children, one of the tibia, one of the femur, as being giant cell tumour or osteoclastoma. Dr. Godfrey Price actually saw one of the cases and he agreed that the appearances were absolutely identical, yet they were different radiologically and in behaviour. In fact they were children before epiphyseal closure; these metaphyseal, or diaphyseal lesions, clearly were non-osteogenic fibromata. I feel that there are not enough differentiating features in a histological section in the same way that there are not in a radiograph. This is the limitation. I know that people meant this anyway:—it's the limitation of the subject, and not the practitioner.

Prof. Sissons I note that my pathological colleagues here have been slow to enter into this discussion of the limitations of pathology or variations of feeling between different pathologists so I think I should do so. I am not commenting on pathologists as a whole, but simply saying something of the experience of one person who has had to do with collaborative studies with other pathologists. I particularly refer to the experience with the British Empire Cancer Campaign Bone Tumour Panel where a number of experienced people have seen the same material. When one speaks of error of diagnosis or difference of diagnosis, these certainly exist; we are all aware of them from our own experience either in seeing cases or in collaborative studies. But there are many different types of opinion. Sometimes these are serious, and sometimes they are over highlighted. For instance, on our Bone Tumour Panel we can spend sometimes very considerable periods of time discussing whether the label chondrosarcoma or osteosarcoma should be applied to a particular lesion. Quite obviously we agree that we are dealing with a rapidly growing highly malignant tumour. This is quite a different type of error from the one where, say a lesion which is subsequently decided to be aneurysmal bone cyst is mis-diagnosed on biopsy as an anaplastic sarcoma. So I, as a pathologist, accept a variety of different types of differences of opinion. But I would like to emphasize one circumstance which I think is very important in assessing lesions, and that is the circumstances under which a pathological opinion is sought and the information that is available to the pathologist. Sometimes what seems to be a conflict in opinion or a flagrant error in diagnosis can be explained by the fact that the material seen by one pathologist was not the same as the material seen by another; or the background information provided to one man being either absent or even incorrect. And I come back to Dr. Murray's opening remarks about the need for careful discussion and collaboration between clinicians, radiologists and pathologists in achieving an accurate diagnosis.

Mr. Robbins   Dr. Murray was emphasizing the problems of diagnosis between infection and neoplastic bone. I would just like to ask him whether he would consider that tuberculosis, particularly where it affects the distal joints, i.e. the bones in the hands rather than the more common sites, does give a particular problem on occasions?

Dr. Murray   I think the tuberculous infections in my experience have rarely caused me difficulty in separating them from tumours. You see in tumours we are talking mainly about purely osseous lesions. This happens with staphycoccal infections, but most of the tuberculosis lesions are articular. But I think I know what you are talking about. Some of the disseminated tuberculosis lesions in children, such as tuberculous dactylitis, occasionally can simulate a tumour—for example, a benign osteoblastoma. But I can't recollect tuberculosis for me causing confusion with an aggressive malignant tumour.

Mr. Webb   Speaking with due humility amongst so many people with such knowledge, I would just like to say one thing about the histological problems. Having been a member of the Bone Tumour Registry for now 3 years or so, and for much longer than that having an interest in tissue cytology, I have studied breast tumours and lymph nodes to a considerable degree. I would just like to say one thing. I have the impression that the histologists often have created difficulties for themselves by the manner in which they obtain, fix and render their material available for examination. Certainly in other fields there is a lot to be gained by having the additional benefit of a cytological view of your tissue together with the histology. I just wonder whether if this process was pursued rather more vigorously than it is at the moment, a lot of problems over the classification and form of neoplasms or pseudo-neoplasms of bone and soft tissue might in due course be solved.

Prof. Middlemiss   I am going to ask people not to pursue that comment at this particular moment, as I want to bring this discussion to a close, but I am quite certain that this particular point about cytology will come up again.

In closing the discussion on these five papers we have had this morning, I would like to look perhaps on the positive side, rather than on the negative side. We have heard of the difficulties; I think these have been rightly emphasized, but I think also that we should not over-emphasize them. The point has been made that in clinical management of this type of problem the collaborative approach should be that the surgeon is in charge and that the pathologist and the radiologist are of service in arriving at a diagnosis.

But I would like also to come back to the point that emerged from Professor Edling's paper—and that is that we must as soon as possible establish a uniform terminology in this field. So that when we have collaboration between colleagues in one centre, this collaboration can be compared with similar collaborative studies in others. Otherwise we shall get nowhere.

The problems of biopsy in the
Westminster Hospital experience

by

E. STANLEY LEE

SUMMARY

The technique of pre-operative supervoltage radiotherapy with delayed selected amputation as practised at the Westminster Hospital has shown a crude 5-year survival rate of 21%. Whilst this method does not demand urgent definitive histological diagnosis as does immediate ablation, accuracy in histopathological assessment is desirable. The therapeutic regime however may be impeded by certain complications of an open biopsy—haematoma, sepsis, fungation or by fracture and flexion contracture. As an alternative, therefore, a trial was made of needle or drill biopsy which did not always provide an adequate sample for conventional histology. This was discarded in favour of a simple punch method sometimes with preliminary use of a trephine. In a series of over 60 tumours including 40 osteosarcomas satisfactory material has almost always been obtained and a number of examples are illustrated. Punch biopsies are reliable, less damaging and avoid delay in initiating treatment.

MANY HERE will know that at Westminster Hospital we have, for 20 years, followed a policy of supervoltage radiotherapy and delayed ablation for osteosarcoma.[1] Till 1966 this policy was applied in all cases, with only a handful of exceptions. The overall, crude and uncorrected 5-year survival rate was 21%.[2] Our view was—and is—that many futile and cruel amputations can thus be avoided, without compromising the patient's chance of survival.

Clearly a positive histological diagnosis is just as indispensible for radiotherapy as it is for immediate surgery, though in one way the task of the pathologist is easier: he can take his time.

However, this conservative management does call into question the usual techniques of "open" biopsy—i.e. exploration of the tumour through an incision which may be 10 cm or more long. Understandably, the pathologist likes to have as much material as he can get, on which to base his opinion—who shall blame him? But in this particular situation I think some compromise for the sake of the patient is desirable. Devotees of the "open" biopsy claim that it gives greater certainty but it does have disadvantages if the limb is to be retained and irradiated.

I don't think that anyone has shown that opening up the tumour by open biopsy shortens the patient's life. As we watched a 6-year old boy with an osteosarcoma of his tibia come hurtling along the corridor towards us one day on a toy tricycle, a colleague exclaimed: "Here comes Keith on his metastasis pump!"—a remark which embodies a profound truth. These are for the most part massive and advanced tumours, and it seems likely that (so far as promoting metastasis goes) nothing we do to the tumour will equal the day-to-day insult and trauma already inflicted on it by the normal vigorous activities of a child or adolescent. To quote Crile: "By the time these tumours are detectable by our present clinical methods, their biological characteristics have sealed the patient's fate."

The disadvantage of "open" biopsy, therefore, is not so much the risk of bloodstream dissemination, as the local damage. More than half of the patients arriving at Westminster for treatment have already had biopsies, almost always by incision and sometimes three or more weeks before, and we have often been dismayed by the disastrous effects of the procedure. These include haematoma formation and infection leading to wound break-down and tumour fungation (Fig. 1); joint damage leading to flexion contracture (Fig. 2); and fracture or collapse of frail bones, so that healing, if it is obtained, fails to result in a comfortable, useful limb.

These side-effects sadly interfere with radiotherapy, and may stultify its whole objective, which is to leave the patient comfortable and mobile. In some few cases radiotherapy has had to be abandoned in favour of prompt amputation; in many others the patient's suffering has been increased or the local result marred. We now tend to opt for immediate surgery rather than radiotherapy if there is gross fungation, marked flexion deformity or severe pathological fracture.

To avoid these ill-effects, we tried at first needle or drill biopsies, but in quite a proportion the material obtained was inadequate. Perhaps if we had practised cytological techniques instead of concentrating on histology we might have done better. But around 1960 we turned to the use of a simple punch technique—usually nowadays a Henckel punch (Down Bros.—diameter across blades 6 mm), inserted into the tumour via a 1 cm skin incision through a trocar and cannula of inside diameter about 7 mm (Thackray: 22 F.G. gauge). If the tumour is entirely endosteal, and covered by hard cortical bone, this may first be trephined, using the Royal National Orthopaedic Hospital trephine for iliac crest biopsy, to obtain easy access to the tumour. I have used this simple biopsy, procedure now at least 60 or 70 times on various bone lesions, including 40 osteosarcomas, often under image intensifier control or using guide pins to locate the exact spot: and have almost always managed to obtain sufficient material, without inflicting the kind of damage that can spoil the chances of the radiotherapist.

Admittedly the method is a compromise, but without fail it has enabled us to answer the question "is this a malignant tumour of bone?" correctly. Occasionally, later events have modified our opinion as to (for example) the differentiating potential of a tumour or, in the case of a giant-cell tumour, its grading. But in our hands the technique has proved much more reliable than drill or needle biopsy, and much less damaging than open incision.

Where the lesion is clinically an undoubted malignant tumour, and only its precise label is in doubt, we have usually given a pre-biopsy initial dose of irradiation, 1,000 rads, the same or the preceding day. It is reasonable to hope that this will reduce the risk of local tumour implantation or spread, though the point is difficult to prove. Probably the really important thing is to avoid delay between the biopsy and the start of radiotherapy. After a punch-biopsy treatment can, of course, begin the same or the next day. My plea to referring surgeons is, therefore, "please don't be tempted to do a biopsy, leave it to us!"

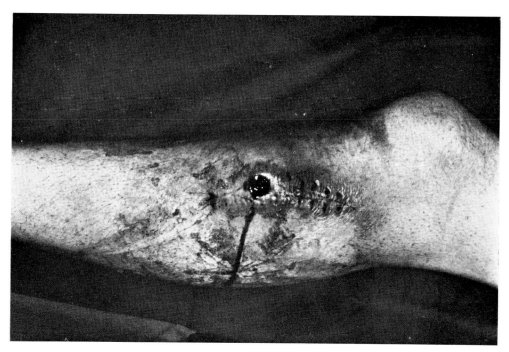

Fig. 1. Incision biopsy. Osteosarcoma of tibia fungating through wound.

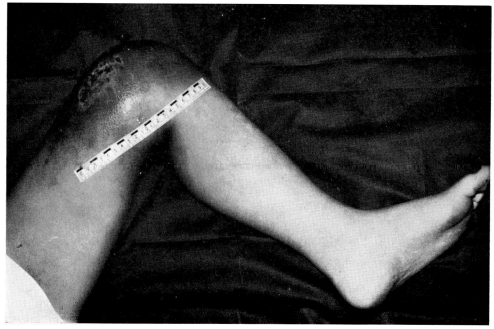

Fig. 2. Incision biopsy. Pyrexia, severe pain, fixed flexion. Radiotherapy is useless in such circumstances.

166

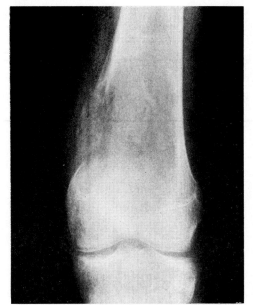

Fig. 3. Male, 14. Telangiectatic osteosarcoma (see text).

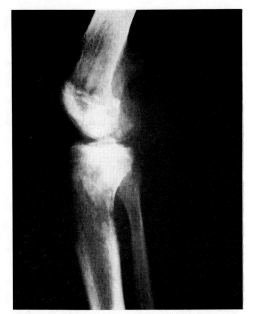

Fig. 5. Familial incidence of bone sarcoma. Male, 19; brother of patient seen in Figs. 3 and 4. Osteosarcoma of tibia.

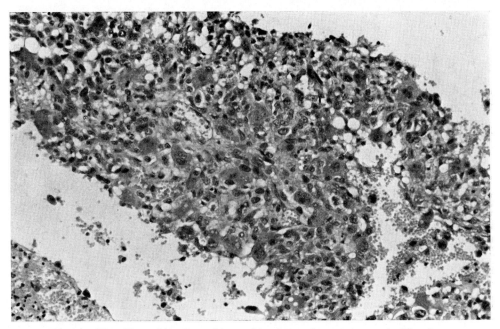

Fig. 4. H & E × 140. Open biopsy histology of tumour seen in Fig. 3.

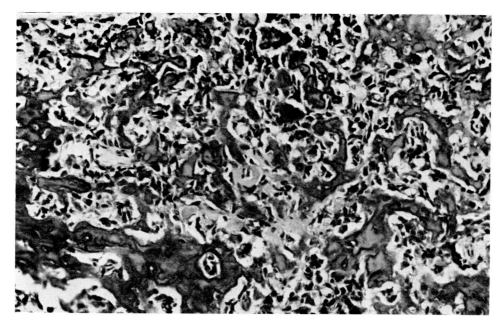

Fig. 6. H & E × 140. Punch biopsy material from tumour seen in Fig. 5.

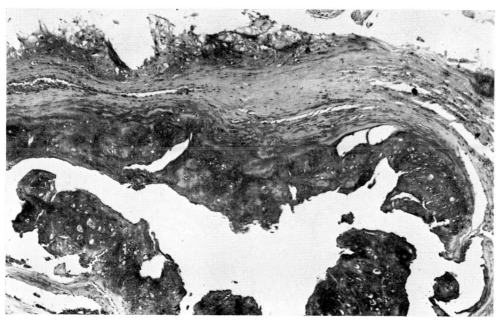

Fig. 7. H & E × 60. Female, 49. Punch biopsy material. Chondrosarcoma.

There are few tumours which could be called (in the words of a speaker yesterday) *Pure*-osteosarcoma. Most have considerable fibroblastic and even chondroblastic potential and the diagnosis of osteosarcoma usually rests on finding osteoid formation, Occasionally the biopsy has not achieved this and the case has been treated as "sarcoma. presumed osteosarcoma", to be sorted out at a later stage.

The same applied to some aggressive giant-cell tumours, but these are notoriously difficult, even with large masses of curettings.

This lesion in a boy of 14 (Fig. 3) had been called a giant-cell tumour on open-biopsy material (Fig. 4). It proved so aggressive and destructive that radiotherapy was abandoned after 2 weeks and the limb disarticulated. He died very soon from chest metastases. Even with ample material the diagnosis was in the balance but the final diagnosis was a telangiectatic osteosarcoma. That was in 1960. It is of great interest that 11 years later, his brother, aged 19, developed a malignant tumour of the upper end of the tibia (Fig. 5): it was an osteosarcoma (Fig. 6) and this patient too has died of

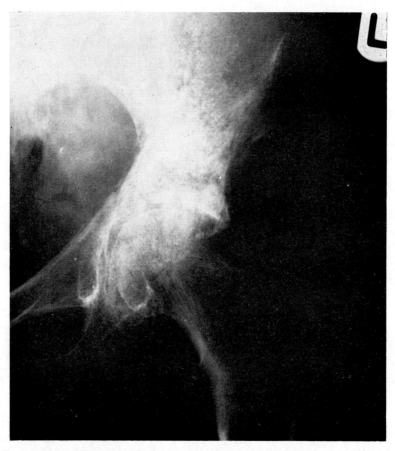

Fig. 9. Female, 72. Tumour of left hip bone 20 years after radiotherapy for carcinoma corporis uteri.

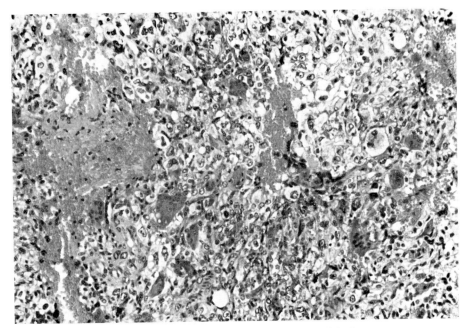

Fig. 8. H & E × 140. Female, 15. Punch biopsy material. Osteosarcoma.

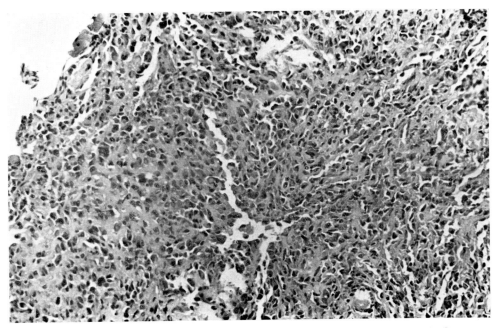

Fig. 10. H & E × 140. Punch biopsy material of tumour shown in Fig. 9. Osteo-sarcoma.

G

metastases. This is the second example we have had of what appears to be familial incidence of the disease.

On the other hand, this tumour in a woman of 49 defied diagnosis on the open-biopsy material submitted to us. A punch-biopsy was then done, and the tumour appeared to consist entirely of malignant cartilage (Fig. 7). A firm diagnosis of chondrosarcoma was made. The patient died in 18 months with widespread metastases.

This girl of 15 had a very destructive tumour of the femur, X-Rays suggestive of osteosarcoma; and on punch-biopsy we entered a cavity with much bleeding and very little solid tissue. Yet a satisfactory diagnosis of osteosarcoma was made (Fig. 8). Subsequently in the disarticulated limb no recognizable tumour could be found, but the patient died in a year with multiple metastases.

One last case is of interest (Fig. 9). This 72-year-old lady had had a carcinoma of the body of the uterus in 1952, with 250 kV X-rays to the whole pelvis by opposed A & P fields to a centre dose of 2,750 rads. She now came with increasing pain in the left hip (only) and was found to have a tumour involving the ilium and displacing the ureter. Was this a late recurrence? How much was radiation change?

A punch-biopsy via the groin was made in this area, and a firm diagnosis of osteosarcoma, presumably post-radiation, has been made (Fig. 10).

Clearly there are important factors for a successful biopsy routine, in addition to the mere size of the piece! The pathologist should be experienced and if possible be present at the biopsy procedure. We at Westminster are fortunate in having Professor Mackenzie, who gives an enormous amount of time and care to these cases, and to whom I am indebted for the photomicrographs. And the surgeon, too, must be prepared to take the necessary trouble, for it is my firm belief that open incision biopsy almost always can, and should, be avoided.

REFERENCES

1. Lee, E. S. & Mackenzie, D. H. Osteosarcoma: A Study of the Value of Preoperative Mega-voltage Radiotherapy. *Brit. J. Surg.*, **51**, 252–274, 1964.
2. Lee, E. S. Treatment of Bone Tumours, *Proc. roy. Soc. Med.*, **64**, 1179–1180, 1971.

Discussion

Professor Schajowicz   I believe that the paper read by Mr. Lee is so important, especially for pathologists, that we need to clear up many points. The first point is about open biopsy and I would like to hear later the opinion of Dr. Dahlin who is the champion of frozen sections of open biopsies, which Mr. Lee did not mention at all.

I wish to speak mainly about the puncture biopsy. It can be an aspiration by means of a simple needle or trocar biopsy and of this I can speak with considerable experience. Actually we have collected around 5,000 cases of aspiration biopsies of bone and articular lesions and in *Cancer* in 1968[1] I reported 4,050 of these and now want to show you our results.

In this group of 4,050 cases 4 years ago we had positive results in 76%. By positive I mean not only that the material was from a tumour or even a malignant tumour. We only call the result positive when we can make an exact diagnosis of a primary tumour or a metastatic tumour because this is important in the treatment for the orthopaedic surgeons.

When we exclude lesions of the cervical, thoracic and lumbar spine we are left with 2,776 cases with positive results in 78%. In 941 punctures of the spine (excluding sacro-coccygeal lesions) positive results were attained on 76% in the cervical spine and 71% for the thoracic and lumbar regions. You can see how important it is to do an aspiration or puncture biopsy of the vertebrae as these methods avoid a big operation and save the patient a lot of time and money. It may sound a little dangerous, but we have had no adverse complications except two cases of haemorrhage which were not severe.

Wherever possible I am present when the puncture is performed. Many are of course done by orthopaedic surgeons of other departments as we get biopsy material from all over South America. We use a 2 mm needle with a special guide for vertebral punctures with differing points of access according to the site of the lesion. In the thoracic spine, which we first avoided, we thought it might be dangerous to push a needle in so far. However, after a study on the cadaver we found it was safe to insert the needle at 4 cms distance from the spinous process. By this means we got exactly into the vertebra and have now carried out over 40 biopsies in this way without complications.

When material is thus obtained we examine it by combined methods of smear cytology and histology, sometimes also using histochemical techniques. This is very important. A number of cases showing the applications of these three related but different methods of studying aspiration biopsy material are illustrated in the paper which I have already mentioned.

Puncture biopsy is of use not only for the spine but also for the lesions in the long bones and is used for these also by many American pathologists, although not universally accepted in this wider field.

It is necessary to add that this is an easy and safe method, but the quality of the material obtained will depend upon the experience of the operator. When it comes from the centre where I work with Ottolenghi at the Italian Hospital, where we have developed this method, aspiration biopsy results are 90% positive, but this drops to only 60% where material is collected by an inexperienced surgeon.

If there is insufficient material for examination we may say—repeat the puncture, and this has been done two or three times without any danger. If on the other hand it is a sclerotic lesion or one where the surgeon cannot get in perfectly we advise an open biopsy. There is no contraindication for an open biopsy if a puncture biopsy has been unsatisfactory.

Mr. Fitton   I would like to raise a point as a clinician. In our region a fair number of biopsies of this type are done, and I notice that in the spine the results are not always positive at the time, the positive results follow later. As a clinician one is really like a shepherd with sheep—it is not the ones that are in the field that are obviously nice— they may be alright if you have a solution quickly. It is the ones that you don't diagnose and have to wait three weeks, then another three weeks, before you can tell those anxious parents what the situation is. I would just like to ask Mr. Lee if he could tell us if he used the same instrumentation on the vertebral bodies and what results he gets there.

Mr. Lee   We haven't done very many vertebrae. We use the same trephine to get into the vertebrae, and then we put a small punch through it or even a needle. But the results are, as we have heard, more difficult.

Professor Dahlin   I think it is very fine when Dr. Schajowicz can use enough South American finesse to make the diagnosis most of the time by needle biopsy, but I think we have to bear in mind the surgical pathologist normally has the final responsibility for giving a judgement on which the therapy is to be based. If our surgeons use the punch biopsy they are quite prepared to go ahead with an open biopsy unless we can provide them with a definitive histologic diagnosis, and I think this tag is probably useful. I think we should also bear in mind that nowadays when certain chemotherapeutic agents are employed along with radiotherapy or with surgery—it is important that our initial specimen should be adequate so that we have a definitive classification. Else we might end up with such things as indeterminate small round cell malignancy that Dr. Suit cures with some magic chemical, and we don't quite know what he has cured. *Let me make a plea that however we get the material, we make sure it is adequate.*

Professor Campbell   Mr. Lee gave the impression that one would have to do an enormous incision to do an open biopsy. I would tend to disagree with this in principle. I think that if one carefully plans the biopsy depending on the clinical manifestations and the roentgenograms, one can go through a relatively small incision, and do much more adequate tissue biopsy by open methods, using about an inch or two in length in most places. Our results are, I believe, superior to those shown here by Dr. Schajowicz of Argentina and we also do a frozen section as Dr. Dahlin does with a high percentage of accuracy initially.

Dr. Marcove   As far as the first reference goes to just doing smears, it is the Memorial Hospital routine to examine blocks and sections as well as smears. Getting away from needle aspirations and thinking of small open biopsies, examples of flexion contractions and so forth must be a great rarity, especially if one does not put a drain into a vein and the bleeding and just sew them up tight.

Whether or not to treat an osteogenic sarcoma with radiotherapy is I think a point of great controversy. If you say it is cruel to amputate and not to irradiate, we can all pull out cases to show the cruelty of this latter method of treatment with multiple pathological fractures, flexion contractions and useless limbs. It has been the teaching of Coley and Higinbotham and everyone I have worked with, including Henry Jaffe, to amputate early. Irradiation is not used any longer.

Professor Enneking I would like to make one point in the use of open as opposed to trocar and needle biopsy. The results in terms of dissemination of tumour locally are essentially the same. If you examine amputated limbs following either method of biopsy, carefully making cross-sections of the entire limb, you will see tumour spread up and down the fascial planes where the biopsy was done. We have very carefully examined 76 such limbs, and you can find tumour as far up as the inguinal ligament from an open biopsy done around the femoral condyles, and as high as the middle of thigh in punch biopsies from the tibia metaphysis. The interval between the time of biopsy and the definitive procedure is frequently delayed either by irradiation, or by consultation or by geographical limitations in seeking surgical care; so these cases give an opportunity to see what the result is—which you can't appreciate early on in the course of the disease. I have no doubt that the same thing happens to the spine, that tumours spread along the paravertebral musculature from any kind of biopsy. The suggestion that a trocar biopsy is less likely to cause local dissemination of the tumour is I think a fallacious attitude.

Mr. Lee I really don't find myself getting hot under the collar on any of these points which have been made. I regard the question of radiotherapy versus surgery as one which is largely a matter of one's attitude to the patient and one's ethics and so on. I think the outcome is the same. When I said amputations are cruel, I didn't mean that the amputation itself is cruel. But to do it when a patient has a 5 to 1 chance of lung metastases within a very few months and therefore the amputation is of no avail, this is what I consider to be such a pity. As regards to the dissemination of the tumour, I am most interested in this study. I, of course, have merely gone by the fact that a breakdown of the biopsy wound for example or some damage done to the joint is much more likely to happen with an incision. Admittedly, the longer the incision the greater the danger; and therefore again it is perhaps a distinction without much difference between a very small biopsy incision and the kind of 1 cm puncture we make. The actual breakdown of the wound which hinders the radiotherapy we haven't seen with the tiny punch biopsies. We have seen it with the longer incisions.

REFERENCE

1. Schajowicz F. & Derqui J.C. Puncture Biopsy in Lesions of the Locomotor System. *Cancer* **21**, 531. 1968.

Malignant round-cell tumours in bone

Chairman: PROFESSOR LAUREN V. ACKERMAN

A critique of Ewing's tumour of bone

by

C. H. G. PRICE

SUMMARY

Past confusion in the classification and diagnosis of the malignant round-cell tumours in bone has been largely resolved by biochemical, ultrastructural and tissue culture studies which have revealed intrinsic differences between Ewing's tumour, reticulosarcoma and metastatic neuroblastoma. Nevertheless, careful autopsy reports of the two former are still urgently required. A histological review of 129 round-cell tumours established the three main groups, but in 22% no certain diagnosis was possible and six tumours of structure intermediate between Ewing's tumour and reticulosarcoma were encountered. Forty-two reticulosarcomata showed no intracellular glycogen which was demonstrated in 59% of the Ewing group and in 18% of the neuroblastomata.

A separate observer error exercise on selected sections of round-cell tumours indicates the wide divergence of interpretation for many specified features and their relative value in differential diagnosis. Disregarding controversial nomenclature, most long-term survivors are patients whose tumours are composed of rather pleomorphic cells with ample reticulin and no intracellular glycogen.

EVERYBODY HERE must be familiar with the controversy which has been associated with the non-osteogenic so-called "round-cell" sarcoma in bone. This neoplasm was first described by Lücke[26] in 1866 and amplified in subsequent publications, but it was not until 1921 that the celebrated paper by James Ewing[13] appeared in which he applied the term "diffuse endothelioma of bone", the "endothelioma" designation persisting as late as 1949 (Coley).[6] During the 20 years after Ewing's paper a voluminous literature accumulated which was noteworthy for three main features:

1. The more precise characterization of a progressive destructive tumour in bone composed of rather featureless masses of small round or oval cells. The nature and histogenesis was regarded as uncertain hence by many the eponymous title Ewing's sarcoma was preferred.

2. A large measure of agreement about the age, sex and site distribution and usually lethal outcome.

3. Alleged confusion between primary round-cell sarcoma of bone and metastatic neuroblastoma—this of course stemmed from the well-known papers of Colville and Willis 1933,[9] and Willis 1960.[45] The last writer in fact strongly questioned the very existence of such a tumour entity, referring to the "Ewing Syndrome"—a view which he still maintained in 1967,[46] That occasional mistakes occurred in this respect was generally accepted, although Willis's adverse criticism was based upon the results of only two autopsies in which lesions thought to be osseous primaries were shown to be metastatic.

During the last 20 years large series of Ewing's Sarcoma have been reported by a number of authors.[4,5,8,10,18,23,37,43] These papers largely confirm the features already mentioned, and are in broad agreement even to the infrequency of autopsy reports, thus still leaving somewhat unsilenced the essential misgivings of Willis.

Contributions from the United Kingdom have been notably few but I may mention those of Magnus and Wood (1956),[28] Lumb and Mackenzie (1956),[27] Marsden and Steward (1964)[30] and Ball (1970).[2] Comparing the two former papers the most interesting aspect is the uncertainty expressed of the relationship of Ewing's Sarcoma and reticulosarcoma of bone. The differences, both clinical and pathological, between reticulosarcoma and Ewing's Sarcoma were emphasized by the 1939 paper by Parker and Jackson[36] who also drew attention to the former's better prognosis. Further papers on reticulosarcoma of bone confirmed these results.[7,12,15,21,32] Coming to the most recent work, Shoji and Miller (1971)[40] reported a 5-year survival rate of 44·2%, and 64% of those cases given combined treatment was reported by Miller and Nicholson (1971).[33] The better prognosis for reticulosarcoma may be compared with the situation for Ewing's tumour where the 5-year survival rate of 646 cases collected from the literature by Bhansali and Desai (1963)[4] was a meagre 8·7%, and the even worse response for osseous metastatic neuroblastoma of 9% alive at 3 years reported by Marsden and Steward (1968).[31] These wide prognostic differences, and the clinical need to distinguish between the primary bone tumour and the metastatic, together with the possible future developments of divergent forms of treatment make it imperative to attempt accurate differential diagnosis between reticulosarcoma, Ewing's Sarcoma and neuroblastoma. The criticism levelled by Willis regarding the existence of Ewing's tumour as an entity has been largely answered in four ways:

1. By autopsy examinations; few but suggestive (only one in the present series) Stout 2/42 (1943),[41] Geschickter and Copeland 12/167 (1949),[18] Lichtenstein and Jaffe 4/17 (1947),[25] Marsden and Steward 7/21 (1964),[30] Lumb and Mackenzie 3/10 (1956).[27] Whilst there might be good reasons why post-mortem examinations are unusual in young adults, a cynic would obviously point out that this infrequency of autopsy records could be due to revelation on the autopsy table of the metastatic nature of lesions thought to be primary in bone.

2. There are a small number of patients who have long survivals > 20 years—there are two such in the Bristol series. Regression of a primary tumour after ablation of a metastasis is not unknown, but is nevertheless very unusual.

3. During the last decade the study of the increased and deranged metabolism of the pressor amines has been shown to be a characteristic feature of the large majority of tumours of the sympathetic nervous system including neuroblastoma and ganglioneuroblastoma.[3,19,29]

4. Tissue culture methods and electron microscopy have demonstrated ultrastructural and cultural differences between reticulosarcoma, Ewing's tumour and neuroblastoma and cultural differences between reticulosarcoma, Ewing's tumour and neuroblastoma.[16,17,20,24,34,35,44]

It is stated by Jacobson (1971) that the existence of Ewing's tumour and reticulosarcoma is uncertain in animals, although in certain species (bovines and dogs) lymphosarcoma is not uncommon. Moreover, in sub-human species, neuroblastoma metastatic in bone has not been reported.[22]

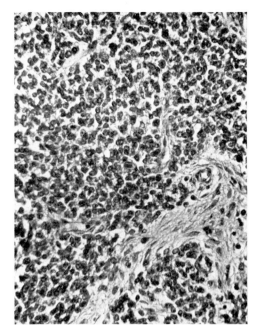

Fig. 1. H & E × 200 (BTR/245). Ewing's tumour. The characteristic rather uniform pattern of closely packed oval or round cells, 10–15 μ in size.

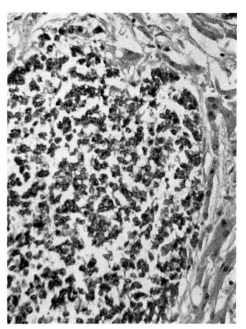

Fig. 2. H & E × 200 (BTR/3117). Ewing's tumour. Metastatic in liver. The cells are here more pleomorphic and variable in size.

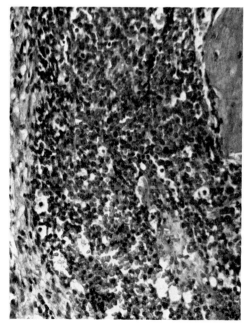

Fig. 4. H & E × 200 (BTR/2637). Ewing's tumour. Some cells lie in vacuolar spaces simulating the "starry sky" appearance of a malignant lymphoma.

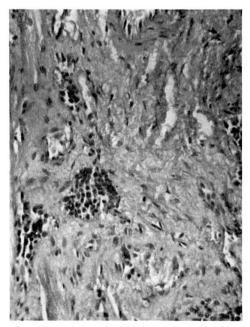

Fig. 4. H & E × 200 (BTP/L). Ewing's tumour. Scanty nests of tumour cells dispersed through an extensive fibrovascular reactive stroma which may be the predominant feature.

Despite the extensive advances already mentioned which support the concept of Ewing's Sarcoma as a primary tumour, the day-to-day problem of differential diagnosis is still largely a matter for morbid anatomy, so to provide confirmation of lesions suspected by the clinician and radiologist.

Perusal of many descriptive texts of the round-cell sarcomata, gives the impression of frequent repitition of certain histological features and less information about the range of structure, with but little indication of the relative diagnostic value of the specific points which may be observed. Photomicrographs are often confined to areas of typical well-preserved pure tumour tissue (Fig. 1) and seldom show cells invading other tissues or mingled with the more or less vascular reactive fibrous tissue where cell morphology and arrangement may be modified and atypical (Figs. 2, 3 and 4). My personal experience indicates that in terms of cell arrangement and morphology of the three main types of round-cell tumour in bone, there is greater variation in each one than between them. In some instances multiple blocks of tissue for study increases the diagnostic dilemma, whilst in the small biopsy with less than 10 high-power fields of well-preserved tumour tissue, no firm diagnosis other than malignant round-cell tumour is usually attainable. Moreover, the histological appearances my be modified by differing methods of fixation and processing. I do not think that this possibility has ever been adequately investigated. These anomalies are the crux of the histological problem—at least for myself.

The pathologist members of the Bristol Registry were not unique in their early diagnostic error in accepting as Ewing's tumour some which were otherwise. This was however corrected in December 1955 when former cases were reviewed and re-classified some as neuroblastoma, some reticulosarcoma, some as malignant round-cell tumour unspecified. After this episode the majority of such lesions were classified as malignant round-cell tumour with or without any further designation, unless the Registry Panel were unanimous, or a rider was added stating the majority opinion.

As one part of the work reported here, I have reviewed all the histology of about 160 round-cell tumours, sections being of tissues fixed in 10% formal saline or alcoholic Bouin's fluid, embedded in paraffin wax and stained by haematoxylin and eosin, or by haematoxylin, phloxin and tartrazine. The silver impregnation methods of Gömöri, and Gordon and Sweets have been used to demonstrate reticulin. Glycogen has been demonstrated on duplicate sections of the same paraffin blocks by means of the P.A.S. and diastase P.A.S. method.[38,39]

After eliminating examples of Hodgkin's Disease, primitive myeloma and leukaemia, and a small group of soft tissue round-cell tumours, I accepted 129 as being round-cell tumours in bone within my terms of reference.

The breakdown of this series is shown in Table 1. The initial step was separation of all reticulated tumours to be regarded as reticulosarcoma, but also including a number which are lymphosarcoma. These numbered 48 and subsequent study of the case notes divided them into three groups:

1. A solitary osseous primary tumour (22).
2. Lesions involving multiple bones *ab initio* or bones and groups of lymph nodes (16).
3. Bone invasion by an adjacent soft tissue tumour (4).

A second review showed a small group of five tumours which were positive for intra-cellular glycogen. These had originally been regarded histologically as reticulosarcoma, but on review it was noted that this small series has more of the cyto-morphology and

TABLE 1

ROUND CELL TUMOURS IN BONE (129) DECEMBER 1971

Type	Metastatic neuro-blastoma	Group "X"	Ewing's tumour	Group "Y"	Reticulosarcoma 1	2	3	Unspecified M.R.C.T.
Number	29	14	29	6	22	16	4	9
Age range	3M–33	1–25	6–45	5–21	7–85	2–71	23–83	11–71
Median age—years	10	8	20	15	50	46	56	21
Survival—								
5 years	4%	nil	17%	20%	47%	nil	33%	25%
Average—months	14	12	25	12	22	10	30	34
Still living	?1	1	7	2	10	nil	1	1
Presenting in long bones	28%	43%	52%	50%	52%	—	—	55%
Autopsy	19/28	1/13	1/22	1/4	4/12	6/16	0/3	2/7
Glycogen positive	5/27	7/14	16/27	5/6	nil	nil	nil	3/6

Histologically undiagnosed tumours—29/129 = 22%

pattern of Ewing's sarcoma, [14] and contained a less marked or patchy reticulin network. On a third examination of the reticulated tumours one further example was added to this group making a total of six—this being Group "Y" of the table. These tumours I believe to be intermediate in their structure between reticulosarcoma and Ewing's tumour which they resemble in their age distribution and behaviour. These six may resemble other tumours mentioned by Dahlin (1965)[11] and by Lumb and Mackenzie (1956).[27] One tumour in particular was of special interest, B.T.R./1374, male, 15 years, tumour of scapula, as one block of four showed reticulosarcoma whilst the other three had the morphological pattern of Ewing's Sarcoma. Intracellular glycogen was found only in the tissue resembling Ewing's tumour where the reticulin network was diminished or absent (Figs. 7 to 12).

Twenty-nine examples of neuroblastoma were confirmed (Fig. 5); of the residual 52 tumours, 29 showed the characteristic uniform and featureless non-reticulated pattern of Ewing's Sarcoma. In 14 other tumours I think the histological diagnosis is either neuroblastoma or Ewing's Sarcoma, but I am unsure as to which. There was also a residual group of nine tumours where for various reasons I can make no diagnosis beyond malignant round-cell tumour unspecified. Following the histological study of the non-reticulated group, sections were examined where available for the presence of intracellular glycogen. 5/27 neuroblastomata were positive (4 being cases confirmed by autopsy material (Fig. 6): 16/27 Ewing's sarcomata were positive as also were 7/14 in the Group "X"—tumours of questionable nature. The demonstration of glycogen in a proportion of the neuroblastomata amply confirms the results reported by Arthur *et al.* (1970).[1] In Table 1 the general features which emerge for neuroblastoma, for Ewing's tumour and for reticulosarcoma are similar to those from other sources in spite of the modest number of cases presented. It will be noted, however, that there are 29/129 tumours undiagnosed on the sections available, i.e. 22%, and I feel that this is probably

182

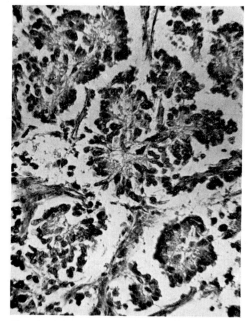

Fig. 5. H & E × 200 (BTR/1189). Metastatic neuroblastoma: numerous well-formed rosettes are seen with central neurofibrils.

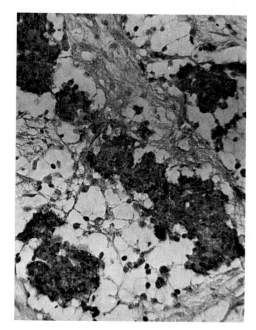

Fig. 6. P.A.S. × 200 (BTR/1189). Metastatic neuroblastoma. Clumps of cells some of which contain glycogen granules.

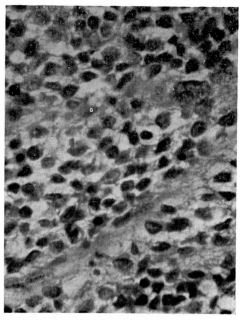

Fig. 7. H & E × 400 (BTR/1374. Block B). Tumour of mixed structure (Group Y—Table 1). The cell pleomorphism and nuclear features resemble reticulosarcoma: cf. Fig. 8.

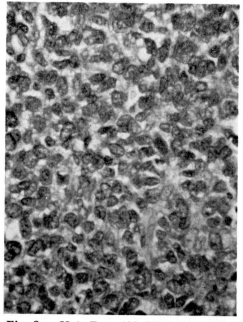

Fig. 8. H & E × 400 (BTR/1374 Block C.). In this field the appearances are those of Ewing's tumour with several rosette-like structures visible.

TABLE 2

C.R.C. BONE TUMOUR PANEL 1969–1970. OBSERVER ERROR STUDY—M.R.C.T.
6 members—12 sections (11 tumours)

Good agreement, over 90%: Rosettes, giant cells, calcification.
Fair agreement, 75–90%: Glycogen, reticulin, fibrous septae, conspicuous eosinophilic nucleoli.
Poor agreement, 50–75%: Nuclear characteristics, cell size and arrangement.
Bad agreement, under 50%: Mitoses per square mm of tumour tissue.
Overall diagnostic score agreement −66% (4 of 6 members)

the measure of the residual diagnostic puzzle as it would confront the working pathologist. This no doubt may be reduced in size by reviewing each case in the light of clinical, radiological and biochemical findings, thus improving the overall diagnostic accuracy. This problem I feel certain is not mine alone.

In this survey the search for intracellular glycogen was not used as a diagnostic criterion[38,39] except in separating the five tumours of six in my Group "Y". Using only formalin or alcoholic Bouin fixed material I may well have some false negative results, especially in the Ewing's Sarcoma group, nevertheless, I deny that there are any pseudopositives. Many of my sections contained muscle fibres which although only partially reactive for glycogen provide a useful positive control. I have also seen three examples of autopsy proven Ewing's Sarcoma, which in well-preserved formalin fixed material were glycogen negative, and I have one soft tissue tumour of buttock in a girl of 15 (B.T.R./2025) which shows the Ewing type structure and is glycogen positive.

The histological difficulties I have outlined have for many years been a source of controversy amongst the members of the Cancer Research Campaign Bone Tumour Panel. It was therefore proposed by Dr. Ball that we should attempt to evaluate observer error and degree of diagnostic divergence within the Panel. A protocol was therefore devised in which members were required to record certain features.

Professor Sissons organized this exercise and selected 12 blocks from 11 round-cell tumours for this study in which he participated together with Drs. Ball, Byers and Catto, the late Dr. W. Goldie and myself. The results were analysed by Professor Sissons with the following results (Table 2):

Good agreement between observers was found for cell arrangement, i.e. presence or absence of "rosettes", acini, giant cells etc. These were mainly negative findings.

Fair agreement appeared in respect of intracellular glycogen, "star" cells, nucleoli, reticulin and fibrous septae. All other results were poor (<75% agreement) whilst evaluation of mitotic activity was frankly bad. The average diagnostic score was 66%, i.e. 4/6 members in accord. It was clearly noted that discordant results obtained for observations which required quantitative judgement, and judgement in histology is difficult to acquire and coloured by personal experience. For example, it was noted that for several parameters certain participants in this work were quite consistent in their disagreement from others. This rather tedious but nevertheless interesting exercise has since been extended to a larger number of round-cell tumours, and will when completed be reported elsewhere. The value of this type of work lies in clearly demonstrating two points:

(a) The magnitude of differences between observations, concepts and interpretations of several trained histologists.

(b) The unequal significance to be attached to certain specified characteristics in the interpretation of histological preparations. Obviously more reliance should be placed on features with a high observer agreement, or on those which are constantly noted or which are pathognomonic. The controversial or indefinite should be given low or limited credence.

In my review of the histology of the 129 Bristol tumours I relied upon cell arrangement and morphology, and the patterns of necrosis and reticulation when these were present. The intracellular glycogen study was an ancillary investigation not regarded as a diagnostic criterion except as mentioned in the segregation of the five Group "Y" tumours, which I regard as intermediate in their nature between reticulosarcoma and Ewing's tumour (Figs. 7 to 12). From this Group "Y" I derive a unifying concept of three related types of primary marrow sarcoma—other than myeloma and the leucoses. These are reticulosarcoma, lymphosarcoma and Ewing's Sarcoma, the position being analogous to the skeletogenic series where we have the three main types of osteosarcoma: fibrosarcoma and chondrosarcoma. Within the two classes of marrow and bone tumours we may encounter examples which have an intermediate or mixed structure, those in which there is uncertainty in recognition of their cell or matrix differentiation or evolutionary changes, which I have certainly observed amongst the bone sarcomata. This I believe is the view most widely accepted at present. Beyond this, for the clinician it is clear that the presence of ample reticulin and absence of glycogen in a solitary tumour are good prognostic features, irrespective of the name actually applied to a given lesion. Such features in conjunction with clinical, radiographic and biochemical findings are relevant to behaviour and prognosis.

Lastly, to summarize my conclusions:

1. There can be no doubt that the majority of tumours reported as Ewing's Sarcoma are primary in bone.

2. Nevertheless, I believe that up to one-fifth may be histologically mis-diagnosed and confused *inter alia* with metastatic neuroblastoma and reticulosarcoma.

3. Ewing's Sarcoma is allied to, but usually distinct from reticulosarcoma and lymphosarcoma—although intermediate forms may be encountered.

4. In the evaluation of histological sections certain specific features are more trustworthy than others. Estimates of cell size, depth of nuclear staining and mitotic activity can be deceptive and controversial.

5. With formalin fixed material a large proportion of Ewing's tumours show intracellular glycogen, as also do about one-fifth of neuroblastomata metastatic in bone.

   The majority of tumours in which an extensive reticulin network exists are glycogen negative.

6. This histological study of the Bristol series of round-cell tumours in bone indicates two dominant but related types of primary marrow malignancy—apart from myeloma and the leucoses:

   (a) The non-reticulated rather uniform small round-cell pattern, often with intracellular glycogen. This neoplasm appears in older children or young people and has an ominous prognosis.

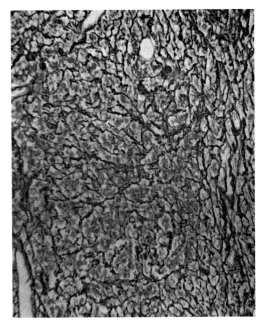

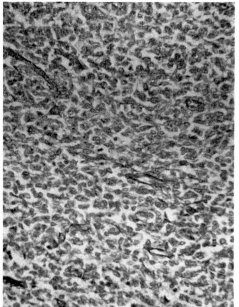

Fig. 9. Gömöri Reticulin × 200 (BTR/1374 Block B). There was a well-marked reticulin network throughout this sample of the tumour. cf. Fig.10.

Fig. 10. Gömöri Reticulin × 200 (BTR/1374 Block C). The scanty reticulin present is mainly around small blood vessels.

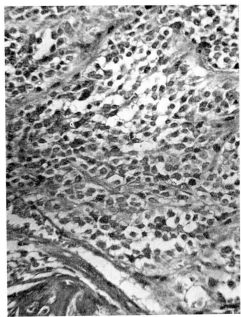

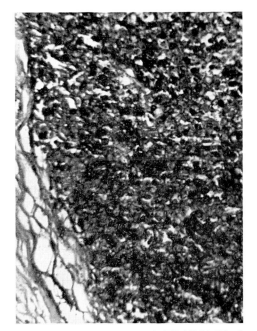

Fig. 11. P.A.S. × 200 (BTR/1374 Block B). The tumour cells contain no glycogen where the reticulated pattern seen in Fig. 9. was found.

Fig. 12. P.A.S. × 200 (BTR/1374 Block C.). An area having the appearance of Ewing's tumour with cells rich in glycogen.

(b) The reticulated more pleomorphic glycogen-free sarcoma more characteristic of older persons. When monostotic this responds to treatment in about 40% of cases.

These are the essential facts irrespective of diverse nomenclature or histogenetic speculation.

ACKNOWLEDGMENTS

The author's thanks are due to the members of the Bristol Bone Tumour Registry and numerous colleagues who have referred the cases included in the histological survey. The author is also indebted to the Cancer Research Campaign Bone Tumour Panel for authorizing the presentation of the preliminary findings of the observer error study. Likewise, the technical aid of Mr. A. Wilson and Mr. J. E. Hancock are acknowledged together with much clerical assistance from Mrs. J. E. Nutt. This work, and also the Bristol Bone Tumour Registry, are financially supported by the Cancer Campaign for Research.

REFERENCES

1. Arthur, J. F., Bennett, M. H., Jelliffe, A. M., Kendall, B. E., Millett, Yvonne L. & Tucker, Audrey K. Small Round-Cell Tumours of Bone. *Symposium Ossium*, p. 186. Ed. by A. M. Jelliffe & B. Strickland. Livingstone, Edinburgh & London, 1970.
2. Ball, J. Ewing's Tumour *and* Reticulum-cell Sarcoma. In *Symposium Ossium*, p. 184. Ed. by A. M. Jelliffe & B. Strickland. Livingstone, Edinburgh & London 1970.
3. Bell, M. In *The Clinical Chemistry of Monoamines*, p. 82. Elsevier, Amsterdam, 1963.
4. Bhansali, S. K. & Desai, P. B. Ewing's Sarcoma. *J. Bone Jt. Surg.*, 45–A, 541, 1963.
5. Bone Tumour Committee of the Netherlands. *Radiological Atlas of Bone Tumours*. Williams & Wilkins, Baltimore, 1966.
6. Coley, B. L. *Neoplasms of Bone*, p. 297. Hoeber, New York, 1949.
7. Coley, B. L., Higinbotham, N. L. & Groesbeck, H. P. Primary Reticulum Cell Sarcoma of Bone—Summary of 37 Cases. *Radiology*, 55, 641, 1950.
8. Coley, B. L., Higinbotham, N. L. & Bowden, L. Endothelioma of Bone (Ewing's Sarcoma). *Ann. Surg.*, 128, 533, 1948.
9. Colville, H. C. & Willis, R. A. Neuroblastoma Metastasis in Bones, with Criticism of Ewing's Endothelioma. *Amer. J. Path.*, 9, 421, 1933.
10. Dahlin, D. C., Coventry, M. B. & Scanlan, P. W. Ewing's Sarcoma. A Critical Analysis of 165 Cases. *J. Bone Jt. Surg.*, 43–A, 185, 1961.
11. Dahlin, D. C. Ewing's Sarcoma and Malignant Lymphoma (Reticulum-cell Sarcoma of Bone). In *Tumors of Bone and Soft Tissue*, p. 179. Year Book Medical Publishers, Chicago, 1965.
12. Dahlin, D. C. *Bone Tumors*, 2nd Ed., p. 156. Thomas, Springfield, Ill., 1967.
13. Ewing, J. Diffuse Endothelioma of Bone. *Proc. N. Y. Path. Soc.*, 21, 17, 1921.
14. Ewing, J. Neoplastic Diseases, p. 360. 4th Ed. Saunders, Philadelphia & London, 1940.
15. Francis, K. C., Higinbotham, N. L. & Coley, B. L. Primary Reticulum Cell Sarcoma of Bone: Report of 44 Cases. *Surg. Gynec. Obstet.*, 99, 142, 1954.
16. Friedman, B. & Gold, H. Ultrastructure of Ewing's Sarcoma of Bone. *Cancer*, 22, 307, 1968.
17. Friedman, B. & Hanaoka, H. Round-cell Sarcomas of Bone. A light and electron microscope study. *J. Bone Jt. Surg.*, 53–A, 1118, 1971.
18. Geschickter, C. F. & Copeland, M. M. *Tumors of Bone*, p. 387, 3rd Ed. Lippincott, Philadelphia, London & Montreal, 1949.
19. Gitlow, S. E., Bertani, Laura M., Rausen, A., Gribetz, D. & Dziedzic, S. W. Diagnosis of Neuroblastoma by Qualitative and Quantitative Determination of Catecholamine Metabolites in Urine. *Cancer*, 25, 1377, 1970.

20. Goldstein, M. N. & Pinkel, D. Long-term Tissue Culture of Neuroblastomas. *J. nat. Cancer Inst.*, **20**, 675, 1958.

21. Ivins, J. C. & Dahlin, D. C. Malignant Lymphoma (Reticulum Cell Sarcoma) of Bone. *Proc. Mayo Clin.*, **38**, 375, 1963.

22. Jacobson, S. A. *The Comparative Pathology of the Tumors of Bone*, p. 334. Thomas, Springfield, Ill., 1971.

23. Japanese Bone Tumour Registry. K. Iribe. Personal communication, 1970.

24. Kadin, M. E. & Bensch, K. G. On the Origin of Ewing's Tumor. *Cancer*, **27**, 257, 1971.

25. Lichtenstein, L. & Jaffe, H. L. Ewing's Sarcoma of Bone. *Amer. J. Path.*, **23**, 43, 1947.

26. Lücke, A. Beit. 2. Geschwülstlehre III. *Virchows Arch. Path. Anat.*, **35**, 524, 1866.

27. Lumb, G. & Mackenzie, D. H. Round-cell Tumours of Bone. *Brit. J. Surg.*, **43**, 380, 1956.

28. Magnus, H. A. & Wood, H. L.-C. Primary Reticulo-sarcoma of Bone. *J. Bone Jt. Surg.*, **35–B**, 258, 1956.

29. Marsden, H. B. In *The Clinical Chemistry of the Monoamines*, p. 76. Elsevier, Amsterdam, 1963.

30. Marsden, H. B. & Steward, J. K. Ewing's Tumours and Neuroblastomas. *J. Clin. Path.*, **17**, 411, 1964.

31. Marsden, H. B. & Steward, J. K. Tumours in Children, pp. 131, 315, *Recent Results in Cancer Research*. Springer-Verlag, Berlin, Heidelberg, New York, 1968.

32. Medill, E. V. Primary Reticulum-cell Sarcoma of Bone. *J. Fac. Radiol (Lond.)*, **8**, 102, 1956.

33. Miller, T. R. & Nicholson, J. T. End Results in Reticulum-cell Sarcoma of Bone treated by Bacterial Toxin Therapy alone or Combined with Surgery and/or Radiotherapy (47 cases) or with Concurrent Infection (5 cases). *Cancer*, **27**, 524, 1971.

34. Murray, M. R. & Stout, A. P. Distinctive Characteristics of the Sympathicoblastoma Cultivated *in vitro:* Method for Prompt Diagnosis. *Amer. J. Path.*, **23**, 429, 1947.

35. Murray, M. R. & Stout, A. P. The classification and diagnosis of human tumours by tissue culture methods. *Tex. Rep. Biol. & Med.* **12**, 898, 1954.

36. Parker, F., Jnr. & Jackson, H., Jnr. Primary Reticulum-cell Sarcoma of Bone. *Surg. Gynec. Obstet.*, **68**, 45, 1939.

37. Poppe, H. Reticulumzellsarkome und Ewing Sarkome. *Symposium Ossium* p. 178. Ed. by A. M. Jelliffe & B. Strickland. Livingstone, Edinburgh & London, 1970.

38. Schajowicz, F. & Cabrini, R. L. Histochemical Studies of Bone in Normal and Pathological Conditions. With special reference to Alkaline Phosphatase, Glycogen and Mucopolysaccharides. *J. Bone. Jt. Surg.*, **36–B**, 574, 1954.

39. Schajowicz, F. Ewing's Sarcoma & Reticulum-cell Sarcoma of Bone. With special reference to the Histochemical Demonstration of Glycogen as an Aid to Differential Diagnosis. *J. Bone Jt. Surg.* **41–A**, 349, 1959.

40. Shoji, H. & Miller, T. R. Primary Reticulum-cell Sarcoma of Bone. Significance of Clinical Features upon the Prognosis. *Cancer*, **28**, 1234, 1971.

41. Stout, A. P. A Discussion of the Pathology and Histogenesis of Ewing's Tumor of Bone Marrow. *Amer. J. Path.*, **50**, 334, 1943.

42. Wang, C. C. & Fleischli, D. J. Primary Reticulum Cell Sarcoma of Bone with Emphasis on Radiation Therapy. *Cancer*, **22**, 994, 1968.

43. Wang, C. C. & Schulz, M. D. Ewing's Sarcoma—Study of 50 cases treated at Massachusetts General Hospital, 1930–52 inclusive. *New Eng. J. Med.*, **248**, 571, 1953.

44. Weinberger, M. A. & Banfield, W. G. Fine Structure of a Transplantable Reticulum Cell Sarcoma. I. Light and Electron Microscopy of Viable and Necrotic Tumor Cells. *J. nat. Cancer Inst.*, **34**, 459, 1965.

45. Willis, R. A. Metastatic Neuroblastoma in Bone Presenting the Ewing Syndrome, with a discussion of "Ewing's Sarcoma". *Amer. J. Path.* **16**, 317, 1940.

46. Willis, R. A. *Pathology of Tumours*, p. 702, 4th Ed. Butterworths, London, 1967.

Differential diagnosis of Ewing's sarcoma

by

FRITZ SCHAJOWICZ

SUMMARY

A comparative clinico-radiological and pathological study, including cytological histological and histochemical investigations of malignant round cell sarcoma was carried out.

One hundred and seventy-three cases were classified as Ewing's sarcoma, 78 cases as malignant lymphoma of bone (including 75 cases of primary and secondary reticulo-sarcoma and three cases of lymphosarcoma) and 38 cases as metastatic neuroblastoma.

The differential diagnosis of these processes is discussed in detail confirming the value of the demonstration of glycogen in tumour cells of Ewing's sarcoma and its absence in reticulosarcoma and metastatic neuroblastoma.

THE DIFFICULTIES of differential diagnosis within the group of malignant round-cell tumours of bone, and specifically of separation between Ewing's sarcoma, malignant lymphoma (reticulo- and lymphosarcoma) and metastatic neuroblastoma (sympathico-blastoma) are well known. Myeloma, because of its specific cytologic and clinical features with the associated protein disturbances, usually is easily distinguished from the other malignant round-cell tumours.

Primary reticulosarcoma ("reticulum-cell sarcoma") of bone was first distinguished from Ewing's sarcoma by Parker and Jackson (1939) as a separate clinical and patholo-gical entity. Although most authors, including Ewing, accepted their criteria there are still several authors who feel that it is impossible or very difficult to separate these entities.

Although certain cases may be distinguished by clinical and roentgenographic exam-ination, the definite diagnosis must fundamentally be based on the histopathological study. Proper differentiation between the two entities has more than academic interest because of the vastly better prognosis of reticulo-sarcoma compared with that of Ewing's sarcoma.

In a previous paper (1959) we showed that the histochemical demonstration of glyco-gen granules in the cytoplasm of tumour cells of Ewing's sarcoma and its absence in reticulosarcoma proved to be an easy and efficient method of differential diagnosis, provided the specimens were properly fixed (alcohol 80% or Rossman's fluid, which is an alcoholic picric solution) and stained. The periodic acid Schiff stain (P.A.S.) in McManus's or Hotchkiss's modification has been satisfactory. Eight cases of Ewing's sarcoma were positive for glycogen and the nine cases of reticulosarcoma of bone, which were fixed by the methods described, were negative. In older material, fixed in formalin, glycogen was found in about half of the 43 cases of Ewing's sarcoma, but in none of those of reticulosarcoma, myeloma and a number of other lesions of the marrow, for example, eosinophilic granuloma and malignant lymphomata (Hodgkin's disease and lymphosarcoma). Concluding this paper we stated very briefly: "The histological differential diagnosis of neuroblastoma may also present difficulties. Although the few cases studied by formalin fixed material *lack glycogen, these results are not considered conclusive.*"

During the last years the material studied in our laboratory has increased notably and the results obtained by us and many other workers confirmed our previous findings with the routine light microscope techniques. More recently several electron microscopic studies were reported (Friedman and Gold 1968, Kadin and Bensch 1971, Friedman and Hanaoka 1971, and Hou-Jensen *et al.*, 1972) confirming the presence of abundant glycogen in Ewing's sarcoma and its absence in malignant lymphoma and metastatic neuroblastoma (Friedman and Hanaoka).

The purpose of this paper is to report the results of the comparative clinico-radiological and pathological study, including cytological, histological and histochemical investigations, of the cases studied in our laboratory during the last 31 years (up to December

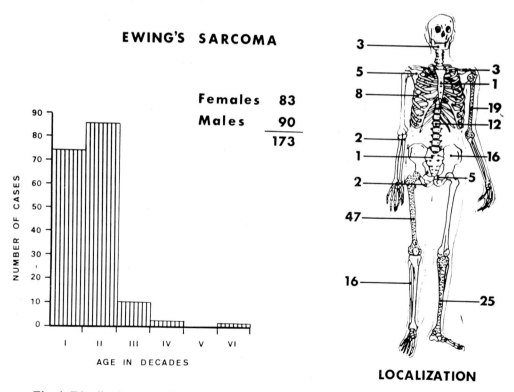

Fig. 1. Distribution according to age, sex and location of 173 cases of Ewing's sarcoma seen in the osteoarticular pathology centre up to December 31, 1971.

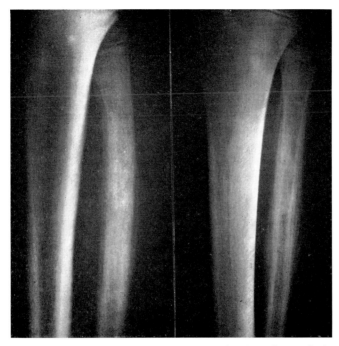

Fig. 2. Lateral and antero-posterior radiograph showing the typical radiological appearance of Ewing's sarcoma located in the fibula diaphysis with the "onion skin" periosteal bone reaction.

1971) actually filed at the Latin-American Registry of bone pathology. Only those cases with sufficient clinico-pathological data were included in this review. In the last 10 years the urinary catecholamines were determined in most cases suspicious of metastatic neuroblastoma.

EWING'S SARCOMA

It is not the purpose of this report to discuss the histogenesis or to present in detail the clinical or pathological aspects of Ewing's sarcoma which are well described in several textbooks and papers. As Fig. 1 shows, the distribution according to age, sex and location, coincides with slight variations with the findings of other authors. The preferred locations were the metadiaphysial region of long limb bones (femur, tibia, humerus and fibula), as also some flat bones, especially the pelvis. The predominant age was between 5 and 15 years, being exceedingly rare after the third decade. Males were affected slightly more than females. The radiological appearance, showing an "onion-skin" periosteal bone new formation, may be a frequent and characteristic, also non-diagnostic finding, in long limb bones (Fig. 2), but a typical pattern is lacking in flat or short bones (Figs. 3 and 4). Some benign lesions and eosinophilic granuloma or osteomyelitis may simulate radiographically the appearance of Ewing's sarcoma. There is a striking tendency for this tumour to involve other bones so that a multi-centric origin has been suspected.

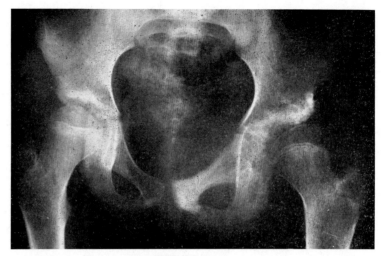

Fig. 3. Radiograph of Ewing's sarcoma of pubis lacking characteristic features.

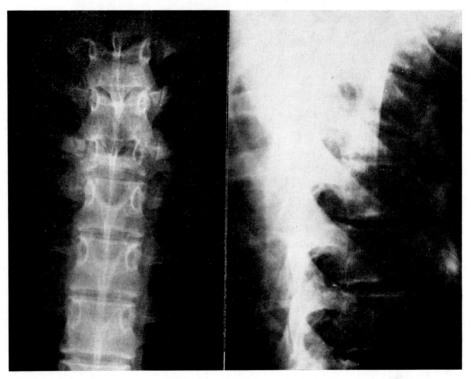

Fig. 4. Antero-posterior and lateral radiographs of Ewing's sarcoma of the ninth thoracic vertebra, showing vertebra plana, very similar to that observed in eosinophilic granuloma.

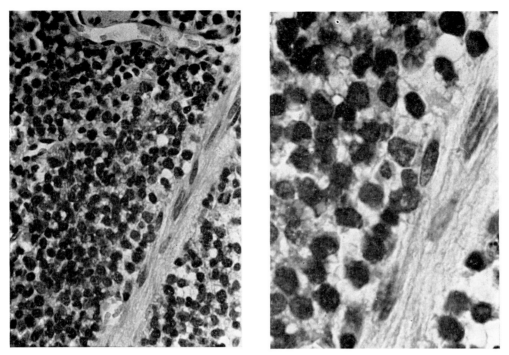

Fig. 5. Photomicrograph showing at lower (H & E × 250) and higher (H & E × 800) magnification the uniform appearance of the tumour cells in Ewing's sarcoma with regular round nuclei and indistinct cytoplasmic borders.

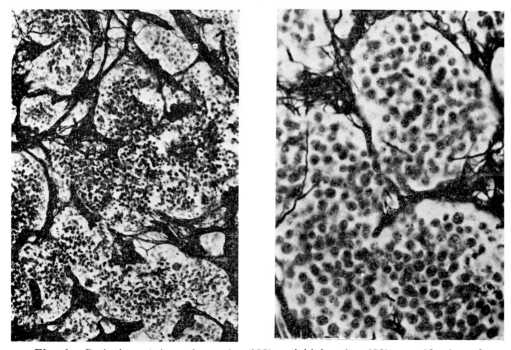

Fig. 6. Reticulum stain at lower (× 100) and higher (× 400) magnification of Ewing's sarcoma, showing the reticulin fibres circumscribing large lobules of tumour cells (Del Rio Hortega's silver technique).

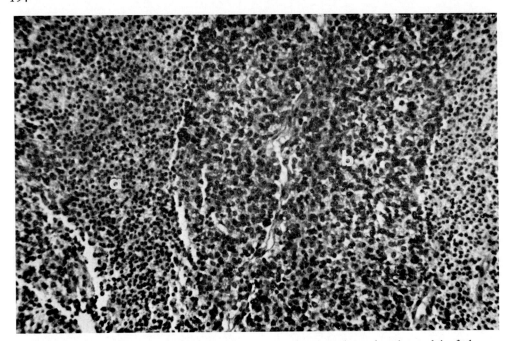

Fig. 7. Photomicrograph of Ewing's sarcoma showing the pyknotic nuclei of the necrobiotic tumour cells (a), the blood vessels separated by strands of well preserved cells (b) (H & E × 250).

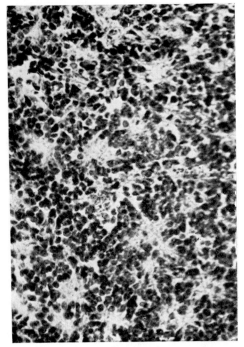

Fig. 8. Photomicrograph showing rosette-like structures in a Ewing's sarcoma (H & E × 250).

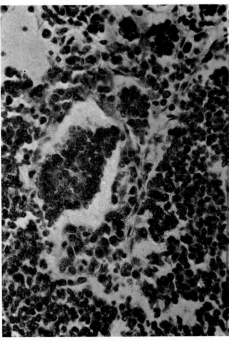

Fig. 9. Photomicrograph of another Ewing's sarcoma in which the autopsy findings confirmed the diagnosis (H & E × 300). In both cases (Figs. 9 and 10) abundant glycogen was present.

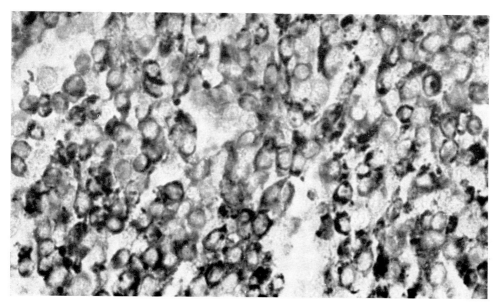

Fig. 10. Photomicrograph showing darkly stained glycogen granules in the cytoplasm of Ewing's sarcoma cells. The nuclei appear as clear disks since no counterstain has been used (80% alcohol fixation, McManus stain, ×600).

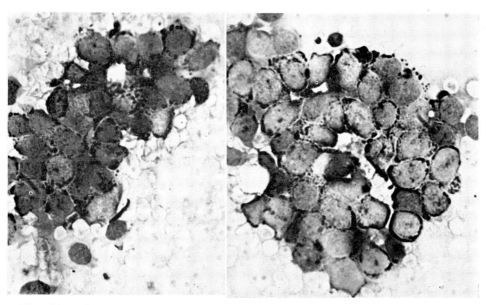

Fig. 11. Photomicrograph of smear of Ewing's sarcoma, obtained by aspiration biopsy, stained by means of the McManus method (P.A.S.). Numerous darkly stained cytoplasmic glycogen granules are clearly visible, (×800).

Histologically the tumour is characterized by a tissue with a rather uniform histological appearance, made up of densely packed cells with round nuclei about two or three times the size of a lymphocytic nucleus, without clear cytoplasmic outlines or prominent nucleoli (Fig. 5) and by the absence of intratumoural reticular fibres (Fig. 6) and tumour bone formation. The tumour is divided into irregular strands or lobules by conspicuous septa of fibrous tissue. Mitosis are present but infrequent. Haemorrhages and extensive areas of necrosis are common producing sometimes an apparent perithelial arrangement of the viable cells (Fig. 7(b)) due to the necrosis of the tumour tissue which was at some distance from the blood vessels. In the zones of necrobiosis, the nuclei were often small and pyknotic, about the size of a lymphocyte (Fig. 7(a)). These fields are particularly prone to be mistaken for malignant lymphoma of lymphocytic type (lymphosarcoma). Sometimes the tumour cells surround small necrotic foci, or yield alveolar-like (Fig. 8) and ganglion-like (Fig. 9) formations which resemble the rosettes of neuroblastoma.

In 27 cases in which the specimens were fixed in 80% alcohol or Rossman's fluid and stained by McManus's and Hotchkiss's techniques (P.A.S.) more or less abundant glycogen in granular form was found, filling the cytoplasm, the granules varying in size from fine to coarse. Most of the tumour cells contained granules regularly, but some areas, apart from the necrotic zones existed in which glycogen was lacking. Previous digestion by ptyalin or Takadiastase caused the P.A.S. positive granules to disappear, thus confirming that they were indeed glycogen. P.A.S. staining, without nuclear counterstain, is preferable because the glycogen granules are more clearly visible with this technique (Fig. 10). The demonstration of glycogen is specially helpful in the small specimens obtained by aspiration biopsy which was used in many of our cases, and could be applied to the staining of smears prepared in these cases (Fig. 11). Fixation with 80% alcohol had the advantage of preserving alkaline phosphatase and gave a little more satisfactory result than Rossman's fluid. Formalin only inconstantly preserves

TABLE 1

EWING'S SARCOMA: 173 CASES

	PAS: +	−	Total
Fixation			
Formalin	67	48	115
Rossman or Alcohol 80%	27	—	27
Without P.A.S.			20
Doubtful			11
Total			173

glycogen, but in about half of the cases (58%) it could be demonstrated also in formalin fixed material, being always lacking in specimens decalcified with nitric or other strong acids. Therefore the absence of glycogen in incorrectly treated material does not exclude the diagnosis of Ewing's sarcoma (see Table 1).

In none of the 38 cases classified as metastatic neuroblastoma (sympathicoblastoma) was glycogen found in the tumour cells. Many of these cases were fixed for a long time in formalin but in nine cases the P.A.S. stain was performed on material fixed in 80% alcohol.

TABLE 2

Neuroblastoma: 38

Histochemical Study
Fixation:

Formalin	P.A.S. Negative	17	26
Alcohol		9	
Without P.A.S.			9
Doubtful			3
			38

Catecholamine Excretion: 11

	Increased	Normal
Without metastasis	2	
With osseous metastasis	8	1

Although the histological distinction from Ewing's sarcoma and malignant lymphoma is often difficult or impossible in formalin fixed specimens of poorly differentiated neuroblastoma (sympathogonioma or sympathicoblastoma) in which rosette-like structures are lacking, with special silver stains nerve fibrils can be sometimes demonstrated, and the biochemical study of urinary catecholamine excretion is positive in about 80% of the cases. On the other hand, metastatic neuroblastoma occurs generally in a younger age group (under 5 years of age) and the roentgenographic aspect frequently shows a radiolucent lesion located in the metaphyseal region of a long bone and permits its correct diagnosis. However, the most specific and diagnostic features are observed with the electron microscope (Friedman and Hanaoka 1971), showing the presence of neurosecretory granules and neural processes, containing neurofilaments, which help to distinguish the cells of this tumour from the other round cell sarcomas.

There are only a few bone tumours that may present diagnostic difficulties due to an abundance of glycogen in their tumour cells. In undifferentiated areas of osteosarcoma, when the cells are uniform, they may contain glycogen. In these cases the intense alkaline phosphatase activity of the tumour cells permits differentiation from Ewing's

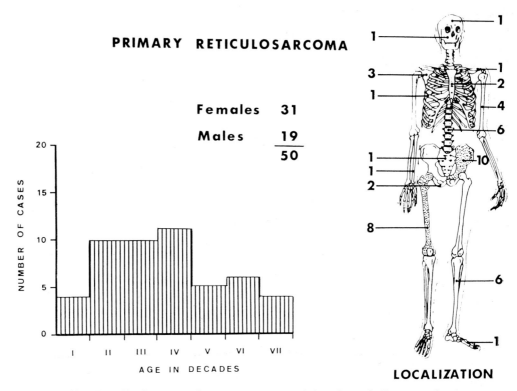

Fig. 12. Distribution according to age, sex and location of 50 cases of primary reticulosarcoma of bone.

sarcoma, in which such activity is absent. In two cases of mesenchymal chondrosarcoma we could observe more or less numerous glycogen granules in the undifferentiated areas of mesenchymal aspect in which the tumour cells were very similar to those of Ewing's sarcoma. However, the presence of cartilage areas, which in our experience are always lacking in Ewing's sarcoma, permitted the correct diagnosis. Another tumoural process of soft tissue origin, which sometimes may invade bone secondarily may show abundant cytoplasmic glycogen granules and a similar histologic aspect, is the alveolar or embryonal rhabdomyosarcoma. In one of our cases, with invasion of the fibula a wrong diagnosis of Ewing's sarcoma was made, which was rectified after examination of a metastasis in the neck occurring one year later, and which showed an evident myoblastic differentiation.

MALIGNANT LYMPHOMA (RETICULOSARCOMA) OF BONE

Seventy-eight cases were classified as malignant lymphoma including 75 cases of primary and secondary reticulosarcoma (reticulum cell sarcoma) and three cases of lymphosarcoma, primary in bone.

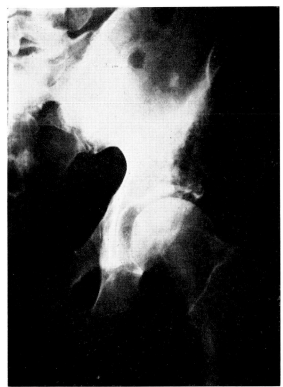

Fig. 13. Radiograph showing primary reticulosarcoma of ilium.

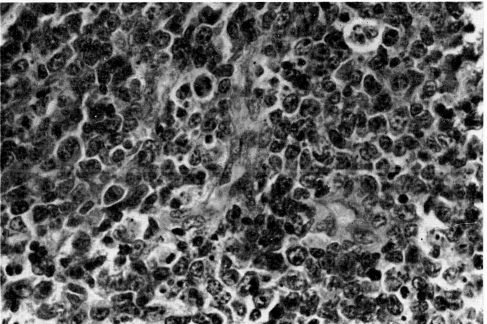

Fig. 14. Photomicrograph of a case of reticulosarcoma, constituted predominantly of histiocytic cells. (H & E ×600).

200

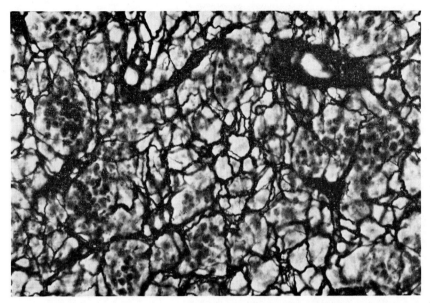

Fig. 15. Photomicrograph of primary reticulosarcoma (mixed-cell type) stained with Del Rio Hortega's silver impregnation technique. Abundant reticulin fibres, forming a dense network surround individual cells or small groups of cells ($\times$ 250).

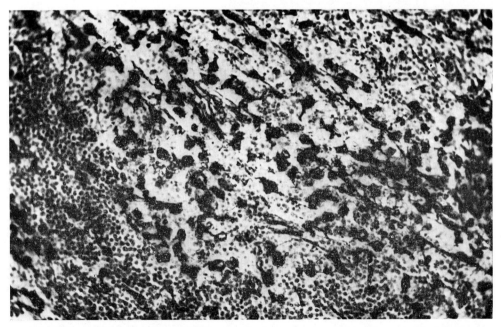

Fig. 16. Photomicrograph of primary reticulosarcoma, mixed-cell type, (histiocytic-lymphocytic) stained with Del Rio Hortega's technique, specific for reticuloendothelial elements showing the rhomboid and stellate aspect of the histiocytic tumour cells, the lymphocytes remaining unstained ($\times$ 300).

TABLE 3

MALIGNANT LYMPHOMAS OF BONE (RETICULO- AND LYMPHOSARCOMA)

Primary in Bone	50
Secondary or multiple	18
Doubtful	10
Total	78

The age, sex and skeletal distribution of 50 cases of reticulosarcoma, primary in bone, is shown in Fig. 12. We classified as such only those cases in which at the time of onset no evidence of other lesion could be revealed by an extensive clinical and radiological study. In the remaining 25 cases there was involvement of other portions of the skeleton and other organs or a known malignant lymphoma was present in other tissues, the bone lesion being obviously secondary. Hodgkin's disease, which only exceptionally involves bone primarily, was excluded from our study. Primary reticulosarcoma of bone can occur at any age but is more common after the second decade and is rare in young children, thus differing from Ewing's sarcoma. The roentgenologic features of malignant lymphoma are not characteristic, showing a generally predominantly ill-limited osteolytic appearance (Fig. 13), sometimes accompanied by irregular zones of bone sclerosis. The *histological* structure is rather variable. The tumour cells are usually rounded and rather pleomorphic and have usually, but not always, well-defined cytoplasmic outlines many of their nuclei are indented or horseshoe shaped and have one or more prominent nucleoli (Fig. 14). Often an evident lymphoblastic–lymphocytic differentiation may be observed. In most cases numerous reticular fibres are present and are distributed rather uniformly between the tumour cells which always lack glycogen (Fig. 15).

The majority of this group correspond to the original description of Parker and Jackson, and belong, in our experience, to the histiocytic reticulosarcoma and the mixed cell (histiocytic–lymphocytic) type of malignant lymphoma, according to Rappaport's classification of lymphnode lymphomas; but a few cases of undifferentiated reticulosarcoma ("Stem cell") may also occur in bone. The distinction between this variety and Ewing's sarcoma may be extremely difficult and can only be established by the presence of glycogen in the latter, both entities lacking reticulin fibres. Although it is true that these tumours often contain a mixture of cells and this mixture may vary in samples taken from the same case, many tumours have a relatively homogenous cellular composition of reticulum cells, histiocytes or poorly and well-differentiated lymphocytes. Therefore, like Dahlin (1965) we have tried to classify the malignant lymphomata of bone following the criteria of Rappaport (1966). As already mentioned most cases corresponded to the histiocytic and mixed cell type, the undifferentiated reticulosarcoma and lymphosarcoma being extremely rare.

As in reticulosarcoma, this last type, is to be distinguished from examples of bone involvement by secondary deposits of lymphosarcoma, although in advanced cases separation between the two types may be difficult. Frequently it may be associated with leukaemic changes in the peripheral blood.

H

TABLE 4

MALIGNANT LYMPHOMAS OF BONE

	Primary	Secondary	
Undifferentiated	4	1	= 5
Histiocytic (reticulum cell sarc.)	9	6	=15
Mixed cell (reticulo-lympho sarc.)	28	6	=34
Lymphosarcoma	3	3	= 6
Unclassified	6	2	= 8
	50	18	68

Finally, we want to emphasize that the *cytological* investigation of smears (in material obtained by puncture biopsy) or imprint preparation from the tumour tissue, was very useful in all examples of round-cell tumours of bone, especially in the precise diagnosis of the different types of malignant lymphoma.

REFERENCES

Dahlin, D. C.   Ewing's Sarcoma and Malignant Lymphoma (Reticulum cell sarcoma) of bone. In *Tumors of bone and soft tissues*, pp. 179–190. Year Book Medical Publishers Inc., Chicago, 1965.

Dahlin, D. C.   *Bone Tumors*, 2nd ed. Charles C. Thomas, Springfield, Ill., 1967.

Friedman, B. & Gold, H.   Ultrastructure of Ewing's Sarcoma of Bone. *Cancer*, 22, 307–322, 1968.

Friedman, B. & Hanaoka, H.   Round-cell Sarcoma of Bone. A light and Electronmicroscopic Study. *J. Bone Jt. Surg.*, 53–A, 1118–1136, 1971.

Gitlow, S. E., Bertani, Laura M., Rausen, A., Gribetz, D. & Dziezic, S. W.   Diagnosis of Neuroblastoma by Qualitative and Quantitative Determination of Catecholamine Metabolites in Urine. *Cancer*, 25, 1377–1383, 1970.

Hou-Jensen, K., Priori, E. and Dmochowski, L.   Studies on Ultrastructure of Ewing's Sarcoma of Bone. *Cancer*, 29, 280–286, 1972.

Kadin, M. E. & Bensch, K. G.   On the Origin of Ewing's Tumour. *Cancer*, 27, 257–273, 1971.

Parker, F. Jr. & Jackson, H. Jr.   Primary Reticulum Cell Sarcoma of Bone. *Surg. Gynec. Obstet.*, 68, 45–53, 1939.

Rappaport, H.   Tumors of the Hematopoietic System. *Atlas of Tumor Pathology*, Section III, Fasc. 8. Armed Forces Institute of Pathology, Washington, D.C., 1966.

Schajowicz, F.   Ewing's Sarcoma and Reticulum Cell Sarcoma of Bone: With Special Reference to the Histochemical Demonstration of Glycogen as an Aid to Differential Diagnosis. *J. Bone Jt. Surg.*, 41–A, 349–356, 1959.

Vohra, V. G.   Roentgen Manifestations in Ewing's Sarcoma. A study of 156 Cases. *Cancer*, 20, 727–733, 1967.

Willis, R. A.   Ewing's Tumour, pp. 702–703. In *Pathology of Tumours*, 4th ed. Butterworths, London, 1967.

Discussion

Dr. Friedman   I think that we owe Prof. Schajowicz a debt of gratitude for pointing out the value of the presence of intracellular glycogen as shown by the P.A.S. stain by light microscopy. We have shown also by electron microscopy that there is no doubt that there is glycogen in the cytoplasm of Ewing's sarcoma cells. I'm interested to hear Dr. Price say that glycogen was found in some of his neuroblastoma cells as well. This is I think the first that I've heard of this. The only comment I would like to make is in reference to your comment in describing the two types of cell. We referred to the typical Ewing's cell in electron microscopy. The second is a type of cell which is questionable as to whether this is a necrotic cell or whether it is a form of reticulum cell. I stick to my guns that this is a cell of a different stage in maturation and for this reason that necrotic cells are known to appear and there is no question about this. At least in ultrastructure the necrotic cells are quite different in appearance, particularly in view of the fact that this second type of cell contains a larger number of organelles—particularly a larger number of mitochondria and many dilated sacs of endoplasmic reticulum which are not present in the Ewing's cell.

Then there are transitional forms between that more mature cell (at least I consider it to be a more mature cell) and the much more primitive Ewing's sarcoma cell. On the other hand a necrotic cell by electron microscopy at least shows destruction of the cell membrane and all the intracellular material. The nucleus becomes clumped into smaller aggregates, in contrast to the nucleus which remains intact in the darker type of cell. This is I suppose an academic point, although it was the impression of Dr. Gold my co-author in this paper[1] and myself that the more transitional forms, possibly with a better prognosis of the tumour, might tend to fall into the group of transitional tumours which Dahlin has pointed out are between Ewing's and reticulum cell sarcoma arising in bone.

Prof. Van Rijssel   I am not quite happy with the term "round cell sarcoma". Only the lymphosarcoma and the myeloma have round cells: in the Ewing's sarcoma the nuclei are round but the cytoplasmic borders cannot be seen. My impression is that many of these cells have cytoplasmic threads going to other cells—just as in the reticulum cells which are not round either.

Dr. Lloyd   Dr. Price has already told you the story about how the Bristol Bone Tumour Registry met on an evening in December 1955 and had in front of them 11 cases with the category of Ewing's tumour. By the end of that evening the category was empty: we had classified them all under other headings. I can assure Dr. Price that if he likes to bring these 29 cases along to two or more meetings of the Bone Tumour Registry we will succeed in emptying this category for him again and putting them into others. Probably the one which would gain most from the cases he has been showing this afternoon would be neuroblastoma. After all a great many of you know how difficult it is to find rosettes even in cases of neuroblastoma which you know to be that. Sometimes you may search the primary for rosettes and find none and yet they may be obvious in the metastases. The opposite is also the case sometimes. Therefore in any particular tumour the finding of rosettes is not essential for the diagnosis of neuroblastoma, provided all the other features are there.

The other possible objection to being neuroblastoma is this question whether there is a primary in bone or not. Well now, this to a considerable extent as you know, Mr. Chairman, is unanswerable unless you have a post-mortem examination afterwards. But I would draw your attention to the fact the neuroblastoma is one of those tumours which sometimes undergoes spontaneous regression. This was in fact mentioned.

I am very familiar indeed with another kind of tumour which also undergoes spontaneous regression—namely the malignant melanoma. What we find there is that it is particularly likely to do so in one place—particularly in the primary—if it is becoming more malignant in another place. If part of the primary becomes very malignant then other parts of the primary which were less malignant undergo regression; or if it metastasizes, which is another demonstration of greater malignancy, then sometimes the entire primary undergoes regression. I wouldn't be at all surprised if the same thing was the case for neuroblastomas, and because the bone tumour one may be more malignant than the primary, the primary may be encouraged to undergo regression. Finally, Mr. Chairman, if I may I would like to tell a little story that I heard 30 years ago from Robb-Smith which may be apocryphal, but is very notable really. It is about Ewing in his old age who became less and less inclined to make the diagnosis of Ewing's tumour. People used to send him sections and ask, "Is this Ewing's Tumour?" and the answer used to come back more and more often—"No, it is not". So they then said, "We really want to learn about these things, please send us a section of a genuine Ewing's tumour." So he did that; and they took off the label and put on another one, sent it back to Ewing and said, "Is this a Ewing's tumour?" and the reply came back, "No, it is not"!

Professor Schajowicz   I want to say that I don't use the name "round-cell sarcoma" but only the "so-called round-cell sarcoma." Price uses the term, but I say Ewing's sarcoma. I would like to reply to Dr. Friedman. How do you know in Ewing's sarcoma that the second type of cell is not necrotic but is a reticulum cell? If you are sure that it is in fact a reticulum cell we should accept that a Ewing's sarcoma is a form of reticulum cell sarcoma. But we don't know what Ewing's sarcoma is—nobody knows!

Professor Ackerman   There is one other point that I don't believe has been mentioned that we have used tissue culture for neuroblastoma which works quite well. The electron micrograph is quite definitive too in the differential. So that I don't believe that you have to rely just on this glycogen business all the time.

Dr. Price   Concerning glycogen in neuroblastomata, I have found five positive out of 27 where I had material for the P.A.S. and the diastase P.A.S.

Professor Ackerman   May I ask if in these cases that you said were neuroblastoma do you have other evidence that they were neuroblastoma—for example, in the adrenal and things like that?

Dr. Price   Four of these cases came to autopsy and they were done by my esteemed colleagues at the University. In the one I showed you a primary tumour in the left thoracic sympathetic chain was found I believe, although it originally presented as a tumour of the femur.

Professor Ackerman   I think that you should show those sections to Dr. Schajowicz.

REFERENCE

1. Friedman, B. and Gold, H. Ultrastructure of Ewing's sarcoma of bone. *Cancer*, **22,** 307, 1968.

Primary malignant lymphoma (reticulum cell sarcoma) of bone

by

DAVID C. DAHLIN

SUMMARY

A study of 110 cases reaffirms that malignant lymphoma (reticulum cell sarcoma) apparently can be primary in a bone. The prognosis is considerably better than in cases of the more common Ewing's sarcomas and osteosarcomas. The tumor's definite tendency to become disseminated and to kill should govern studies of the patient before and after initial therapy.

MORE THAN 40 YEARS have elapsed since Oberling[1] suggested the existence of reticulum cell sarcoma of bone. Although it was established as an entity by Parker and Jackson[2] in 1939, some authors[3] have questioned the validity of separating this tumor from Ewing's sarcoma. When studying Ewing's sarcoma at the Mayo Clinic in 1952, McCormack and co-workers[4] separated a group of tumours that was histologically distinct and different. Sections from these tumours were like sections from Parker and Jackson's original tumors, which we were privileged to study.

It has become apparent that "reticulum cell sarcoma" is a misnomer for the "round-cell" tumors of bone that differ histologically and cytologically from Ewing's sarcoma and from myeloma. Although many of them contain a predominance of reticulum cells, the majority contain lymphoblasts and lymphocytes in variable numbers; a few are purely lymphoblastic or lymphocytic, and a few have the Sternberg–Reed cells of Hodgkin's disease. "Malignant lymphoma" is a more correct term for the general group.

Classic Ewing's sarcoma is readily distinguished from malignant lymphoma on cytologic grounds. Some tumours, however, are difficult to classify because they have histologic characteristics similar to both Ewing's sarcoma and lymphoma. We call such tumors "Ewing's sarcomas" when they are not clearly lymphomas cytologically, even though the nuclei in them are somewhat larger and less regular in outline than those in conventional Ewing's sarcoma. Since the cytologic criteria cannot be absolutely quantitated, the distinction is not always clear-cut. Reticulum stains are of little value in these problem cases, because the reticulin component varies in different parts of the tumors. The periodic acid-Schiff (P.A.S.) stain for glycogen on tissue fixed in 80% ethanol, championed by Schajowicz,[5] may help. He stated that Ewing's tumor cells contain glycogen and that lymphoma cells do not. This glycogen also has been identified by electron microscopy.[6]

Malignant lymphoma can be considered primary in bone if thorough examination, preferably including roentgenologic skeletal survey, does not reveal evidence of disease other than the skeletal focus in question. Most authors have permitted regional nodal involvement. A few cases have features such as distant, "somewhat enlarged" nodes, a questionable abdominal mass, and ill-defined backache that make absolute exclusion of distant disease impossible. An arbitrary rule has been that there should be a 6-month interval between onset of symptoms of the primary focus and the appearance of metastatic lesions.[7] When metastasis is found, or has existed, in a patient whose major problem relates to an osseous focus of lymphoma, the bone lesion cannot be presumed to be primary and the prognosis is worse.

PRESENT STUDY

This study included 192 patients whose malignant lymphoma was first diagnosed from tissue taken from an osseous lesion. Metastasis was found or became evident within 6 months of onset of symptoms from the osseous lesion in 82 cases. In the remaining 110 patients the lesion was considered to be primary lymphoma of bone. These lesions comprise about 5% of the primary malignant skeletal tumors encountered at the Mayo Clinic, excluding cases of disseminated myeloma.

AGE AND SEX

The 110 patients included 68 males and 42 females, a ratio of 1·6 : 1. The age distribution for patients with malignant lymphoma is contrasted with that for those with Ewing's sarcoma (Table 1). The peak incidence was in the sixth decade of life. Only 15% of the 110 patients were less than 20 years of age whereas 70% of those with Ewing's sarcoma were in that age group.

TABLE 1

PERCENT OF PATIENTS WITH MALIGNANT
LYMPHOMA AND EWING'S SARCOMA BY DECADES

Decade	Malignant lymphoma	Ewing's sarcoma
1	1	22
2	14	48
3	13	19
4	11	7
5	16	3
6	26	1
7	14	0
8	5	0

ANATOMIC SITES

A wide variety of bones was involved (Table 2). The femur and humerus accounted for 37 cases and the innominate bone and sacrum, for 27. The 11 lesions in the sacrum included a few tumors that involved the adjacent ilium also. This tumor rarely originates in the peripheral portions of the skeleton; only two of the lesions under study were beyond the elbow or knee. Lesions of the maxilla and of vertebrae above the sacrum were excluded because of the difficulty of determining whether they arose in bone or in contiguous soft tissues. Lymphomas originating in each of these two sites present complex clinicopathologic problems because of encroachment on and involvement of contigous structures and they are logically analyzed separately.

SYMPTOMS

Local pain, sometimes intermittent, was the main complaint of more than 90% of the patients. In only 13 cases was the duration reported to be less than 3 months before diagnosis; 40 patients had had pain for more than a year and 11 for more than 3 years. Swelling of the part was frequent; with lesions of the skull and mandible it was the predominant symptom. Pathologic fracture had occurred in four cases. Local regional nodes were enlarged and probably involved in six cases. As has been noted by others,[2] patients often have extensive local disease with a contrasting feeling of well-being and lack of significant systemic signs. Laboratory studies are rarely helpful in the diagnosis, but evidence of leukemia should be sought, especially in younger patients whose apparently primary bone lesions show prominent lymphoblastic differentiation.

ROENTGENOLOGIC ASPECTS

Irregular areas of cortical and medullary destruction and variable amounts of reactive proliferation of bone were common (Fig. 1). Considerable density within the lesion may occur as in some metastatic carcinomas. Periosteal reaction is absent or moderate and

TABLE 2

SKELETAL DISTRIBUTION (110 LESIONS)

Femur	21
Tibia	8
Fibula	1
Humerus	16
Ulna	1
Skull	8
Mandible	11
Sternum	2
Scapula	8
Ribs	7
Sacrum	11
Innominate bone	16
Total	110

H*

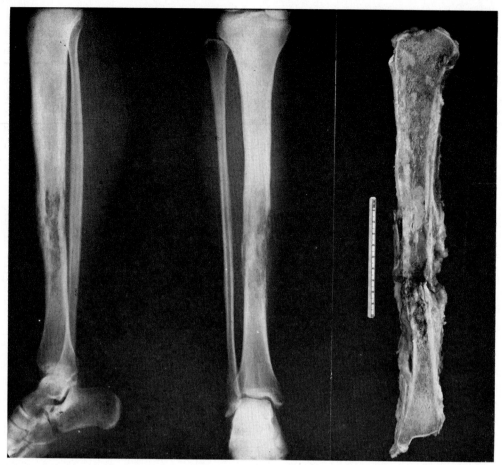

Fig. 1.   Primary lymphoma of tibia in a 43-year-old woman who had noted pain and swelling for 14 months.

Fig. 2.   Same case as Fig. 1. The specimen showed most of tibial shaft permeated by tumor. There was little extraosseous extension. (From Dahlin D.C. *Bone Tumors*, 2nd ed. Charles C. Thomas, Springfield, 1967. By permission.)

there is usually a contiguous mass of soft tissue (Fig. 3). Wilson and Pugh,[8] after studying material from the Mayo Clinic, concluded that the appearance varies too much to be characteristic, but the radiologist may suspect the diagnosis. The possibility of osteogenic sarcoma, Ewing's tumor, eosinophilic granuloma, and chronic osteomyelitis cannot always be excluded with certainty.

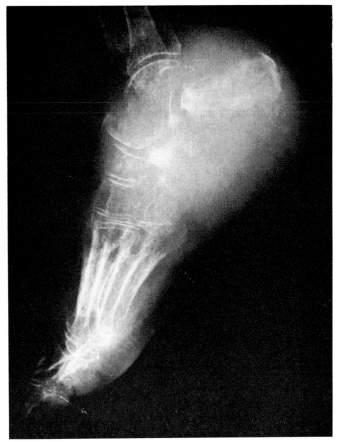

Fig. 3. Malignant lymphoma with destruction of several tarsal bones. The case was excluded from the series because of massive enlargement of ipsilateral inguinal nodes and another osseous lesion that developed within 6 months from onset of symptoms. (From Dahlin D.C. *Bone Tumors*, 2nd ed. Charles C. Thomas, Springfield, 1967. By permission.)

PATHOLOGIC FINDINGS

GROSS PATHOLOGY

The gross appearance of tissue is not pathognomonic. Usually the material is soft and the tumors, both in the bone and in adjacent soft tissues, have indistinct margins. In bone, residual trabeculae are frequently present imparting a firm and gritty quality. Nearly white areas of necrosis and zones of rather dense sclerosis may be seen (Fig. 2). Involvement in bone is often more extensive than is indicated by roentgenograms. Tumors in long bones are usually located near one end.

HISTOPATHOLOGIC ASPECTS

Reticulum cells with their grooved or folded nuclei, prominent nucleoli, and indistinct cytoplasmic boundaries are the most characteristic cells of these tumors (Fig. 4). Of the

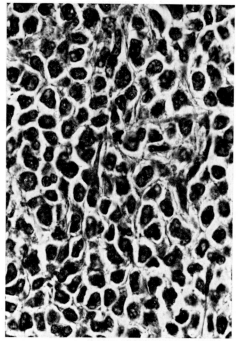

Fig. 4.   Same case as Fig. 1. Microscopic appearance of tumor showing malignant lymphoma composed almost exclusively of reticulum cells. (H & E ×650). (From Dahlin D.C. *Bone Tumors*, 2nd ed. Charles C. Thomas, Springfield, 1967. By permission.)

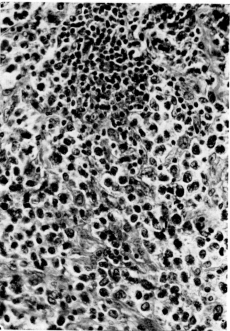

Fig. 5.   Common type of lymphoma of bone with reticulum cells showing differentiation to lymphoblasts and lymphocytes. (H & E ×300). (From Dahlin D.C. *Bone Tumors*, 2nd ed. Charles C. Thomas, Springfield 1967. By permission.)

110 tumors studied, only 17 had no significant numbers of other types of cells; 80 had a significant admixture of lymphoblasts and lymphocytes and were called "mixed" (Figs. 5 and 6), five were composed almost exclusively of rather mature lymphoblasts or lymphocytes, and eight contained a mixture of proliferating elements, including Sternberg–Reed cells, and were regarded as Hodgkin's lymphoma (Fig. 7).

A typical reticular framework was visible in frozen or paraffin sections. This pattern can be exaggerated by silver impregnation techniques, which are rarely necessary in establishing the diagnosis. P.A.S.-positive material in the form of glycogen is typically absent, a finding that may help in differentiating Ewing's sarcoma (Figs. 8 and 9). More clinicopathologic correlations are in progress, however, and hopefully they will establish the validity of this stain in problem cases in which the cytologic characteristics of lymphoma and Ewing's sarcoma overlap.

TREATMENT AND RESULTS

The complex combinations of radiotherapy, chemotherapy, and surgery are under investigation and additional follow-up is being obtained. Data obtained from this study are forthcoming from this clinic. Radiation is currently the treatment of choice with

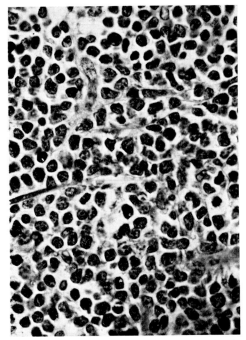

Fig. 6. Osseous lymphoma with predominant cell type showing lymphoblastic differentiation. (H & E ×600). (From Dahlin D.C. *Bone Tumors*, 2nd ed. Charles C. Thomas, Springfield, 1967. By permission.)

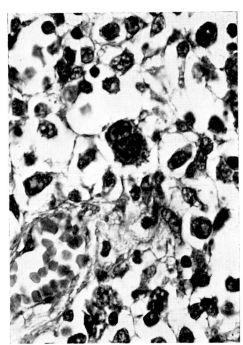

Fig. 7. Hodgkin's lymphoma manifesting itself first as a destructive tumor of sternum with invasion of structures behind and in front of manubrium. (H & E ×700). (From Dahlin D.C. *Bone Tumors*, 2nd ed. Charles C. Thomas, Springfield, 1967. By permission.)

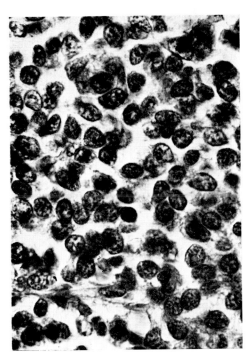

Fig. 8. Typical Ewing's tumor with round and oval nuclei all of approximately the same size. (H & E ×800.) (From Dahlin D.C. *Bone Tumors*, 2nd ed. Charles C. Thomas, Springfield, 1967. By permission.)

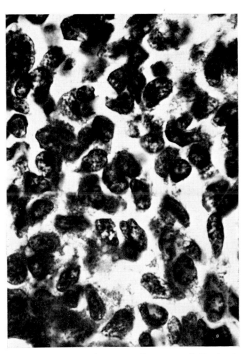

Fig. 9. The larger-cell type of Ewing's tumor which may be confused with reticulum cell sarcoma. (H & E × 800). (From Dahlin D.C. *Bone Tumors*, 2nd ed. Charles C. Thomas, Springfield, 1967. By permission.)

amputation being reserved for recurrent or radioresistant tumors. Chemotherapy has been valuable in the management of some cases in which dissemination has occurred. Coley's toxins[7] have been of some value in a few cases. Radiation for recurrent tumors and for distant foci, sometimes in combination with chemotherapy, has been associated with the prolonged survival of many patients so affected.

Of the 110 patients, 92 had their diagnosis and initial treatment more than 5 years prior to this study, and follow-up was available on 87 of them. Thirty-eight of the 87 (44%) lived more than 5 years, some with evidence of disease at that time. An appreciable number died from the disease after 5 years, but about a third of the 38 lived at least 10 years. These data are surprisingly like the 5-year survival rate of 44·2% for the 43 cases reported by Shoji and Miller[7] in 1971. In Parker and Jackson's[2] study, seven of 17 patients lived at least 10 years, and Wang and Fleischli[9] reported a 5-year cure rate of 50% in a series of 21 cases. Potdar's[10] report on 35 cases was less optimistic. Except for these reports, there is a dearth of significantly large series in the literature.

Thirteen of 37 eligible patients (35%) with tumors primary in the long bones have survived more than 5 years. Eight of 19 (42%) with tumors in the innominate bone or sacrum have survived, an observation that contrasts with the poor prognosis for Shoji and Miller's[7] patients with involvement of the pelvic girdle. Interestingly, four of six patients with primary tumors in the skull and seven of 11 with primary mandibular lesions survived more than 5 years.

Most of the long-term survivors were naturally in the large group with mixed malignant lymphomas in which 64 were eligible for 5-year survival studies. However, four of 13 with "pure" reticulum cell sarcoma, one of four with the lymphocytic variety, and two of six with Hodgkin's disease lived at least 5 years.

The majority of patients with primary lymphoma of bone die from the effects of generalized disease, and an appreciable number of them die even after surviving for 5 years. As Potdar[10] indicated, the tumors have a spectrum of activity varying from a rapidly fatal outcome (that is, within a few months) to survival for many years. No less than 22 of the patients in this study died within 1 year after diagnosis and another 18 died during the second year. Leukemia developed in three of these patients who died in this short period, and two of the three were young patients (10 and 11 years, respectively) with predominantly lymphocytic tumors. Obviously there is a need for detailed study of the patient in a search for systemic disease at the outset of treatment for what is presumed to be a single focus of skeletal lymphoma. At the minimum this study should include a roentgenologic skeletal survey and perhaps sternal marrow and lymphangiographic studies as well.

REFERENCES

1. Oberling, C. Les réticulosarcomes et les réticuloendothéliosarcomes de la moelle osseuse (sarcomes d'Ewing). *Bull. Cancer* (Paris), **17**, 259–296, 1928.
2. Parker, F. Jr. & Jackson, H. Jr. Primary Reticulum Cell Sarcoma of Bone. *Surg. Gynec. Obstet.*, **68**, 45–53, 1939.
3. Magnus, H. A. & Wood, H.L.-C. Primary Reticulo-sarcoma of Bone. *J. Bone Jt. Surg.*, **38–B**, 258–278, 1956.
4. McCormack, L. J., Dockerty, M. B. & Ghormley, R. K. Ewing's Sarcoma. *Cancer*, **5**, 85–99, 1952.

5. Schajowicz, F. Ewing's Sarcoma and Reticulum-cell Sarcoma of Bone: with Special Reference to the Histochemical Demonstration of Glycogen as an Aid to Differential Diagnosis. *J. Bone Jt. Surg.*, **41**–**A**, 349–356, 1959.
6. Friedman, B. & Gold, H. Ultrastructure of Ewing's Sarcoma of Bone. *Cancer*, **22**, 307–322, 1968.
7. Shoji, H. & Miller, T. R. Primary Reticulum Cell Sarcoma of Bone: Significance of Clinical Features upon the Prognosis. *Cancer*, **28**, 1234–1244, 1971.
8. Wilson, T. W. & Pugh, D. G. Primary Reticulum-cell Sarcoma of Bone, with Emphasis on Roentgen Aspects. *Radiology*, **65**, 343–351, 1955.
9. Wang, C. C. & Fleischli, D. J. Primary Reticulum Cell Sarcoma of Bone: with Emphasis on Radiation Therapy. *Cancer*, **22**, 994–998, 1968.
10. Potdar, G. G. Primary Reticulum-cell Sarcoma of Bone in Western India. *Brit. J. Cancer*, **24**, 48–55, 1970.

Discussion

Dr. Suit I would like to ask you if these cases which showed gradation between the Ewing's sarcoma and reticulum cell sarcoma are more frequent in the younger patient than your adult?

Prof. Dahlin I don't know: I haven't looked that up specifically. It is, however, a very good point and should be done.

Prof. Ackerman May I ask you are there any things you recommend, e.g. lymphangiography or bone scanning which have yielded positive results in any cases where you thought the disease was just restricted to a single bone?

Prof. Dahlin I don't believe that any of the total body scanning has yielded positive results but we haven't been doing that for more than about a year or so. Unfortunately, we haven't been doing lymphangiography on very many of these cases where it has been thought to be a primary skeletal tumour. So I don't know that the yield is going to be significant. But I noticed in going over the histories of a fair number of these patients that when the tumour in the bone is treated they develop pain in the back—a strong suggestion that there is dissemination along the spine—and then finally and usually within a few months there is proof that this has occurred. I feel rather strongly that we should be doing it.

Prof. Schajowicz I want to ask you one question. What is the difference in the treatment at your institute between Ewing's sarcoma and reticulosarcoma? Because we treat the Ewing's sarcoma in practically the same way as reticulosarcoma.

Prof Dahlin What way is that?

Prof. Schajowicz First we use radiotherapy on the whole limb, accompanied by chemotherapy, we use Sarcolysin or Melphalan, if it doesn't work then Cyclophosphamide. After several months when the patient is still free of metastasis we perform a segmental resection of the tumour. Because I have seen in irradiated, resected or amputated tumours histologically there is still viable tumour tissue. By this we try to give more safety and a better chance of life. We do the same for Ewing's sarcoma and reticulosarcoma. For Ewing's sarcoma we have now much better results after this combination of treatment than before, when we had less than 3% of 5-year survival.

Prof. Ackerman You mustn't give Dr. Suit's paper!

Prof. Dahlin I feel that malignant lymphoma is a bad enough disease that it ought to be treated vigorously and I suppose that really it's a kind of academic differential that we

216

are talking about anyhow. Dr. Suit has told me before in Houston that he believes that both tumours should be treated about the same. That makes it easier for me because if I make a mistake it won't make much difference to the patient. We have probably even treated a few neuroblastomas that same way, I hope not too many! Do you want to comment on that Dr. Suit?

Dr. Suit   No. I will be speaking later.

Dr. Ball   I must say that I find myself more or less in agreement with much that Dr. Dahlin has said, and indeed with the exception of the transition which Professor Schajowicz doesn't seem to like, much of what he said too, in other words I am a Ewing's man. I have a question for Dr. Dahlin. It has been my impression that the follicular or nodular type of lymphoma doesn't occur in bone. It is curious that although we have these similarities between lymphoma in bone and lymph glands in all other respects apparently, we don't have it in respect of the follicular type of growth. And indeed in those patients I have seen with clear cut follicular lymphoma in the chest with later a solitary lesion in the skeleton, which has turned out to be reticulum cell sarcoma, it has not been the follicular type of growth. I wonder whether you have any comment to make on this curious distinction?

Prof. Dahlin   Only that our experience is the same. We haven't seen a follicular type. I wonder if it may be related to the way that tumours grow in bone. I really have no comment other than that.

Dr. Marcove   I've had some experience with lymphangiography in children and it seems to be quite tricky. Sometimes a lymphangiogram seems positive and the results of the biopsy have turned out negative. So it's a difficult problem. In an earlier publication from Memorial Hospital the poor figures may have been related to the fact that radiotherapy was given merely to one local area. Since then my colleague has changed his plans to treat the whole image complex and we have seen our first cure of Ewing's sarcoma of the pelvis since.

Dr. Lewis   I wonder if any of the cases you have diagnosed as a Ewing's sarcoma have had any leukaemic manifestation? If so, what form of leukaemia did you diagnose?

Professor Dahlin   I had one experience about 15 years ago. I was studying a slide of a femoral tumour and I took a photomicrograph and labelled it "Typical Ewing's Sarcoma". The patient went home and died with fatal manifestations of acute leukaemia within a few months. Leukaemia has been a problem in cases where we have made the diagnosis of malignant lymphoma of lymphocytic or lymphoblastic type. In that group—and they tend to be in the younger people—two or three of that small number developed leukaemia rather shortly after the biopsy had been made.

Dr. Ball   I have seen one case of leukaemia with a large lesion of the upper end of the humerous which, so far as I could see had all the characteristics of reticulum cell sarcoma.

Prof. Dahlin   That points up again the need for total examination including marrow aspiration studies and so forth in these patients.

Radiation therapy and multi-drug chemotherapy in management of patients with Ewing's sarcoma

by

H. D. SUIT, C. FERNANDEZ, W. SUTOW, M. SAMUELS and J. WILBUR

SUMMARY

Results which have been achieved in the management of a consecutive series of 54 patients with localized Ewing's sarcoma (no clinically evident metastatic disease) at the University of Texas, M. D. Anderson Hospital are presented. These patients were seen over the period from 1948 to July 1971. Discussion centers on frequency of local recurrence, frequency and site of appearance of distant metastasis in patients treated in two periods: (1) radiation therapy alone or in combination with single drug and usually single course chemotherapy; (2) a planned treatment featuring radiation therapy of the primary and multiple course Vincristine-Cytoxan chemotherapy. Results appear to be greatly superior in the latter group: local recurrence in one of 14 patients instead of 13 of 40 patients; median time to appearance of first metastasis >15 months instead of 8 months. Certain aspects of this experience are considered in detail.

A MORE OPTIMISTIC and enthusiastic attitude regarding patients with primary Ewing's sarcoma has obtained since a report in 1968 by Hustu et al,[1] that five of five patients treated by radiation therapy and prolonged medication with Cytoxan and Vincristine were alive and well at 12 to 38 months after the start of therapy. There are now other papers which lend support to that early experience.

This report is an account of the results achieved at the University of Texas M. D. Anderson Hospital in the primary treatment of 54 patients who had no clinical evidence of metastatic tumor at the time of treatment for Ewing's sarcoma. These patients were seen during the period from 1948 to July 1, 1971. Other patients were seen after primary treatment at another institution or with clinically evident metastatic disease. In 1963 an analysis[2] of the results obtained in the first 23 cases in this series two conclusions were reached: (1) permanent control of the primary lesion requires high radiation doses; (2) single drug—single course chemotherapy does not affect the time between treatment and first metastasis. Since then our treatment policy has gone through two phases: (1) 1963 to 1969, 17 patients were treated by high-dose radiation therapy with no planned concomitant chemotherapy; (2) 1969 to 1971, 14 patients have been treated by high-dose radiation therapy and concomitant multi-course Vincristine-Cytoxan chemotherapy.

CLINICAL MATERIAL

All patients with primary Ewing's sarcoma who have been referred to the University of Texas M. D. Anderson Hospital have been seen and handled collaboratively by members of the Departments of Radiotherapy, Medicine, Pediatrics and Surgery. Diagnosis of Ewing's sarcoma was established by review of the biopsy material by our Pathology Department. Diagnostic procedures to exclude the presence of metastatic disease were: chest films, long bone radiographic survey, routine history and physical examination. The age and sex distribution and the anatomical distribution of these tumors are consistent with those usually obtained and are not presented here.

RADIATION THERAPY TECHNIQUES AND DOSE LEVELS

The basic treatment plan had been since 1964 to administer $\approx 4,400$ rads* in 22 fractions over a $4\frac{1}{2}$-week period (five fractions per week) to the entirety of the affected bone. At that dose level the fields were reduced so that the clinically and radiographically evident tumor was included with a rather economical margin of apparently unaffected normal tissue for the next 1,600 rads. Then, at the 6,000-rad point the fields were reduced again so as to encompass only the radiographic and clinically evident mass (this was almost invariably much smaller than at the time of treatment initiation) and an additional 500 to 1,000 rads given. Therefore, according to this treatment plan the entire bone received 4,400 rads in $4\frac{1}{2}$ weeks and the area clinically affected by disease received a final dose level of 6,500 to 7,000 rads in $6\frac{1}{2}$ to 7 weeks. In selected anatomical sites and in young children treatment has been stopped at 6,000 rads. There is a definite increase in reaction of normal tissue in patients receiving concomitant Cytoxan and Vincristine; for this reason the final dose is usually 6,500 rads instead of 7,000 rads. An important detail of treatment planning is that even for the first 4 to $4\frac{1}{2}$ weeks of treatment fields are drawn so as to spare normal tissue. For example, if the disease is affecting the upper portion of the femur then the field would be drawn relatively generously around the primary lesion and soft tissue swelling. For coverage of the distal shaft and condyles of the femur, the fields are drawn only wide enough to cover the bony structure. Shaped fields are employed throughout the entire treatment; other appropriate techniques are utilized to minimize irradiation of tissue unintentionally. Irradiation of the full circumference of the limb even for the first portion of the treatment is avoided. If "fall-off" were required on one side of the limb, some normal tissue would be protected on the other side. These special efforts to protect normal tissue permit tolerance of radical dose levels and retain good function in a painless and non-edematous limb.

CHEMOTHERAPY

For the recent 14 cases Vincristine and Cytoxan have been given on a multi-course schedule. The protocol for this treatment plan is shown in Fig. 1. Drug administration begins with the start of radiation therapy. In most patients moderate to severe leukopenia develops by the ninth or tenth day of Cytoxan. The drug is stopped before the tenth dose if the absolute neutrophil count drops below 1,800 cells per mm.[3] This leukopenia recovers promptly. Gastrointestinal upset has not been a problem. Most patients experience signs of Vincristine induced peripheral neuropathy. In all instances this neuropathy

* $\approx$ very nearly equal to.

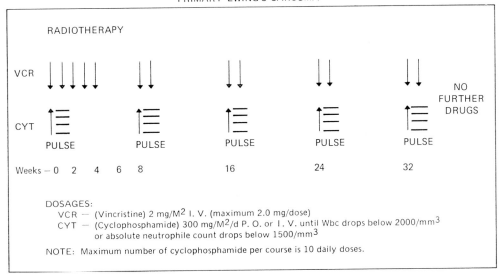

CHEMOTHERAPY SCHEDULE
PRIMARY EWING'S SARCOMA

Fig. 1. Reproduced from *Clinical Pediatric Oncology* (1973), edited by W. Sutow and associates, by courtesy of the publishers, C. V. Mosby Co., St. Louis, Mo.

has subsided following cessation of the medication. During the multi-course chemotherapy the patient develops depilation; full growth of hair occurs as soon as the drug is discontinued. Usually there is a reduction of the Cytoxan dose given during the latter courses. Patients are usually admitted to hospital during the latter portion of the first course, but not at all during subsequent courses. Many patients have the final two, three or four courses administered on an out-patient basis by their local physician.

FOLLOW-UP EXAMINATIONS

The patient is under almost constant medical supervision during the first 6 months. After the chemotherapy has been completed, follow-up examinations are performed at two monthly intervals for the next 12 months. Then the patients are seen at 3-monthly intervals until the thirty-sixth month after start of treatment. At these follow-up visits special attention is paid to the status of the primary lesion and the lungs. Any vague symptoms of bone or joint discomfort are investigated promptly because of the frequency of metastasis to bone.

RESULTS

CONTROL OF THE PRIMARY LESION

Clinically evident local recurrence of Ewing's sarcoma has been observed in 14 of the 54 patients treated. Thirteen of these regrowths appeared in the 40 patients who were treated prior to the institution of the protocol which featured administration of Vincristine and Cytoxan at the time of or immediately following the treatment of the primary lesion. Among these 13 recurrences there is no definite correlation between radiation dose and local control frequency. A clinically important fact is that these recurrences occurred at the site of the primary lesion, i.e. at the location in the bone of the initially radiographically evident tumor. Therefore, these lesions occurred at the site which received the maximum radiation dose. There have been no instances of reactivation of disease in the region of bones treated to 4,000–4,500 rads. This demonstrates that subclinical extensions of Ewing's sarcoma in the marrow cavity are controlled by the dose level of 4,000 to 4,500 rads. In contrast, the central primary tumor is not regularly destroyed by doses of $\approx 7,000$ rads: in this series there have been three instances of clinically evident regrowths following doses of $\geq 7,000$ rads.** In addition to the 13 instances of gross local regrowth of tumor there have been two patients who perhaps should be scored as local failures. One of these had radiographic evidence indicating reactivation of the primary lesion during the terminal phase of his disease. Another patient had histologically demonstrable Ewing's tumor at the site of the primary lesion at necropsy examination. Both of these patients died because of metastatic disease but were asymptomatic of the primary tumor. Accordingly, they have not been included in Table 1 as gross local recurrences.

TABLE 1

CLINICALLY EVIDENT LOCAL RECURRENCE OF EWING'S SARCOMA
(LOCAL CONTROL COUNTED ONLY IN PATIENTS SURVIVING MORE
THAN 12 MONTHS)*

Radiation dose (rads, 60 Co or equivalent)	Local recurrence
< 5,000	4/11
5,000 ≤ 6,000	3/6
> 6,000	6/15†
> 6,000 + Vincristine and Cytoxan	1/11‡

*Ten patients died of metastatic tumor before the twelfth month without evidence of local recurrence.
† One patient had cells present at site of primary on necropsy study and another patient had radiographic changes consistent with regrowth. Both of these patients died of metastatic tumor and neither had symptoms of local disease at time of death. These two patients are not included in this figure of 6/15.
‡ Includes one patient alive and well at 9 months.

Among the 14 patients who received local radiation therapy plus systemic Vincristine–Cytoxan chemotherapy there has been only one local recurrence; this is not a definite recurrence because the distinction between reactivation and necrosis is not clear at this time. Local control results are presented in Table 1 and these strongly indicate that the combination of high dose radiation therapy and intensive multi-drug–multi-course chemotherapy yield an improvement in the frequency of control of the primary lesion. There has been no change in radiation therapy technique during the recent 2 to 3 years (time that the combined treatment approach has been employed) except for an increased sophistication of secondary blocking procedures which result in a more adequate

** ≧—at least as great as.

protection of normal tissue. This is not judged to affect the local control of the primary tumor.

Recurrences have had a median time of appearance of 12 months with a range from 7 to 42 months. The time for appearance of regrowth of tumor has not been appreciably delayed as radiation dose has increased. From these facts we are especially concerned during the follow-up examination over the first 24 months after treatment to give special attention to the status of the primary lesion. Local recurrence of disease has been in our series an ominous prognostic sign; all patients who have had local regrowth have died or are alive with uncontrolled metastatic tumor. The relationship between recurrence and metastatic tumor is unclear. In this series, four of the 14 recurrences were diagnosed prior to the time that the metastasis became evident. In the remaining 10 patients, metastases were diagnosed before the appearance of local regrowth of tumor. The median time between the diagnosis of metastasis and recurrence in these 10 patients was 4 months with a range of 0 to 26 months.

DISEASE FREE SURVIVAL RESULTS

Among the 40 patients treated prior to the institution of the program of combined radiation therapy and Vincristine–Cytoxan chemotherapy, four patients are alive and free of evident tumor. Two of these patients had lesions in the humerus and were treated by radiation therapy alone. The other two patients had tumors in the maxilla; these were treated by combinations of radiation therapy, drug therapy and surgery. In one, the surgery for a lesion of the maxilla was grossly incomplete and radiation therapy was given post-operatively. In the other patient, radiation therapy and Amethopterin were given pre-operatively; the surgical specimen was negative for residual tumor on histological examination. Of the remaining 36 patients metastases have developed in 35; one patient died of intercurrent disease. Accordingly, of the entire group of 40 patients there is a 10% 5-year survival rate (four of 40); if the four lesions of the head and neck were excluded then the 5-year survival figure would be two of 36 patients or approximately 6%. The median time between initiation of radiation therapy and the diagnosis of metastatic tumor in the 36 patients (excluding the four patients whose lesions were located in the maxilla or mandible) was 8 months; the 95% confidence limits around this estimate were 7 to 10 months. Thus this disease ran a highly malignant course in these patients. Fifteen of the first 40 patients received some form of chemotherapy as part of their initial treatment. The median time to metastasis in those 15 cases was 8 months also. In most instances the chemotherapy consisted of single drug and often single dose medication. Two patients, however, were given Vincristine–Cytoxan and actinomycin D at the time of initiation of treatment: metastases were diagnosed at 33 and 41 months and recurrence appeared in one of these patients at 42 months.

Metastases have been diagnosed in only six of the 14 patients treated according to the new protocol (radiation therapy, Vincristine, Cytoxan). One of these patients developed metastatic tumor between the completion of the radiation therapy and the institution of the chemotherapy. Thus of the 13 patients who actually received the drug therapy before the diagnosis of metastasis, five have subsequently developed metastatic disease (7, 12, 14, 15 and 18 months). The median time to metastasis is in excess of 15 months in this group of 14 patients: eight patients are alive without evident disease at 31, 30, 30, 26, 20, 19, 13 and 9 months (Table 2).

TABLE 2

DISEASE-FREE SURVIVAL IN PATIENTS WITH EWING'S SARCOMA

Treatment	Number of patients	Median time to Diagnosis of metastasis (months)
Radiation therapy (with or without chemotherapy)	40	8
Radiation therapy + multicourse of Vincristine and Cytoxan	14	>15

SIGN OF FIRST METASTASIS

The sites of the first detected metastasis among the 40 patients who have developed metastatic disease are listed in Table 3. The lung was much the most common site, i.e. 23 of 40 patients. In 16 patients the first metastasis appeared in the bone. These were most commonly in the vertebral column and then less frequently in the long bones and then the skull. One patient had the first metastasis as a subcutaneous or cutaneous nodule overlying the skull. In this series of patients there was no instance of the first metastasis appearing in the central nervous system.

TABLE 3

SITES OF FIRST DETECTED METASTASIS (40 PATIENTS)

Lung	23	
Bone	16	Metastasis appeared
Skin	1	in Multiple Sites
CNS	0	in three Patients
Unknown	1	

DISCUSSION

The observed difference in local recurrence frequency and length of disease free survival in patients treated by radiation therapy alone versus those treated by a planned schedule of radiation therapy and multi-course Vincristine—Cytoxan therapy is of serious clinical interest. Although the differences as reported here are not significant in the usual statistical sense, they are quite strong clinical indications that the combined treatment approach represents a superior treatment method.

A practical question arises regarding the selection of the radiation dose to be employed. Our own experience has been that permanent control of the primary Ewing's sarcoma requires high radiation dose. An explanation for our observed high frequency of local failures after doses in the range of 6,500–7,000 rads for a tumor which is generally classed as "radiosensitive" is not obvious. A practical explanation may be that we have given more than usual attention in follow-up studies to the status of the primary lesion. However, others have also described local recurrences after high dose levels. At the Institute Gustave Roussy,[3] 55 patients with primary small-cell sarcoma of bone were treated by radiation therapy with the intent to cure (no evident metastatic tumor at time of treatment). Clinically evident regrowth of tumor was observed in 15 patients: in eight of these, the tumor had received ≥ 6,000 rads. Results of radiation therapy in terms of local regrowth of Ewing's sarcoma has been reported from the Princess Margaret Hospital:[4] eight of 24 Ewing's sarcomas recurred following doses in the range of 4,000–6,000 rads in 3 to 7 weeks (three of six patients recurred after doses of 5,000–6,000 rads in 4–5 weeks). D'Angio[5] now advocates 7,000 rads to the entire bone because of his observation of a number of local regrowths following doses in the range of 6,000 rads. In this context the reports of long term control of Ewing's sarcoma following doses of the order of 4,000 rads are of special interest. For example Phillips *et al.*[6] recommended that the total dose should not exceed 4,000 rads. Their results are impressive: 13 of 39 patients treated at Memorial Hospital for localized Ewing's sarcoma survived 5 or more years. Also Wang and Schultz[7] have described a number of 5-year survivors in patients who have received modest dose levels to the primary lesion. The results from most of the centers however, do report a substantial number of local failures after doses in the range of 4,000 to 5,000 rads. From our own experience and that in the literature our conclusion is that the dose response curve is not really a very steep one.

For the present we are continuing on a program whereby the primary lesion receives a minimum dose of 6 500 rads in about 6½ weeks except in those sites where tolerance of adjacent normal structures makes such a dose hazardous. This would apply for lesions in certain portions of the pelvis, vertebral column and certain sites within the skull. Perhaps it is relevant to these considerations to note that the one probable recurrence among the 14 patients who were treated by radiation therapy and Vincristine–Cytoxan chemotherapy received 6,000 rads, *viz.* the lower limit of the dose range now being employed.

The experience to date in the use of combined Vincristine and Cytoxan chemotherapy at the same time as radiation therapy for the primary is too limited to formulate a final evaluation of the efficacy of this approach. Our good results with this method support the earlier reports of Hustu *et al.*,[1] Johnson and Humphrey[8] and others, which describe apparent prolonged disease-free survival of patients with Ewing's sarcoma treated by a combined modality approach: radiation therapy plus multi-course treatment with Vincristine and Cytoxan (also actinomycin D in some patients). There are no reports of a negative result using this basic procedure.

To date, in our experience toxicity of this approach has been acceptable and there have been no fatalities. Table 4 presents the time of appearance of metastasis in six patients in relationship to the chemotherapy in our recent 14 cases. It is noted that one patient developed metastasis between the end of radiation therapy and the start of chemotherapy. During the initial phase of this study, the radiation therapy was completed before the chemotherapy was started because we were uncertain as to the ability of the normal tissues to tolerate a full dose of radiation therapy and the combined drug therapy. It seems now that the concomitant approach may be used if the total radiation dose is kept to something in the order of about 6,500 rads. Exceptions will be in the pelvis or in certain other sites where large volumes of very sensitive normal tissues must be treated. Two patients had

TABLE 4

RELATIONSHIP BETWEEN TIME OF DIAGNOSIS OF DISTANT METASTASIS AND
ADMINISTRATION OF CHEMOTHERAPY.   FOURTEEN PATIENTS WITH EWING'S
SARCOMA

Diagnosis of distant metastasis	Number of patients
After start of radiation therapy and before chemotherapy	1
During chemotherapy	2
After completion of chemotherapy (4, 6 and 6 months)	3
Free of evident metastatic tumor after completion of chemotherapy (at 0–22 months)	8

appearance of metastatic tumor during the course of chemotherapy while three did not show metastatic disease until following the completion of the therapy. Eight patients are at this time alive and without evidence of metastasis.

Currently, consideration is being given to methods of modifying our program with the expectation that such modification would result in improved survival figures. This might feature more than five courses of Cytoxan and Vincristine. This would be feasible for a large proportion of the patients. Another approach would be to place the patient on maintenance Cytoxan therapy.

A more aggressive initial chemotherapy approach would not appear feasible unless the "life island" approach were employed.

There is interest in consideration of the merit of irradiation of the thoracic contents at the time of treatment of the primary and of the chemotherapy as treatment of metastatic disease in the lung fields. Twenty-three of 40 patients had metastasis in lung as the first recognized metastasis. Of special relevance is the fact that of the 16 patients who had their first metastasis in the bone the metastasis was located in the dorsal vertebra in five patients. This same trend has been maintained in the 14 patients treated by the combined radiation therapy–Vincristine—Cytoxan protocol. Of the six patients in this group in whom metastases have appeared the lesions were located in the lung (three patients), lung plus D 12 (one patient), D 7 (one patient), and lumbar spine (one patient). Thus, some 70% of the first metastasis (23 + 5/40) appeared in the lung, mediastinum or dorsal vertebral column. These findings provide a basis for cautious initiation of a program of total thoracic irradiation: coverage of the site of the first metastatic disease in $\approx 70\%$ of the patients. Because of the sensitivity of lung tissue to both radiation therapy and drug therapy this combined approach should be on the basis of starting with a relatively low dose.

Recently Marsa and Johnson[9] have suggested that the cranial contents be irradiated at the time of initial treatment because two of their patients had their first metastatic disease in the brain or meninges. We have not observed initial metastasis in brain or meninges in our patients.

ACKNOWLEDGEMENT

From the Departments of Radiotherapy, Pediatrics and Medicine, the University of Texas M. D. Anderson Hospital, Houston, Texas.

REFERENCES

1. Hustu, H. O. *et al.* Treatment of Ewing's Sarcoma with Concurrent Radiotherapy and Chemotherapy. *J. Pediat.*, **73**, No. 2, 249–251, 1968.
2. Suit, H. D. Ewing's Sarcoma: Treatment by Radiation Therapy. *Tumors of Bone and Soft Tissue*, pp. 191–200. Year Book Medical Publishers, Chicago, 1965.
3. Sarrazin, D., Schweisguth, O. & Hourtoulle, F. G. Radiotherapie Des Sarcomes Osseux Reticulaires. *Annales De Radiologie*, **10**, Nos. 5–6, pp. 401–418, 1967.
4. Jenkin, R. D. T., Rider, W. D. & Sonley, M. J. Ewing's Sarcoma: A Trial of Adjuvant Total-Body Irradiation. *Radiology*, **96**, 151, 1970.
5. D'Angio, G. Personal Communication, 1971.
6. Phillips, R. F. & Higinbotham, N. L. The Curability of Ewing's Endothelioma of Bone in Children. *J. Pediat.*, **70**, No. 3, part 1, pp. 391–397, 1967.
7. Wang, C. C. & Schultz, M. D. Ewing's Sarcoma: A study of 50 Cases at the Massachusetts General Hospital, 1930–1952, inclusive. *New Engl. J. Med.*, **248**, 571–576, 1953.
8. Johnson, R. & Humphrey, S. R. Past Failures and Future Possibilities in Ewing's Sarcoma. *Cancer*, **23**, 161–166, 1969.
9. Marsa, G. W. & Johnson, R. Altered Pattern of Metastasis following Treatment of Ewing's Sarcoma with Radiotherapy and Adjuvant Chemotherapy. *Cancer*, **27**, 1051–1054, 1971.

The management of osteosarcoma and Ewing's sarcoma

by

R. D. T. JENKIN

SUMMARY

A group of 62 patients with osteosarcoma seen in Toronto, Canada, since 1958 are analysed. The treatment plan of radical irradiation followed by selective amputation was unsatisfactory, in that the primary tumour recurred in all patients, and was a major cause of morbidity.

In Ewing's sarcoma early dissemination was the main cause of treatment failure. The value of elective systemic therapy following control of the primary site is assessed to date, particularly in regard to the value of total body irradiation.

THE PRIMARY PURPOSE of this communication is to consider the value of radical irradiation and delayed selective amputation in the management of osteosarcoma[1] and elective total body irradiation in the management of Ewing's sarcoma[2].

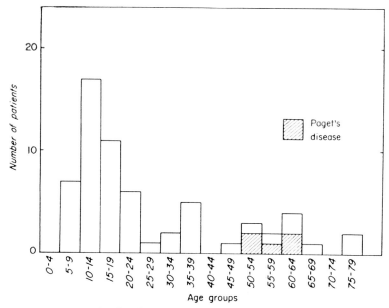

Fig. 1. Osteosarcoma. Age distribution.

229

OSTEOSARCOMA

Sixty-two patients with osteosarcoma were seen at the Princess Margaret Hospital, Toronto, from 1958 to 1970. When we examine the age-incidence of this tumour (Fig. 1) we see that 42 of these patients were less than 30 years old, with a peak incidence at 10–14 years, and 20 were 30 years or older. Five of 10 patients age 50–64 years were known to have coexisting Paget's disease, and in the oldest patient (77 years) the tumour was radiation induced. The site of the primary tumour showed a marked age variation.

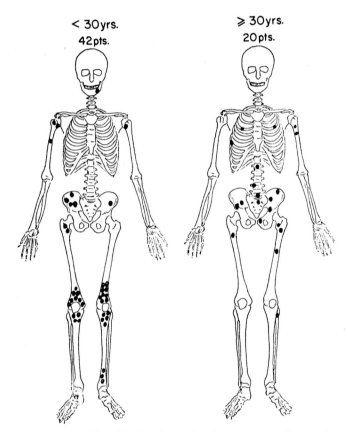

Fig. 2. Osteosarcoma. The distribution of primary sites. Comparison is made between the pattern of involvement in an older group of patients aged > 30 years, and a younger group aged < 30 years.

Thirty of the 42 tumours which occurred in patients less than 30 years old, were in the lower limb distal to the mid-femur (Fig. 2). In comparison only one of 20 tumours in older patients occurred in this part of the leg. Thus in the younger group, in three of every four patients, we were concerned with the management of a distal lower limb tumour. Because of the marked disparity of site and aetiology between these two age groups we analyzed them separately.

PATIENTS AGED < 30 YEARS

SURVIVAL

The crude survival curve and the curve showing the proportion of patients without clinically demonstrable metastatic disease is given for 38 patients followed for more than 6 months from diagnosis (Fig. 3). It is clear that metastases appeared early, most often at the time of diagnosis or within 6 months. Thus of 38 patients treated (36 radically), two remain as possible cures. It is very apparent that we have no good treatment method.

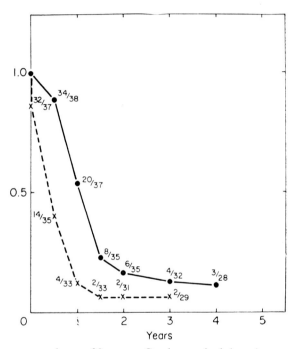

Fig. 3. Osteosarcoma. Age < 30 years. Crude survival (continuous line) and proportion of patients without metastatic disease (dotted line). The number of patients alive or without metastatic disease compared with the number assessable is given for each time interval.

MANAGEMENT

It is generally held that the cure rate in osteosarcoma is the same whether treatment is by immediate radical surgery or by radical irradiation followed by selective radical surgery: at 6 months for the group of patients in whom the primary is controlled and who remain free of metastatic disease, or at an earlier time if there is primary recurrence and no metastatic disease [3,4]. We have most often practised selective surgery on the premise that radical irradiation will provide good local palliation and thus avoid unnecessary amputations for the majority who will succumb to pulmonary metastases during the first year. We have examined our data to see whether this premise is sound.

Of the 42 patients less than 30 years old, 10 were treated by immediate surgery with one apparent cure; 29 were treated by radical irradiation and selective amputation also with one cure, and three with metastases at diagnosis were treated palliatively.

In the group of patients eligible for the combined treatment the volume of tissue irradiated included the whole tumour with a generous margin, particularly along the proximal shaft of a long bone, though only occasionally was the whole bone irradiated. A cobalt unit was utilized in every case.

The response of the primary tumour was classified as complete when there were no residual symptoms and no palpable tumour following irradiation; as partial when there was only a decrease in symptoms and/or tumour size, and as no response when neither symptoms nor size improved.

Data were adequate to assess the response in 27 patients. The response to irradiation was poor (Table 1). A complete response was seen in three, a partial response in 17, and

TABLE 1.

OSTEOSARCOMA. AGE < 30 YEARS. NATURE AND DURATION OF THE
RESPONSE, MEASURED FROM THE DAY OF DIAGNOSIS, FOLLOWING
IRRADIATION OF THE PRIMARY TUMOUR

Response	Number of patients	Duration (months)		
		Range	Mean	Median
CR	3	3–6	4	4
PR	17	1–9	5·5	5·5
NR	7	0	0	0

CR Complete Response; PR Partial Response; NR No Response.

no response in seven. Moreover, the primary tumour recurred in all 27 patients. This was grossly evident in a mean time of 5·5 months for those with a partial response, and in 4 months for the three patients with a complete response. *A distinction between partial response and complete response was therefore not of prognostic value.* The dose used (Fig. 4) in the conventionally irradiated patients ranged from 4,500 rads in 3 weeks to 7,000 rads in 7 weeks, close to tissue tolerance for the chosen time interval. Eight patients with distal limb tumours were treated under hypoxic conditions. All showed a partial tumour response which was not superior to the response in the conventionally irradiated patients. A further increase in dose would not be practical.

Thus, in our experience, radical irradiation offered only temporary growth restraint to these patients, since in all patients there was either failure of control or recurrence at the primary site.

The morbidity associated with primary recurrence was severe. Pain, limitation of joint movement, and the danger of fracture in a weight-bearing bone, were the factors that markedly limited the activity of these patients. Only three of 17 patients with a lower limb tumour had an initially good functional result, and these had recurred within 3 months.

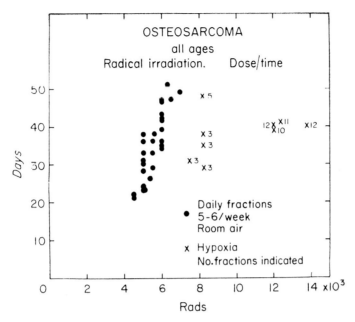

Fig. 4. Osteosarcoma. All ages. Dose/Time relationships for irradiation of the primary tumour.

For the radically irradiated patient, the mean time to recurrence was 3·6 months, to the development of secondaries 4·5 months, and to death 13 months. Pulmonary metastases did not usually produce major functional impairment until the last month or two of life, so that symptoms associated with the recurrence primary site were dominant for most patients.

What then were our indications for ablation of a limb? Twenty-two patients with the primary site in the arm or leg were radically irradiated and followed for at least 6 months Each developed either primary recurrence or metastases or both, during the 6-month follow-up period. Elective surgical ablation at 6 months was therefore appropriate for none. Ablative surgery was carried out in 12 of the 22 patients. In eight, the indication was recurrence of the primary tumour and in the absence of metastatic disease. Three other patients required palliative amputation after the development of pulmonary metastases, and in one patient an elective amputation was performed at 2 months, whilst the patient was asymptomatic and the tumour clinically under control, but pathological examination demonstrated gross tumour.

The retention of a painful limb of limited use, was associated with the early onset of systemic symptoms, particularly loss of appetite and well-being. There was increased use of analgesics, and frequently depression, for the failure of tumour control in a peripheral bone tumour is as evident to the patient as to the physician. In this situation palliative amputation is better undertaken early than late.

PULMONARY METASTASES

In six patients in this series the lungs were treated electively following completion of irradiation of the primary tumour. A dose of 1,500 rads in 14 days (Cobalt 60) was given to the total lung volume and in four of the patients Actinomycin D (single intravenous injection 0·5–1·0 mgm) was given simultaneously. All developed diffuse pulmonary metastases after an interval in the range 2–6 months (mean 4·7 months), compared to a range 0–22 months (mean 5·1 months) for the total series. This procedure was therefore not of value.

In general we do not treat the patient with diffuse pulmonary metastases. When a small number of slowly growing metastases are present these may occasionally be cleared by high-dose "postage stamp" irradiation, but it is this very group of patients that we now treat by multiple local pulmonary resections following the lead of the group at Memorial Hospital[5].

PATIENTS AGED > 30 YEARS

In the older patients osteosarcoma arose predominantly in the trunk bones (13/20) and proximal limbs (6/20). Metastatic disease was present at diagnosis (7/20) more often than in those younger than 30 years (4/42).

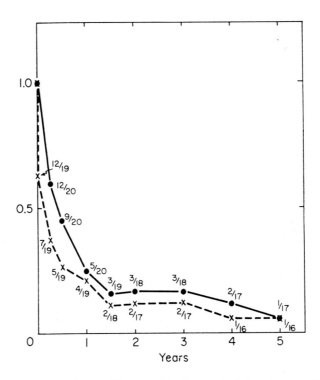

Fig. 5. Osteosarcoma. Age >30 years. Crude survival (continuous line) and proportion of patients without metastatic disease (dotted line). The number of patients alive or without metastatic disease compared with the number assessable is given for each time interval.

SURVIVAL

The crude survival curve (Fig. 5) demonstrates that 15 of the 20 older patients died during the first year after diagnosis. Only two patients remain well.

TREATMENT METHOD

Twelve of the older patients were treated radically, nine by irradiation and three surgically.

In the nine radically irradiated patients the response was judged to be complete in 4 and of average duration 10·5 months; partial in 3 and of average duration 2·3 months and no response was seen in two patients.

Only one patient in this group, with a primary tumour in the upper femur proceeded to surgical ablation when the primary recurred. He remains well 8 years later. The site or the early onset of metastatic disease contra-indicated surgery for the eight other patients.

One of the three surgically treated patients had a prolonged survival to 58 months from diagnosis.

DISCUSSION

In our experience osteosarcoma has been a lethal disease with a 5-year survival rate not greater than 5%.

It is necessary to question whether our poor results might be due in part to our policy of selective delayed amputation of the limb. Certainly, we obtained no more than transient control of the primary tumour by radical irradiation, so that we cannot feel confident that, in the difficult period before surgery, further tumour cell dissemination had been totally suppressed. On the contrary, all of our patients were operated on at a time when the primary was grossly recurrent, and we see no reason to suppose that a recurrent primary should not have recovered its potential for producing viable metastatic cells. It is difficult to estimate the weight to be given to this argument. It may be unimportant in that it is not relevant to the large majority with occult metastases already present at diagnosis, and in the small number without such metastases a low potential for metastases has already been demonstrated, which may well be lowered further for some months after devitalization of the primary tumour by irradiation.

Retrospective reviews show no significant difference in the chance of survival in osteosarcoma whether the primary treatment is immediate amputation or irradiation followed by amputation at about six months for those without metastases.[3] In such studies, it is never clear whether the treatment groups contain similar patients, so there remains no clear demonstration whether or not a delay in amputation is associated with a decreased chance of survival. If there is a risk the published data suggest it must be small.

In the Toronto region irradiation and selective delayed amputation became a common treatment method during the period 1958–1970, because of the poor results obtained with immediate amputation. For example, the tumour registry of the Hospital for Sick Children, Toronto, indicated that of 18 children with osteosarcoma diagnosed at that hospital during the years 1924–1958 there was no 5-year survivor regardless of the treatment method.

Because of the lethality of osteosarcoma in the Toronto region it seemed that initial high-dose irradiation should be given in the expectation of providing reasonable palliation and preserving a useful limb for the majority who will succumb to metastatic disease. The data we have presented clearly indicate that for the young patient with a peripheral primary site, treatment by irradiation did not accomplish either of these aims. The duration of tumour control by irradiation was too short. The mean time to the recurrence of the primary tumour at 3·6 months was even shorter than the mean time of 4·5 months to the development of grossly demonstrable metastatic disease. Therefore, in the group undergoing amputation for primary recurrence, the risk of developing pulmonary metastases had not appreciably declined by the time of amputation and all but two were still to succumb. In this group initial irradiation therefore had no advantage but had the appreciable disadvantage of increasing both hospitalization and the time before local palliation was secured. In the complementary group where primary recurrence followed the onset of metastatic disease there was a natural reluctance to amputate, so that with three exceptions this group of patients faced the terminal misery of both their recurrent primary tumour and pulmonary metastatic disease. In reviewing the files of these patients, the conclusion was inescapable that the late morbidity associated with a recurrent primary was of such degree that its avoidance by early amputation would be fully justified. In this group too, the initial hospitalization for diagnosis and irradiation consumed too much time for a patient who might have only a few months of useful life left to him.

It seems unlikely that our failure to obtain adequate local control was dose-dependent. Cade originally employed a dose-range 7–9,000 rads in 8–12 weeks[6], and in more recent years at the same hospital, Lee reported the results obtained with 6–7,000 rads in 6–7 weeks.[7] McWhirter used 5,000 rads in 4 weeks for peripheral limb tumours.[8] In the United Kingdom similar results were obtained at these varying dose-levels, which overlapped the dose-levels utilized in our conventionally irradiated patients (Fig. 4). That we can hope for little more by increasing the dose is indicated by the equally poor results we obtained in nine patients irradiated under hypoxic conditions. Whilst in these patients the number of fractions was small, the soft tissue changes noted suggested that in some of these patients normal tissue tolerance had been exceeded.

We conclude that pre-operative irradiation used in the manner described has failed, both in its primary role of providing adequate local palliation and as a means by which patients with a good chance of survival could be selected for amputation.

The alternative management by immediate amputation is therefore advocated as offering the best palliation and a small chance for cure.

EWING'S SARCOMA

In sharp contrast to osteosarcoma, Ewing's sarcoma, as a rule, responds rapidly and completely to local irradiation, and there is prompt recovery of any functional disturbance.

It is important that the tissue volume irradiated be adequately large. For limb tumours the whole of the involved bone, together with all its associated soft tissues, is included in the irradiated volume. For tumours involving trunk bones, particularly the pelvic bones, a full radiological investigation, which will often include angiography, is oblig-atory for these tumours are often much larger than indicated by palpation alone. We irradiate the chosen volume to a minimum tumour dose of 5,000 rads in 5 weeks. At the end of such a course the response is usually complete.

The cure rate in this tumour remains moderate because metastases, chiefly to lung and bone, occur early and frequently. The cure rate is the same whether the primary treatment is by irradiation or surgery. Since response to irradiation is rapid and complete this is the preferred treatment in that unnecessary amputations are avoided.

In recent years attention in this tumour has been focused on the systemic management of the metastatic phase of the disease, for it has long been recognized that even in advanced disease good objective remissions can be obtained with chemotherapy, particularly with Cyclophosphamide and Vincristine.

The results obtained at the Princess Margaret Hospital and the Hospital for Sick Children, Toronto, are given (Fig. 6). For 31 patients treated from 1929 to 1959 the primary was most often irradiated, but with no uniformity of dose or volume. Amputa-tion was occasionally performed. Little active treatment was given in the metastatic phase of the disease. These patients serve as a baseline for our subsequent experience. Sixty-eight per cent of these patients died in the first year after diagnosis. Ten per cent were cured. From 1960 to 1965, 16 patients without demonstrable secondaries at diagnosis were treated by irradiation. The volume irradiated was relatively standardized and a dose in the range 4,500–6,000 rads in 3 to 6 weeks was employed. Solitary sites of metastatic disease were managed by local irradiation, commonly 2,000 rads in 4 to 6 days. Chemotherapy, most often using Cyclophosphamide 2·5 mgm per kilogram per day *p.o.* was used for diffuse metastatic involvement or when multiple local sites occurred within a short time. An improvement in the 5-year survival rate was seen in that four of 16 survived 5 years after diagnosis. There was also marked improvement in the control

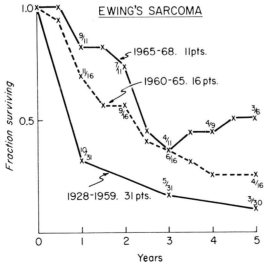

Fig. 6. Ewing's Sarcoma. Crude Survival related to year of diagnosis.

of the early metastatic phase of the disease with approximately two-thirds of the patients being alive at one year.

In 1965 we commenced a trial of adjuvant total body irradiation in Ewing's sarcoma.[2] This was given electively following completion of radical irradiation of the primary tumour. A single dose of 300 rads was used. During these later years irradiation and chemotherapy in the later overt metastatic phase of the disease also became more aggressive. There may well have been further improvement in our results, but the numbers are too small to be sure (Fig. 6).

It is particularly encouraging that two of our three 5-year survivors from this period had single sites of metastatic disease apparent at the time of the initial diagnosis. This is the first time in our experience that such patients have obtained prolonged survival.

Of the 27 patients treated in the period 1960–1968, only one has required amputation for recurrence of the primary tumour whilst still free of metastatic disease. Recurrence at the primary tumour site during the metastatic phase of the disease can usually be satisfactorily managed by palliative irradiation and chemotherapy. Palliative amputation has not been necessary.

Recently it has become apparent that elective systematic therapy with Cyclophosphamide and Vincristine is of value at least in prolonging the initial tumour free interval.[9,10] It may be that the cure rate also in increased. In the last 2 years we have therefore increased our elective systemic therapy to include a 12-month course of Cyclophosphamide (15 mgm per kilogram *i.v.*) and Vincristine (0·05 mgm kilogram *i.v.*) given alternately at weekly intervals. Of six patients treated in this fashion, one has relapsed to date.

In conclusion, and in contrast to osteosarcoma, Ewing's sarcoma responds well to both irradiation and chemotherapy appropriately applied, and there is some promise that energetic systemic therapy of occult metastatic disease may improve the modest cure rate.

ACKNOWLEDGEMENT

Figures 1 to 6 and Table 1 are reproduced by courtesy of the editor of *Cancer* (see reference No. 1).

REFERENCES

1. Jenkin, R. D. T., Allt, W. E. C. & Fitzpatrick, P. J. Osteosarcoma. An Assessment of Management with Particular Reference to Primary Irradiation and Selective Delayed Amputation. *Cancer*, **30**, 393–400, 1972.
2. Jenkin, R. D. T., Rider, W. D. & Sonley, M. J. Ewing's Sarcoma. A Trial of Adjuvant Total Body Irradiation. *Radiology*, **96**, pp. 151–155, July, 1970.
3. Sweetnam, R., Knoweldon, J. & Seddon, H. Bone Sarcoma. Treatment by Irradiation, Amputation or a Combination of the Two. *Brit. Med. J.*, **2**, 363–367, 1971.
4. Editorial: Osteosarcoma. *Brit. Med. J.*, **2**, 355–356, 1971.
5. Martini, N., Huvos, A., Miké, V., Marcove, R. C. & Beattie, E. J. Multiple Pulmonary Resections in the Treatment of Osteogenic Sarcoma. *Annals of Thor. Surg.*, **12**, 271–280, 1971.
6. Cade, S. Osteogenic Sarcoma: A Study based on 133 patients. *J. roy. Coll. Surg., Edin.*, **1**, 79–111, 1955.

7. Lee, E. S. & Mackenzie, D. H. Osteosarcoma: A Study of the Value of Preoperative Mega-voltage Radiotherapy. *Brit. J. Surg.*, **51**, 252–274, 1964.

8. McWhirter, R. On the Management of Osteosarcomata. In *Progress in Radiology: XIth International Congress of Radiology, Rome*, 1965. Amsterdam, Excerpta Medica Foundation pp. 1077–1081, 1967.

9. Pinkel, D., Husto, H. O. & Pratt, C. Treatment of Ewing's Sarcoma with Radiotherapy and Combination Chemotherapy. *Proc. 13th International Congress of Paediatrics*, **Vol. 14**, pp. 53–58, August, 1971.

10. Johnson, R. E., Senyszyn, J. J. & Rabson, R. S. Treatment of Ewing's Sarcoma with Local Irradiation and Systemic Chemotherapy: A Progress Report. *Radiology*, **95**, pp. 195–197, April, 1970.

Discussion

Prof. Ackerman (Chairman)   I think these two papers on Ewing's tumour indicate certainly an advance in results which have been so dismal before. It seems such a reasonable method of treatment to me.

Dr. Cortes   May I report that Palma and associates from our Institute recently submitted a paper to the Cancer Chemotherapy Report about their experience with 12 patients who had metastatic Ewing's sarcoma treated with BCNU (1,3,Bis (β-chloroethyl) -l-nitrosourea). They achieved one complete disappearance of tumour and four objective regressions of over 50%. Although the response was transient, three responding patients were in remission for 6, 8 and 13 months. So Dr. Suit may consider this drug in his combination regimen for a possible more prolonged disease-free period.

Prof. Ackerman   Did these patients have any radiotherapy before other treatment?

Dr. Cortes   Most but not all had prior irradiation to their primary tumour but had relapse or did not respond.

Dr. Brenner   I would like to ask first Dr. Jenkin what he thinks about Dr. Suit's dosage for the radiotherapy of the primary? Secondly, I would like to ask Dr. Suit whether in any of the cases that actually had local recurrence, if systemic chemotherapy did produce local regression, and if so, for what length of time?

Dr. Jenkin   I think it is difficult to know what the right dose of radiotherapy is for Ewing's sarcoma. I think it is very reasonable that around the world there should be two different dose levels being used. The reason why we have stuck to the dose of 5,000 rads is because that is about the maximum dose you can give without getting into the sequelae of high-dose irradiation. It seems to us that the only thing perhaps that matters in Ewing's sarcoma is the number that recur and require amputation before they develop metastatic disease. As I indicated, this has only happened once in our series. That incidentally was the case that we felt most confident that we had controlled. It was a patient with a lesion which was almost invisible on the X-ray—it was so small. Dr. Suit really showed some data which indicated that recurrence still occurs with these higher doses. Because of that, and as in the late phases of the disease, if one gets further symptoms at the primary site, one can give further irradiation normally with good results. It is really very rare to find someone with Ewing's sarcoma who dies in a non-ambulatory state. This is the exact opposite of osteosarcoma.

Dr. Suit   I would like just to follow up that comment. We had four patients who developed recurrence at the time they were free of distant metastases. I have no doubts that it must be a bad prognostic sign or factor for a local recurrence to appear. Every single patient at the Anderson who has developed a local recurrence has succumbed to the disease. This is the basis for our pursuing these higher dose levels. It does appear that the dose-response curve must be relatively flat; it's not steep as it is for some types of lesions. The patients who have had recurrent disease have all had chemotherapy, and there has neither been any major nor significant response other than the primary to chemotherapy. Chemotherapy has been quite effective in causing regression of pulmonary metastases. We've had several patients that are alive and doing quite well 2 or 3 years after diagnosis of opacities and have been managed by intensive chemotherapy.

Prof. Ackerman Dr. Suit, what do you think of adopting the same method of treatment for osteosarcoma as for a Ewing's tumour? I have recently reviewed all the cases of Ewing's sarcoma at the National Cancer Institute. There, the patients who were surviving who entered without evidence of distant disease were something like nine out of 16 for 2 years. There were no cures in patients with lesions of the pelvis. Do you have similar experience?

Dr. Suit No, we have two patients with pelvic lesions who are free of disease at this time, both were treated according to this regime. I am not an enthusiast for treating osteosarcoma by radiotherapy. I have had some experience, but it has been much less discouraging than that described by Dr. Jenkin. I would be most interested if maybe Mr. Lee would comment on the frequency with which the primary is controlled in the very considerable experience they have had at the Westminster Hospital.

Mr. Lee What we heard just now from Dr. Jenkin is what really has been metaphorically called the "other side of the elephant". In other words here is somebody pointing out the bad local results of radiotherapy. I would first of all say this. Since 1966 we've stopped treating all cases indiscriminately in this way and have become much more selective. We wouldn't now I think treat a patient with for instance a fractured tumourous bone. We wouldn't treat a patient with severe contracture of the knee, so that it couldn't be straightened. Neither would we treat a patient with a fungating tumour, because our experience has shown that we don't control the local disease, or at any rate we didn't give the patient a useful comfortable limb—which is the whole object of the exercise. If you can't do this, then I think radiotherapy is useless.

   The other thing is that recurrence of local symptoms does not necessarily mean that it's recurrent disease. Recurrent local symptoms can be due to, for example, cracking through of the tumour or to a haemorrhage, or something of this kind. It hasn't always in our experience been that the tumour was re-activated. Of course from the practical point of view of the patient's comfort, it comes to much the same thing. If the local symptoms recur for any reason then you usually have to amputate or disarticulate forthwith.

Prof. Ackerman Have you some evidence of sterilization of the tumour from the standpoint of the pathology?

Mr. Lee Yes we have. Professor Mackenzie and I wrote this up and I think that it remains about the same. Of the tumours we were able to examine, either in an amputated limb or at post-mortem, 30%, about a third, were totally destroyed, about a third had

I*

what appeared to be quite obviously viable tumour, and the other third had remnants of tumour which were much altered by irradiation. Of course, this is a very obscure picture because much depends on how long after the irradiation you examine the tumour and so on. The only thing I deduce from this is that maybe one shouldn't wait longer than 8 or 9 months before amputating the limb. I think the only risk is an increasing risk of re-activation of the tumour with, I suppose, again the increasing possibility of lung metastases.

Prof. Mackenzie   Yes, I agree with this.

Mr. Lee   Of course, the appearance of viable cells in a microscope slide is again something which is not easy to interpret. It is hard to know whether these cells could in fact survive and multiply. I think we require better techniques. We should try to culture these specimens and see if the things will grow.

Prof. Ackerman   Yes, I agree. I cannot tell when a cell has an evil intention.

Dr. Brenner   I would like to ask Dr. Jenkin a further question about the total body irradiation. I have in fact done two cases of total body irradiation according to his technique. I must say that both cases were widely disseminated disease. I did note temporary regression of tumour but it didn't last for more than about 3 months. Both cases had had previous chemotherapy with Vincristine and Cytoxan given in fairly large doses. They both tolerated total body irradiation. I'm just wondering whether or not the dose should not go up a bit, but I want him to try first.

Dr. Jenkin   We chose to give systemic therapy with total body irradiation in 1965 because of the very good response of the primary tumour to irradiation. And in those days systemic chemotherapy used electively was not well known. We have only treated patients with no evidence of metastatic disease with two exceptions who had a solitary site of metastatic disease at the time of diagnosis. After that dose of irradiation you are going to have a profound pancytopenia about 25–28 days later, when you are going to need hospitalization and treatment certainly with blood, probably with platelets. You are going to encounter a high fever for a few days. Some of these patients are very ill indeed for those few days. However, they pick up very quickly provided they are appropriately managed at the time. The rationale for using total body irradiation I think is that you hope to cure whatever proportion of the patients who have a very small number of metastatic cells. That really is a very small number—probably something less than 100 cells, perhaps less than 10 cells. It may be that the proportion of patients in that situation is vanishingly small. But on the other hand, clearly 20% or so of these patients have no metastatic cells: maybe there is another 20% who have a very small number of metastatic cells. I think there is no point in putting somebody through treatment that has such unpleasant consequences 3 weeks later unless one is doing it for a cure. I'm sure there is no place for palliation with total body irradiation.

Prof. Enneking   I would like to ask Dr. Suit a question. Our few patients roughly fall into two categories. Either the treatment seems to have little effect and they rapidly die, or the benefit seems to be much more long lasting than the curve has shown, with the result that the curve falls somewhere between these two extremes. Admittedly, your group, as with everybody else, is a small group of patients. Has this been your experience? Secondly, I would like to ask if you or Dr. Jenkin has made any measurements of the effect of the treatment on the patient's immunocompetence as to whether the apparent escape from treatment is related to the loss of the patient's immunocompetence as a result of the treatment?

Dr. Suit   I think that our data demonstrates that there is a prolongation of the time between the diagnosis of the primary and diagnosis of the first distant metastasis. There are certainly a couple of patients who have had a metastasis fairly soon, but there are a number who have had a metastasis quite remote in contrast with the number in the very early period. I would say there has been a shift in the number in the two compartments. As more data are accumulated we will be able to say that this is so. In our experience we have not made this assay of immune reactivity of the patient. We are planning to do this in future cases, but we do not have data as of now.

Dr. Jenkin   We have no data either on the effect upon the immunocompetence of the patient. I'm sure that when you use systemic chemotherapy in patients with Ewing's sarcoma you change the survival curve to an "S" shaped curve. The fact that you are delaying tests must make it very unlikely that any temporary immuno-suppression causes chemotherapy to be in any way harmful to the patient or advantageous to the tumour.

Dr. Suit   I would like to take the opportunity to follow up Mr. Lee's paper and state that there are a number of patients who are going to be biopsied with the pre-operative diagnosis based upon roentgenographic findings of osteosarcoma. If one is planning to do an amputation on a patient with osteosarcoma and you do proceed to make one of those generous, or what I would describe as old fashioned, biopsy scars, and the lesion turns out to be a Ewing's sarcoma or perhaps a reticulum cell sarcoma, the patient has I think been subjected to some significant detriment. I would therefore encourage that any kind of biopsy being performed for a primary tumour of bone should be made through a very small incision, even if an osteosarcoma is suspected and an amputation is planned. We have had several patients at the Anderson that were diagnosed categorically by roentgenologists as osteosarcoma. We've had this agreement with the surgeons performing even on these cases a very small biopsy. We were thus able to initiate the radiotherapy straight away.

Prof. Ackerman   That's a very good point. You are pro-Schajowicz I can see.

Mr. Lee   Could I ask Dr. Suit—he had some very important experience with irradiating anoxic limbs for osteosarcoma—has he tried this same technique for the Ewing's tumours?

Dr. Suit We treated one patient and he was about the first that we treated. He developed necrosis. This was due to the fact that we did not leave the tourniquet in place a sufficiently long time. I have stopped treating the patients with osteosarcoma with this method, but we did find that we gave a sufficient dose to eradicate the neoplasm. The changes in the normal tissue were not acceptable, so we discontinued it.

Circulating tumour cells in osteosarcoma

by

I. O. BRENNHOVD, VIVI ROGER and KARI HÖEG

SUMMARY

In 19 of 22 patients with osteosarcoma of the limbs living tumour cells similar to those of the tumour biopsy were identified in the circulating blood. In five patients cells were demonstrated before palpation of the tumour, in 19 during palpation, and in 16 during biopsy procedure. The subsequent histories did not indicate that blood-borne tumour cells during tumour manipulation had any prognostic significance; hence no positive evidence was found that palpation or biopsy worsens prognosis. The release mechanism of such cells and their mode of disposal by the body are virtually unknown.

IT IS THE INTENTION of this paper to comment briefly upon the problem of circulating tumour cells in patients with osteosarcoma. These comments are the result of a cooperative study involving the cytological and surgical departments at the Norwegian Radium Hospital.[1,2]

We know from sad experience that bone sarcomas frequently metastasize to the lungs, and consequently that tumour cells at some stage of the disease invade the veins draining the tumour-bearing area. The problem is therefore not a new one.

There is general agreement upon the diagnostic difficulties in the distinction between tumour cells and tumour-like cells, mainly from the haemopoietic system, i.e. the megakaryocyte. On the other hand opinions vary when it comes to the interpretation of cells in the blood stream positively identified as malignant.

The release mechanism of tumour cells is not completely understood. It is well documented that cells may enter the circulation due to tumour invasion of vessels, and in connection with mechanical procedures such as operative manipulation, palpation and biopsy. It should be clear, however, that cells found in blood samples reflect the situation for a few seconds only. The possibility exists that cells may be released in bursts and unevenly distributed in the blood.

When cells are positively identified, the next problem is whether they are living or not. By the use of Colcemid, cells can be seen in mitosis—which is a certain indication that they are alive. Figures 1 and 2 demonstrate circulating tumour cells in mitosis, and for comparison the histological specimen from the same tumour. We have as yet insufficient experience of the Colcemid technique.

There seems no doubt that the body can destroy these living circulating cells. This brings up the whole problem of host–tumour relationship. The finding of circulating

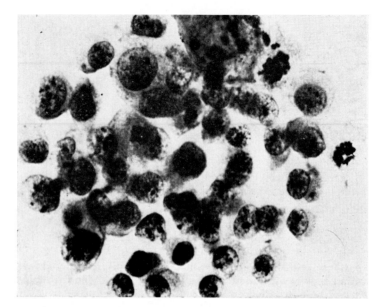

Fig. 1. Papanicolaou × 160. Tumour cells from a case of osteo-genic sarcoma. Three tumour cells in mitoses.

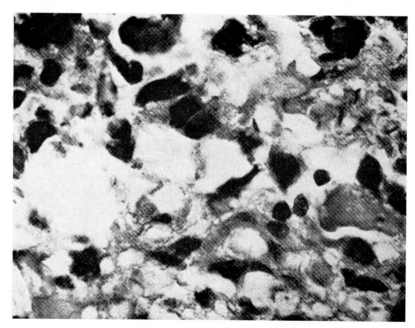

Fig. 2. H & E × 160. Section of the osteogenic sarcoma in tibia. Same case as Fig. 1.

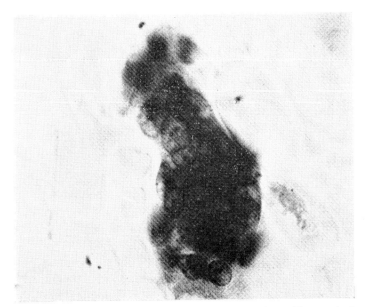

Fig. 3. Papanicolaou ×160. Giant cell from the axillary vein in a case of osteoblastoma.

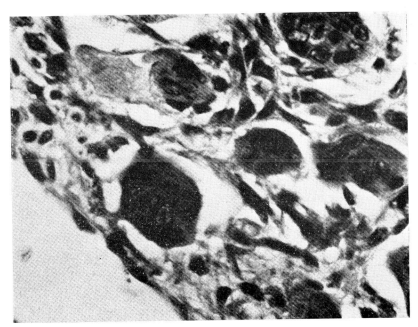

Fig. 4. H & E ×160. Section of the osteoblastoma in humerus. A vascular channel is seen in the lower left corner. Same case as Fig. 3.

cells in *benign* bone tumours is interesting, and may well illustrate our lack of knowledge of the release mechanism of cells and the capacity of our body to destroy them in the circulation. Figure 3 shows a circulating giant cell and Figure 4 the histologic specimen from the tumour. In this case the finding may be explained by the fact that only a fine layer separates the tumour cells from the lumen of the vessels.

The clinical controversial aspects of circulating tumour cells can be concentrated in one question: Does manipulation of a malignant tumour during operation, biopsy or palpation cause dissemination of the disease and thus worsen prognosis?

MATERIAL AND METHODS

We have between 1966 and 1971 investigated 22 patients suffering from osteosarcoma. Only patients with tumours in the extremities were examined, because the axillary and femoral veins were easily accessible for blood sampling. In each case four separate samples, each of 5 ml blood, were taken from the draining veins as follows:
1. Before the tumour was touched.
2. During palpation.
3. During biopsy.
4. Five to 10 minutes after the procedure.

The tumour cells were isolated from the blood on millipore or nucleopore filters according to a technique previously reported, and stained by the *Papanicolaou* method. The cells were always compared with the cells in the biopsy specimen. In most cases many clusters of cells with malignancy criteria were found.

TABLE 1

NINETEEN PATIENTS WITH OSTEOGENIC SARCOMA AND WITH
TUMOUR CELLS IN BLOOD

5 patients showed tumour cells before palpation
19 patients showed tumour cells during palpation
16 patients showed tumour cells during biopsy
13 patients showed tumour cells after the procedure

RESULTS

Tumour cells were found in the blood in 19 out of the 22 patients with osteosarcoma located to the extremities (82 per cent). Table 1 gives details about the frequency of cells in the different four blood samples. It is noteworthy that tumour cells were demonstrated *during palpation in all patients*, while this was not the case in connection with the more traumatic biopsy procedure.

Table 2 shows that of the 19 patients with identified circulating cells six are alive and 13 either dead or alive with metastatic disease. It also demonstrates the high mortality rate in the patients without circulating cells.

TABLE 2

TWENTY-TWO PATIENTS WITH OSTEOGENIC SARCOMA. FOLLOW-UP TIME $\frac{1}{2}$–5 YEARS

Tumour cells in blood	A. Patients alive without metastases	B. Patients with metastases, dead and alive
Tumour cells demonstrated	6	13
Tumour cells not demonstrated	1	2

CONCLUSION

This study has shown that in osteosarcoma tumour cells frequently occur in the veins draining the tumour. They may be found spontaneously, and more frequently in connection with manipulation of the tumour. It is astonishing that cells seem to occur more frequently during palpation as compared with the biopsy procedure.

It is an important finding that tumour cells occurring in the blood during manipulation of the primary seem to have no prognostic significance. This should to a certain degree be a comfort to the surgeon who has to biopsy these tumours.

The importance of circulating tumour cells can, however, not be neglected. Too many patients die of metastatic disease to allow a conclusion like that. This study therefore only has the limited value that it demonstrates the need for further research in the release mechanism of both benign and malignant tumour cells and the defence mechanism of the human body against these cells.

ACKNOWLEDGEMENT

From the Surgical Department, Norwegian Radium Hospital, Oslo, and Norsk Hydro's Institute for Cancer Research, Oslo.

REFERENCES

1. Foss, O. P., Brennhovd, I. O., Messelt, O. T., Efskind, J. & Liverud, K. Invasion of Tumour Cells into the Bloodstream caused by palpation or Biopsy of the Tumour. *Surgery*, **59**, 691, 1965.
2. Roger, Vivi, Brennhovd, I. O. & Höeg, Kari. The Prognostic Significance of Tumour Cells in Blood during Palpation and Biopsy. *Acta Cytol.* In press.

Discussion

Prof. Ackerman (Chairman)   Have you any information about the presence or absence of tumour cells after radiation therapy. Do you think the same thing about finding tumour cells in relation to that? Have you made any attempt to grow the tumour cells?

Dr. Brennhovd   All these patients are treated like Mr. Lee's patients. They had a pre-operative course of irradiation before biopsy, 1,200 rads, a very small dose. So this does seemingly not affect the findings. We have not tried to culture these cells, and I should say that this is partly due to the difficulties in coming into contact with people working in basic science.

The cytological diagnosis of round-cell tumours

by

A. JOHN WEBB

SUMMARY

The value of combining cytological studies with conventional histology in the differential diagnosis of malignant "round-cell" tumours of bone is briefly indicated. Three examples illustrate features which may help to distinguish between Ewing's sarcoma and lympho-reticular malignancy.

THE HISTOLOGICAL elucidation of "round-cell" tumours is a problem and the general diagnostic label of "round-cell sarcoma of bone" is often used by the Bristol Bone Tumour Registry. Cytological assessment from air-dried Giemsa-stained smears obtained by fine needle aspiration (Webb, 1969) or imprints from formal biopsies has been made in an attempt to clarify the morphology.

To begin with, the connotation "round-cell" is imprecise; many of the neoplasms to be considered—neuroblastoma, Ewing's sarcoma, "oat cell" carcinoma, reticulosarcoma—display a nuclear form which is more oval than round. The term "spheroidal" would seem more appropriate. Cardozo (1967) has indicated the help afforded to him by Bamforth is distinguishing reticulum cell sarcoma within this group; the cells and nuclei are distinctly oval!

Probably the most serious attempt to define the cyto-morphological features of these varied neoplasms was presented by Cardozo (1964). Despite his detailed descriptions and illustrations they remain a problem and certain other cytological pointers are worthy of note.

Soderstrom (1966) has described the fragments of cast-off cytoplasm seen lying between the cells in smears from benign and malignant lympho-reticular entities; especially the latter. The terms "lympho-glandular bodies" and "golf ball bodies" have been invented by him and in air-dried Romanowsky films they are distinctive, not being found in other neoplasms such as neuroblastoma. Three recent examples will serve to illustrate these "bodies" and two other cytological aspects.

CASE 1. A 46-year-old psychiatrist presented with a large mediastinal mass seen radiologically and a widened carina at bronchoscopy. Endoscopic biopsy led to a report of probable anaplastic lung carcinoma. The lesion responded swiftly and completely to irradiation. Six months later he deteriorated and probable "malignant" splenomegaly was found. Fine needle aspiration produced smears of undoubted lympho-reticular sarcoma

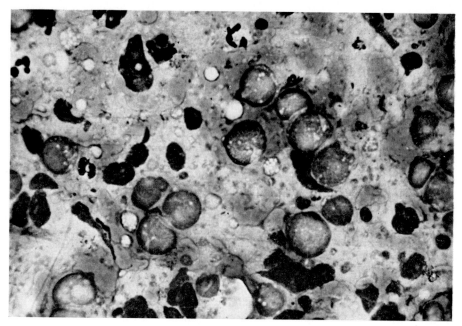

Fig. 1. Giemsa × 700. Case 1. Male age 46 years. Reticulum cell sarcoma—disseminated. Fine needle aspiration of spleen. Light and darkly staining cells are seen together with numerous lympho-glandular bodies.

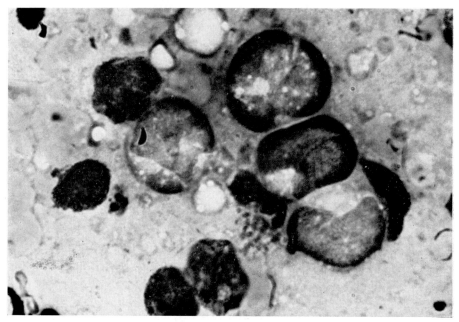

Fig. 2. Giemsa × 1,400. Case 1. Radial splitting and segmentation of the nuclei is evident.

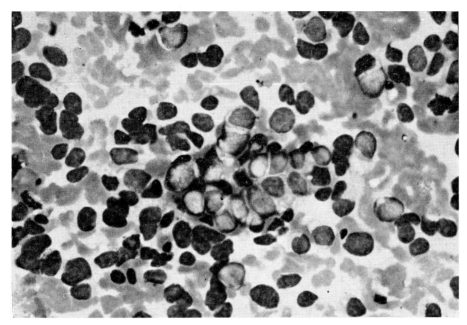

Fig. 3. Giemsa × 375. Case 2. Woman age 20 years. "Malignant round-cell tumour" of chest wall—probably Ewing's sarcoma. Fine needle aspiration smear showing both light and darkly staining cells with no suggestion of lympho-glandular bodies.

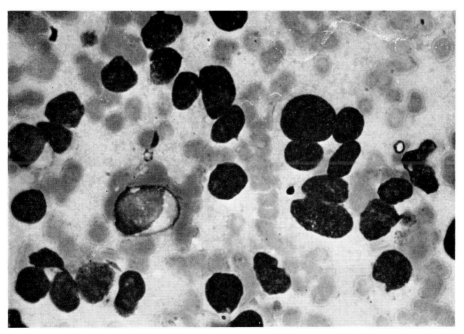

Fig. 4. Giemsa × 1,400. Case 2. Confirms how red cell form differs from lympho-glandular bodies.

254

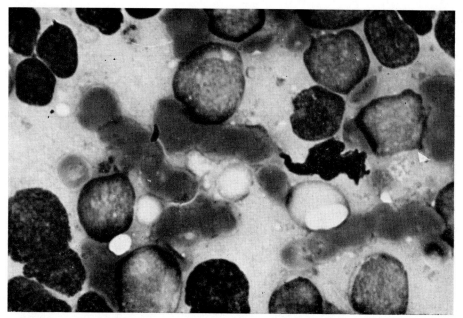

Fig. 5. Giemsa × 1,400. Case 3. Male age 3 years. "Malignant round-cell tumour" of several bones. Fine needle aspiration biopsy of femoral deposit. Exact type uncertain, but smears show light and darkly staining cells with clear lympho-glandular bodies.

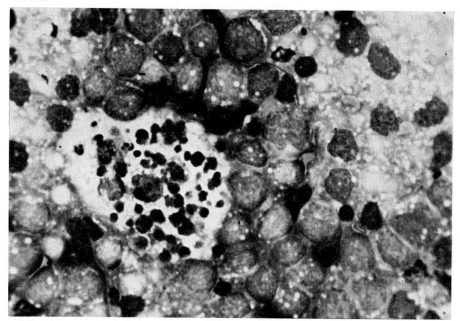

Fig. 6. Giemsa × 700. Girl age 14 years. Lymphoblastic lymphosarcoma presenting in abdominal lymph nodes. Node imprint preparation showing malignant lymphoblasts, "starry-sky" histiocyte and many small lympho-glandular bodies.

(Bessis 1956, Zach 1972) with clear "lympho-glandular" and "golf ball" bodies (Figs. 1 and 2). He failed to respond to chemotherapy.

CASE 2. A 20-year-old woman found a mass in the region of her left breast but refused consultation until 6 months later when a large mass was evident arising from the chest wall deep to the breast. There was a complete left pleural effusion. Fine needle aspiration revealed a "spheroidal" cell sarcoma probably Ewing's sarcoma (Figs. 3 and 4). The smears did not show distinctive "lympho-glandular" bodies but "starry sky" histiocytes were present. Subsequent histology and other relevant investigations (intravenous pyelography, urine catecholamine/creatinine levels) excluded neuroblastoma. The Bristol B.T.R. majority opinion favoured Ewing's sarcoma. In company with neuroblastoma and lympho-reticular malignancy both light and darkly staining nuclei were discerned; the latter seem perfectly viable on cytological grounds. In lymphoid aspirates they are known as "nuclear packets" (Soderstrom 1966).

CASE 3. A 3-year-old boy was taken to a dentist with maxillary and palatal masses associated with loose teeth; radiology revealed also a lesion in the left femoral metaphysis. Fine needle aspiration of these lesions was succeeded by open femoral biopsy and smears were made (Fig. 5). The child was painstakingly treated, and having failed to respond, followed to death and autopsy. A clinicopathological conference failed to establish an agreed diagnosis. Deposits of tumour developed within a testis and the central nervous system—clinical events suggestive of lympho-reticular malignancy. The urinary catecholamine levels were normal and neuroblastoma was not found postmortem. The cytology did show marked "lympho-glandular bodies" and "starry sky" histiocytes—cells seen in Burkitt's lymphoma (Wright 1964) and lympho-reticular malignancy in general (Fig. 6). An additional feature seen in some nuclei is "radial splitting" (Fig. 2), a detail reported by Soderstrom (1966) as specific also for lympho-reticular neoplasia, and the cytological aspects of this case would certainly support this diagnosis.

It is the opinion of the author that cytology and histology are appropriately combined in the elucidation of "spheroidal" cell malignancies and the identification of "lympho-glandular" and "golf ball" bodies together with radial splitting of the nuclei would favour the diagnosis of lympho-reticular malignancy.

REFERENCES

Bessis, M.   *Cytology of the Blood and Blood-Forming Organs*. Grune & Stratton, New York and London, 1956.
Cardozo, P. L.   Die Moderne Klinische Zytologie in der Krebs diagnostik. *Regensburger Jahrbuch für ärtzliche Fortbildung*, Band XII, Heft **3**, 1–8, 1964.
Cardozo, P. L.   Paper to Dutch Cytological Society Meeting. Unpublished, 1967.
Soderstrom, N.   *Fine-Needle Aspiration Biopsy*. Almqvist and Wiksell, Stockholm, 1966.
Webb, A. J.   *Lancet*, **2**, 249, 1969.
Wright, D. H.   Malignant Lymphoma in Uganda, M. D. Thesis, Bristol, 1964.
Zach, J.   *Praktische Zytologie für Internisten*. Georg Thieme Verlag, Stuttgart, 1972.

Metastatic and residual sarcoma

Chairman: DR. BRENDAN T. HALE

The problem of metastatic and residual sarcoma

by

BRENDAN T. HALE

SUMMARY

There is a wide range of survival rates for the different types of sarcoma found in and adjacent to bone. Attention is drawn to this and possible reasons discussed taking into account current modes of treatment and research developments. Suggestion is made that we should not only consider why we fail to control so many cases but should in particular pay more attention to those who survive without recurrence. With improved methods of investigation and alert minds, it is perhaps from these patients that we might eventually come to a better understanding of the whole problem.

SINCE THE PREPARATION of this paper I have been given the honour of being invited to act as Chairman for this session. I will, therefore, attempt to set the stage for our consideration of the "Problem of Metastatic and Residual Sarcoma".

There can be no doubt that there is a "problem" as the crude 5 year survival rate for all types of sarcoma in bone, taken collectively and including myeloma, is under 10%. The actual figure varies considerably with different tumours as we see from cases in the Bristol Bone Tumour Registry[1] (Table 1).

It is well known that the chondroblastic type of osteosarcoma and Paget's sarcoma have poor prognoses. Hence, one should always note the proportion of such cases in published series, when considering survival figures of osteosarcoma. There must also be caution when looking at chondrosarcoma because this is a most unpredictable tumour. We frequently find 5-year survivors but often with disease present. This may be in the form of a slowly progressing localized lesion in some inoperable site, or in some instances metastases will be present. These secondary deposits vary considerably in their rate of growth in different individuals. Sinkovics[2] and colleagues reported that only 16 of 83 cases had a recurrence free 5-year survival.

Let us now consider the 5-year survival of certain types of malignant round-celled tumours in bone (Table 2). The figures are again based on the cases in the Bristol Bone Tumour Registry. In this table "Group X" represents a category of tumour which is either a Ewing's or neuroblastoma, but is has proved impossible to classify further. Similarly "Group Y" represents cases probably intermediate in type between Ewing's tumour and reticulosarcoma. They have the uniformity of cell pattern found in Ewing's tumours and sparse reticulin but a higher glycogen content than is normally found in a reticulosarcoma. They behave as Ewing's tumours.

TABLE 1

FIVE-YEAR RESULTS

Bristol Bone Tumour Registry

Osteosarcoma
   including 64 Chondroblastic
         33 Paget's sarcoma } 134 cases. 15% (recurrence free)

Chondrosarcoma
      60 cases   52% (one third with recurrence)

Fibrosarcoma
      65 cases   28% (recurrence free)

TABLE 2

ROUND-CELL TUMOURS IN BONE (129) DECEMBER 1971

Type	Metastatic neuro- blastoma	Group "X"	Ewing's tumour	Group "Y"	Reticulosarcoma 1	Reticulosarcoma 2	Reticulosarcoma 3	Unspecified M.R.C.T.
Males	17	11	15	2	13	13	2	6
Females	12	3	14	4	9	3	2	3
All	29	14	29	6	22	16	4	9
Age range—years	3M–33	1–25	6–45	5–21	7–85	2–71	23–83	11–71
Mean age—years	10	9	20	13	49	41	55	35
Survival								
3 years	11%	Nil	32%	20%	53%	Nil	33%	38%
5 years	4%	Nil	17%	20%	47%	Nil	33%	25%
Average—months	14	12	25	12	22	10	30	34
Still alive	?1	1	7	2	10	Nil	1	1
Presenting in long bones	28%	43%	52%	50%	52%	—	—	55%
Autopsy	68%	8%	5%	25%	33%	37%	Nil	28%
Glycogen positive	18%	50%	59%	83%	Nil	Nil	Nil	50%

Histologically undiagnosed tumours 29/129 = 22%

Here we note a 47% figure for the 5-year survival of 22 cases of reticulosarcoma presenting with an apparently solitary lesion in one bone. In our figures the survival of Ewing's tumour is probably a false high due to the small numbers. The figure of 8·7% average from the world's literature, reported by Bhansali and Desai[3] is obviously more accurate as this was based on 646 cases. We should also note that in our Registry one in five cases of malignant round-celled tumours remains histologically unclassified in spite of reviewing regularly as more information becomes available.

Note Reticulosarcoma:
  1. Solitary osseous primary tumour.
  2. Lesions of multiple sites ab initio—bones and lymph nodes.
  3. Bone invasion by adjacent soft tissue tumour.

Two thirds of bone sarcomata will have metastasized at the time of, or shortly after, presentation. Those which appear to be still localized after all routine investigations probably do so for one or more of the following reasons:

(a) The tumour may have been present for only a short time.
(b) It may have been present for longer but may also have a longer cell cycle time.
(c) It may have been restrained by anatomical barriers.
(d) Local immune defence mechanisms may be active.
(e) Cells may be disseminated but fail to produce clinical metastases because of generalized host defence mechanisms.

In the sphere of local defence mechanisms there has been interesting work by Underwood and Carr[4] in Sheffield. This conceives permeability changes in tumour vessels and the role that this plays in rendering tumour cells accessible to possible mediators of anti-tumour immunity.

There are reports from various centres regarding generalized immune reactions to certain primary malignant bone tumours. A high degree of cross reactivity between tumour-associated antigens and the sera of patients with many types of sarcoma has been demonstrated.[5,6] In particular this has been found with osteosarcoma and liposarcoma. It may prove possible that antibody titres may be used to monitor the progress of the disease and perhaps help in the management.

Virological aspects are being studied by many workers. In our own Registry there have been no significant findings of any viral particles in human bone sarcomata. However, Miller and Nicholson[7] in New York have been considering the effects of superimposed viral and bacterial infections which may boost the immunological defences against these tumours. Coley type toxins have been used and reticulum celled sarcoma of bone is amongst cases reported as showing favourable response. Toxins given before radiotherapy seem more effective than if administered after radiation.

Pre-operative radiation for osteosarcoma as practised in many centres is a compromise attempt at preventing unnecessary amputation in cases where metastases subsequently become apparent. It is postulated that the radiation will prevent viable tumour cells escaping from the primary site and if no metastases appear after 6 to 8 months, then amputation is indicated. There is, however, no evidence that this procedure affects the 5-year survival figures and about one third of the operation specimens appear to contain viable tumour cells. It is nevertheless worth noting that radiation is capable of producing a 5-year survival of 12·9%. This figure is quoted from a composite table of the results of 143 cases of various authors by Friedman and Carter.[8] Tudway[9,10] in Bristol compared radiotherapy for upper limb lesions with radiation and amputation for those with lower limb lesions. The forequarter amputation, being regarded as a much more mutilating procedure than a leg amputation, suggested a trial of this nature to be worthwhile. It is interesting that some of our long-term survivors were treated in this manner. However, for osteosarcoma the overall figure of 19·7% for surgery alone,[8] based on the results of 1,337 cases by multiple authors, still makes this the treatment of choice when operation is acceptable. It is possible that the overall figure of 12·9% for radiotherapy might be improved with sole use of megavoltage radiation and thus radiotherapy should not be forgotten in inoperable cases. It will also be interesting to see if radiation under conditions of hyperbaric oxygen which renders anoxic cells more radiosensitive might prove beneficial.

We must also remember the appropriate use of surgery for some metastatic, radio-resistant tumours. These metastases may be causing pain, pressure symptoms or otherwise troublesome masses. There have been reports of lobectomy or pneumonectomy having resulted in long-term survivals, although as we know metastases confined to one lung are rare. One of our Ewing's tumour cases had a pneumonectomy, survived over 5 years and is still recurrence free. This is indeed unusual and we should consider whether reduction of tumour volume by surgery, radiation or other means does in certain cases enable the host's defence mechanisms to regain control. Even in the presence of metastases local removal or amputation of a primary lesion which has failed to respond to radiation might be indicated for pains or unpleasant ulceration.

Kuehn[11] and his colleagues have advocated laparotomy for lower limb osteosarcoma and if all appears clear then ligature of the iliac vein before amputation. It is suggested that this might reduce blood borne metastases due to manipulation during amputation.

Cytotoxic drugs, with or without surgery if indicated are proving of interest in the management of certain bone tumours. These have been used by Jenkin[12] and Suit[13] et al in the management of Ewing's tumour. Vincristine with 5–Fluorouracil and Cyclophosphamide has produced limited but definite remissions in metastatic osteosarcoma.[14] Infusion of the bronchial artery has been employed for metastatic osteosarcoma in Japan.[15]

Finally, I would like to mention one particular patient in order to make a particular point.

A young boy of 16 was referred to me by one of my orthopaedic colleagues because of a reticulosarcoma involving the pubic ramus and pulmonary metastases. The pelvis was treated with megavoltage radiation and he was subsequently maintained on oral Cyclophosphamide. Two years later he unfortunately killed himself on a motor cycle. At post-mortem no evidence of tumour was found anywhere in spite of extensive examination. It would, I fear, have recurred eventually, but I mention this case as I feel we must always pay particular attention to the case which does not behave true to form. With improved methods of investigation and alert minds it is from these exceptional cases that we might eventually come to a better understanding of the whole problem.

REFERENCES

1. The Bristol Bone Tumour Registry, The Royal Infirmary, Bristol. Hon. Secretary, C. H. G. Price, 1972. Personal communication.
2. Sinkovics, J. G., Shirato, E., Martin, R. G. & White, E. C. Chondrosarcoma. *J. Med. Exp. Clin.* **1**, 15–25, 1970.
3. Bhansali, S. K. & Desai, P. B. Ewing's Sarcoma. *J. Bone Jt. Surg.*, **45–A**, 541, 1963.
4. Underwood, J. C. E. & Carr, I. The Ultrastructure and Permeability Characteristics of the Blood Vessels of a Transplantable Rat Sarcoma. *J. Path.* 107, 157, 1972.
5. Morton, D. L., Malmgren, R. A., Hall, W. T. & Schidlovsky, G. Immunologic and Virus Studies with Human Sarcoma. *Surgery*, **66**, 152, 1969.
6. Moore, M. Tumour Specific Antigens—Their Possible Significance for the Aetiology and Therapy of Malignant Disease. *J. Bone Jt. Surg.*, **53–B**, 13, 1971.
7. Miller, T. R. & Nicholson, J. T. End Results in Reticulum Cell Sarcoma of Bone Treated by Bacterial Toxin Therapy Alone or Combined with Surgery and/or Radiotherapy (47 cases) or with Concurrent Infection (5 cases). *Cancer*, **27**, 524, 1971.

8. Friedman, M. & Carter, S. K. The Therapy of Osteogenic Sarcoma—Concurrent Status and Thoughts for the Future. *Journal Surgical Oncology*. In press.
9. Tudway, R. C. The Place of External Irradiation in the Treatment of Osteogenic Sarcoma. *J. Bone Jt. Surg.*, **35**-**B**, 9–21, 1953.
10. Tudway, R. C. Radiotherapy for Osteogenic Sarcoma. *J. Bone Jt. Surg.*, **43**-**B**, 61–67, 1961.
11. Kuehn, P. G., Tamoney, H. J. & Gossling, H. R. Iliac Vein Occlusion Prior to Amputation for Sarcoma. *Cancer*, **26**, 536, 1970.
12. Jenkin, R. D. T. Management of Osteosarcoma and Ewing's Tumour. The Colston Papers, No. 24, *Bone—Certain Aspects of Neoplasia*, Ed. C. H. G. Price & F. G. M. Ross. p. 229, Butterworths, London, 1973.
13. Suit, H. D., Fernandez, C., Sutow, W., Samuels, M. & Wilbur, J. Radiation Therapy and Multi-drug Chemotherapy in Management of Patients with Ewing's Sarcoma. The Colston Papers, No. 24. *Bone—Certain Aspects of Neoplasia*, Ed. C. H. G. Price & F. G. M. Ross, p. 219, Butterworths, London. 1973.
14. Allen, B. L. & Frenster, J. H. Low-dose Combination Chemotherapy of Disseminated Human Neoplasms. *Lancet*, **2**, 1324, 1971.
15. Ohno, T. Bronchial Artery Infusion with Anti-cancer Agents in the Treatment of Osteo-Sarcoma. *Cancer*, **27**, 549, 1971.

Chemotherapy of advanced osteosarcoma

by

ENGRACIO P. CORTES, JAMES F. HOLLAND, JAW J. WANG and
LUCIUS F. SINKS

SUMMARY

A report is presented of 17 patients with osteosarcoma of long bones treated by Adria-mycin. All except one had had previous treatment, 14 by amputation. Objective regression of pulmonary metastases occurred in seven patients with survivals from 4 to 20 + months: among the eight non-responders the median survival was 3·5 months—range 0·5 to 5 months. Metastasis shrinkage over 50% was seen in five patients, and in one there was complete disappearance. The behaviour of lung metastases suggested more susceptibility to Adriamycin anti-tumor effect and diminished malignancy in those with delayed manifestation. Multiple drug courses were beneficial. Drug toxicity was noted: temporary alopecia, pancytopenia, stomatitis, deranged liver function and there was fatal cardiomyopathy in two patients. Anti-tumor effects were all accompanied by myelosuppression.

INTRODUCTION

THE 5-YEAR SURVIVAL RATE of osteogenic sarcoma regardless of primary therapy (surgery, radiation or the combination of the two) ranges from 5 to 23%.[1-12] The efficacy of chemotherapy in the disseminated stage has always been low. Among the alkylating agents cyclophosphamide and phenylalanine mustard achieve response rates of 11·5 and 14·2% in 26 and seven cases respectively.[13-16] No series were reported using nitrogen mustard, Thiotepa, chlorambucil, or busulfan. Vincristine has shown no responses in eight cases.[17-18] Few data are reported on antimetabolites. 5-Fluorouracil has been reported in only two cases but one had complete remission.[19] There are no available published data on 6-mercaptopurine, 6-thioguanine, or cytosine arabinoside. Trials of high-dose methotrexate with citrovorum factor rescue have stimulated a great interest because of recent evidence of activity in osteosarcoma.[20]

Among the cytotoxic antibiotics Mitomycin C has been the most extensively studied of all chemotherapeutic modalities in osteosarcoma. Its response rate is almost identical to that observed with the alkylating agents with 16% responses.[21-23] Actinomycin D, one of the most active agents in osteosarcoma in animal studies[24,25] has unfortunately not been evaluated as a single agent. Combination chemotherapy has also not been extensively tested in this disease.

Adriamycin is a cytotoxic antibiotic derived from streptomyces peucetius variant caesius[26] found to have a broad spectrum of anti-tumor activity.[27-32] It is a hydroxy-methyl analog of Daunorubicin and its chemical structure is shown in Fig. 1.

The subject of this report is our updated data on Adriamycin in advanced osteosarcoma which is presently in press.[33]

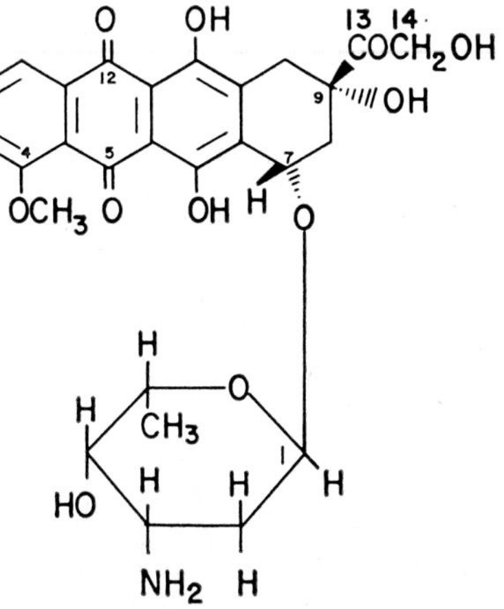

Fig. 1. Structural formula of Adriamycin

MATERIALS AND METHODS

Seventeen patients with pulmonary metastases from osteosarcoma, 14 of whom had amputation of the tumor as the primary treatment were treated with Adriamycin at various doses. All subjects were patients at Roswell Park Memorial Institute during the period of evaluation and treatment. This report is limited by definition to those tumors in which tumor osteoid or bone arise in direct apposition to neoplastic cells. No effort was made to subclassify osteosarcoma further into chondroblastic, fibroblastic, and osteo-blastic subtypes. None of our patients belonged to a subdivision of parosteal osteogenic sarcoma, chondrosarcoma, fibrosarcoma, radiation induced osteosarcoma or osteogenic sarcoma following Paget's disease, all of which have an entirely different course and prognostic implication.

The extent of disease was carefully defined by clinical measurement, roentgenologic study, and biochemical examination. Hematologic, biochemical and electrocardiographic tests were conducted before and during therapy as a measure of the tumor function, response of the tumor to therapy, and toxicity of the drug.

Evaluation of response to therapy was based on objective and subjective changes. Well defined pulmonary metastases were measured in three dimensions. The criteria for evaluation of an objective response were: (a) complete remission—100% disappearance of objective signs of cancer, (b) partial remission—tumor regression of 50 to 99% by volume in the absence of the appearance of new lesions or tumor progression elsewhere, (c) improvement—tumor regression between 25 to 49%, (d) no change—change in tumor size $\pm 25\%$, and (e) progression—unambiguous increase in tumor size of more than 25%.

Drug and dosage

Adriamycin was obtained from Farmitalia, Milan, Italy, through the National Cancer Institute, U.S.A. It is supplied as an orange-red crystalline material readily soluble in water. Each vial contains 10 mg powder dissolved in 10 ml of 0·9% saline at a concentration of 1 mg/ml. The calculated dose was injected directly into the tubing of a running intravenous infusion. Care was taken to avoid extravasation of the drug which might cause chemical cellulitis and necrosis.

Dose schedules used ranged from 17·5 to 35 mg/m²/day for 3 or 4 days. The course was then repeated at 4-week intervals if hematological toxicity had cleared.

RESULTS

Seventeen patients with pulmonary metastases from osteosarcoma whose ages ranged from 8 to 37 years were treated with Adriamycin. Tables 1 and 2 show the clinical data of

TABLE 1. CLINICAL DATA OF PATIENTS BEFORE ADRIAMYCIN THERAPY

Case No.	Age, Sex	Interval from onset of symptoms to diagnosis (months)	Primary Tumor site	Interval from diagnosis to pulmonary metastases	Previous therapy			Interval from pulmonary metastases to Adriamycin treatment
					Surgery	Radio-therapy	Chemotherapy	
1	14F	1	LDF	5	+	0	0	0
2	13F	2	RDF	13	+	0	0	0
3	13M	4	RDF	4	0	+	VCR, CTX	6
4	15M	2	LDF	0	0	0	0	1
5	8M	2	LDR	3	+	0	X-rayed tumor cells	6
6	14F	1	LDF	7	+	0	0	7
7	23M	2	LU	29	+	0	5-FU, MYX CTX	4
8	16F	2	LDF	12	+	0	Dact., CTX VCR	17
9	16M	2	LDF	7	+	0	X-rayed tumor cells	1
10	17M	2	RT	5	+	0	0	1
11	19M	2	LT	6	+	0	L-PAM, Dact.	1
12	15M	1	RT	5	+	0	0	3
13	22M	1	LDF	5	0	+	Dact., CTX, MTX	4
14	17M	1	RDF	3	+	0	0	1
15	20M	2	LT	33	+	0	0	3
16	37F	1	LH	9	+	+	TSPA	4
17	34F	5	RDF	1	+	0	X-rayed tumor cells 5-FU, CTX, MTX	5

LDF—left distal femur; RDF—right distal femur; LDR—left distal radius; LU—left ulna; RT—right tibia; LT—left tibia; LH—left humerus; RPF—right proximal femur; VCR—vincristine; 5-FU—5-Fluorouracil; MTX—Methotrexate; CTX—Cyclophosphamide; Dact.—Actinomycin D; L-PAM—L-Phenylalanine Mustard; TSPA—Thiotepa.

these patients prior to and during Adriamycin therapy, respectively. Objective regression of the pulmonary lesions were observed in seven patients. One had complete remission, five partial remissions, and one improvement by 25%. Of the seven patients responding to treatment, five had objective regression after the first course of therapy. This was detected 2 to 4 weeks after the initial dose. Two patients had an initial increase of their tumor after the first course but tumor regression was evident after the second course of Adriamycin. Repeated courses resulted in continuing regression of the pulmonary lesion, except in one patient whose lesion reached a plateau after the fourth course of therapy.

TABLE 2. CLINICAL DATA OF PATIENTS DURING ADRIAMYCIN THERAPY

Case No.	Adriamycin dose schedule mg/m^2 10	Extent of lung nodules at start of ADM treatment	WBC nadir after first course of Rx 4,000 mm^3	Response	Total ADM dose mg/m^2	Duration of control (months)	Interval from initial ADM Rx to death (months)	Status
1	17·5 × 4	M	3,100	*	105		2·5	Dead, osteosarcoma with massive lung metastases
2	20 × 4	S	3,100	‖	560	20+		NED
3	20 × 4	M		†	160		6	Dead, osteosarcoma with massive lung and liver metastases
4	20 × 4	M		*	160		3·5	Dead, osteosarcoma with massive lung metastases
5	20 × 4	S	3,000	*	160		2·5	Dead, osteosarcoma involving lungs, lymph nodes (thorax, abdomen, pelvis), liver, diaphragm, meninges and bones
6	20 × 4	M		*	240		5	Dead, osteosarcoma with massive lung metastases
7	30 × 3	M	2,600	§	900	10	10	Dead, osteosarcoma with lung metastases, cardiomyopathy from adriamycin
8	30 × 3	M	1,180	§	360	4		Alive
9	30 × 3	M	1,300	§	240	3		Alive
10	30 × 3	M		†	315			Alive
11	30 × 3	M	1,150	*	180		3	Dead, osteosarcoma with massive lung metastases
12	30 × 3	M		*	270		4	Dead, no autopsy
13	30 × 3	M	1,400	*	285		4	Dead, no autopsy
14	35 × 3	M**	2,600	§	1125	12·5	12·5	Pneumonectomy in ninth month, NED. Died from adriamycin induced cardiomyopathy
15	35 × 3	M	1,600	§	650	5	12	Dead, osteosarcoma with massive lung metastases
16	35 × 3	M	800	‡	105		4	Dead, no autopsy
17	35 × 3	M	105	*	105		0·5	Dead, osteosarcoma with massive lung metastases

ADM—Adriamycin; M—multiple bilateral; S—solitary unilateral; * progression, † no change, ‡ improvement.
§ partial remission, ‖ complete remission.
NED—no evidence of disease;
** localized on one lung.

The survival from the start of therapy among the eight non-responders was 0·5 to 5 months, with a median of 3·5 months. In those who achieved objective responses, remission lasted from 4 to 20+ months. Figure 2 shows the relationship of the drug response to survival in months after onset of pulmonary metastases, and the interval in months from the initial diagnosis to metastases. Of the 13 patients whose pulmonary metastases appeared less than 10 months after the initial primary diagnosis, only two had achieved partial remission. Of the four patients whose pulmonary metastases were discovered more than 10 months from the initial diagnosis, all four attained a complete or partial remission. Furthermore, those responding patients with later appearing metastases had a longer survival than those patients whose metastases were noted less than 10 months from onset of diagnosis.

Adriamycin toxicity

The clinical toxicity of Adriamycin in 17 patients is shown in Table 3. All patients treated showed signs of toxicity. Almost total capital alopecia was seen in 17 patients. Hair loss also occurred prominently in all other areas: beard, axillae, eyebrows, eyelashes, pubis and trunk. Hair loss was observed 2 to 3 weeks after therapy and began to grow in 2 to 3 months after Adriamycin administration was discontinued. Repeated courses of

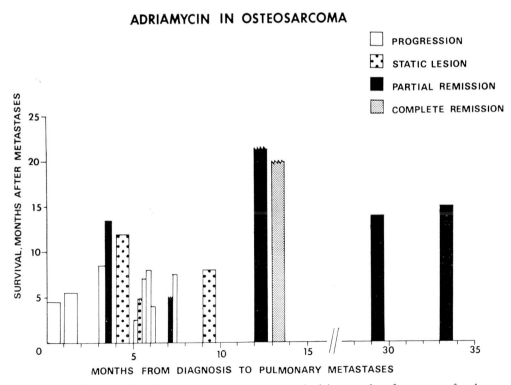

Fig. 2. Relationship of the drug response to survival in months after onset of pulmonary metastases, and the interval in months from the initial diagnosis to metastases.

the drug rendered the patient persistently bald during treatment. Permanent alopecia has not occurred and corporeal hair returned.

TABLE 3. ADRIAMYCIN TOXICITY IN OSTEOSARCOMA

Toxicity	No. of cases	% of Total cases
Alopecia	17	100
WBC < 4000/mm³	12	70
Nausea and vomiting	11	64
Stomatitis	11	64
Hb. drop > 2 gms%	8	47
Platelets < 100,000/mm³	6	35
Elevation of liver enzymes	3	18
Fatal cardiomyopathy	2	12

Twelve patients had leukopenia at their nadir of 4,000 mm³ or less. Eight patients had hemoglobin drop of at least 2 gms% and six had platelet counts below 100,000 mm³. The depression of the hemoglobin, leukocytes, and platelets seemed to parallel one another. The leukocyte nadir usually occurred 8 to 16 days from the initial treatment and recovery of the blood counts was noted 7 to 14 days after the nadir was reached. Figure 3 illustrates the hematological alteration during Adriamycin therapy in Case 2.

Stomatitis with tender tongue and/or ulceration of the buccal mucosa and palate occurred in 11 patients and was usually severe resulting in difficulty of swallowing. These symptoms usually occur 2 to 3 days prior to the nadir of leukopenia. Relief from stomatitis is usually noted 5 to 8 days after its onset. Nausea with or without emesis occurred in 11 patients. It began shortly or 12 to 24 hours after the drug was given and was usually relieved by phenothiazine injections.

Fatal cardiomyopathy appeared suddenly in two patients, 10 and 12·5 months after Adriamycin. The drug was given in cumulative doses of 900 and 1,125 mg/m², respectively. No serial EKG changes or prodromal signs or symptoms were noted prior to the onset of congestive heart failure. These two cases also had LDH and alkaline phosphatase elevation with centrilobular necrosis of the liver ascribed to Adriamycin toxicity. Another patient developed elevated LDH, SGOT, alkaline phosphatase and bilirubin after three courses of Adriamycin. No significant changes in kidney function test were noted that might be ascribed to Adriamycin toxicity.

More severe leukopenia (WBC of 3,000 mm³ and below) was noted in nine patients who had induction dose of 30 to 35 mg/m²/day × 3. Six of these nine patients had tumor regression (one of 25%). Only one of six patients who received Adriamycin at doses of 17·5 to 20 mg/m²/day for 3 or 4 days sustained tumor regression and three of the six had leukopenia. None of the five patients who had no leukopenia responded to Adriamycin therapy, as shown in Fig. 4. Thus, antitumor effects were paralleled by myelosuppressive effects.

Footnote:
  LDH Lactic Dehydrogenase.
  SGOT Serum glutamate-oxalacetate transaminase.

HEMATOLOGIC ALTERATION DURING ADRIAMYCIN THERAPY

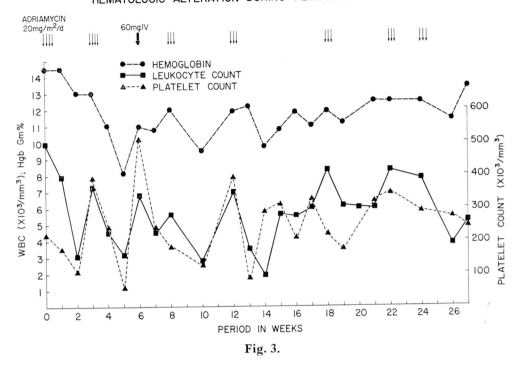

Fig. 3.

OSTEOSARCOMA
DOSE, LEUKOPENIA AND RESPONSE TO ADM

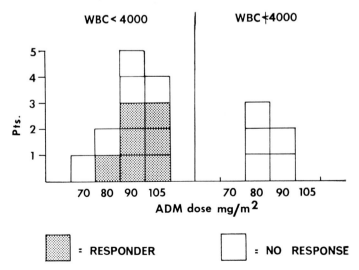

Fig. 4. Relationship of Adriamycin dose (per course), leukopenia and tumor response.

CASE REPORTS

Case 2. J.L., a 13-year-old girl, had a right mid-thigh amputation in June 1969 because of osteosarcoma of the distal femur. In July 1970, a solitary metastatic spherical nodule 1·5 cm in diameter was found in the left lung, (Fig. 5) and Adriamycin treatment was initiated at 20 mg/m²/day for 4 days. A month later, regression of the nodule began. She was maintained on a 3- or 4-day course of Adriamycin at monthly intervals. In October 1970, no appreciable lung lesion could be seen either by regular films or tomogram. Adriamycin therapy was stopped after 9 months in March 1971 after a cumulative dose of 560 mg/m², and she remained free of disease for 20+ months now, 1 year off treatment. (Fig. 5(b).)

Case 7. D.B., a 23-year-old male, had a left supracondylar amputation in September 1968 because of osteosarcoma of terminal ulna. He was found to have pulmonary metastases in November 1970 and was started on weekly 5-Fluorouracil, Methotrexate and Cyclophosphamide for 12 doses in December 1970. Because of disease progression in March 1971 (Fig. 6(a)) Adriamycin was initiated at 30 mg/m²/day for 3 days. He achieved a partial regression of his pulmonary lesions on monthly 3-day courses of Adriamycin (Fig. 6(b)). Ten months after the start of therapy and a cumulative total dose of 900 mg/m² of Adriamycin he was admitted to the hospital because of sudden onset of shortness of breath and orthopnoea of 1 day's duration. His congestive heart failure responded to digitalization and diuretics, but he died of cardiogenic shock 24 hours after admission. Autopsy examination disclosed a heart weight of 425 gms. The heart was dilated and had interstitial edema of the myocardial muscle on light microscopy.

Case 8. M.S., a 16-year-old girl, who had left hip disarticulation in May 1969 because of osteosarcoma of the distal femur. A year later she was given Actinomycin D and Cyclophosphamide because of pulmonary metastases, attaining a partial remission. In

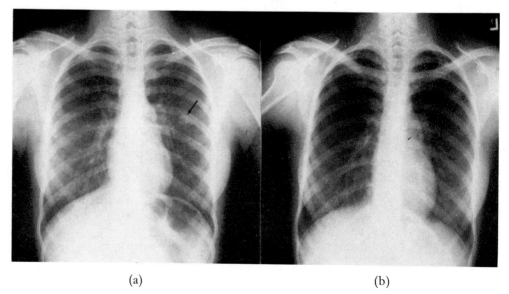

(a)   (b)

Fig. 5. Chest x-ray (a) before and (b) after repeated Adriamycin therapy (Case 2).

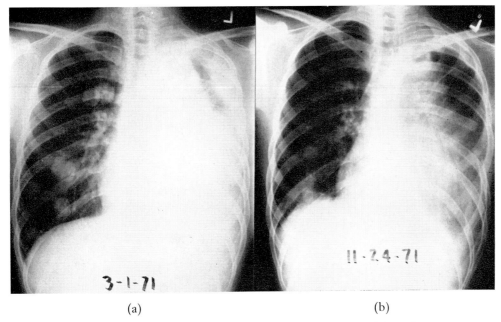

Fig. 6. Chest x-rays of Case 7. (a) before and (b) after repeated Adriamycin treatment.

March 1971 her tumor began to grow and did not respond to Vincristine. In October 1971 Adriamycin was initiated at 30 mg/m²/day for 3 days resulting in a partial tumor regression on repeated monthly 3-day courses. Her pulmonary lesion reached a plateau after 4 courses of Adriamycin, and the drug was discontinued.

Case 9. R.M., a 16-year-old boy, who had left mid-thigh amputation in June 1971 because of osteosarcoma of the distal femur. He was then vaccinated by others with irradiated osteosarcoma tumor cells and BCG monthly for four occasions. In November 1971, pulmonary metastases were noted; he was started on Adriamycin 20 mg/m²/day × 3 in December 1971. Rapid growth of the tumor continued (Fig. 7(a)). A second course of Adriamycin at 30 mg/m²/day × 3 was given in January 1972 and was repeated 18 days later. This resulted in a marked regression of the tumor 7 weeks after the initiation of the higher dose (Fig. 7(b)). No further Adriamycin was given because of abnormalities in liver function tests attributed to Adriamycin administration. The tumor has started to increase in size again.

Case 14. G.D., a 17-year-old boy, had a right hip disarticulation in June 1970 because of osteosarcoma of the distal femur. Three months later three pulmonary masses in the right lung were noted, one only on lateral film (Fig. 8(a) and (b)). Adriamcyin treatment at 35 mg/m²/day for 3 days was started in October 1970 which resulted in disappearance of the two smaller nodules and progression in size of the larger mass a month after the first course of therapy (Fig. 8(c)). Adriamycin administration was pursued in the same 3-day courses resulting in partial regression of the remaining lesion (Fig. 8(d)). A hypothetical total regression curve (Fig. 9) indicated a very long course of chemotherapy probably lay ahead, assuming cumulative drug toxicity and tumor resistance would not

K*

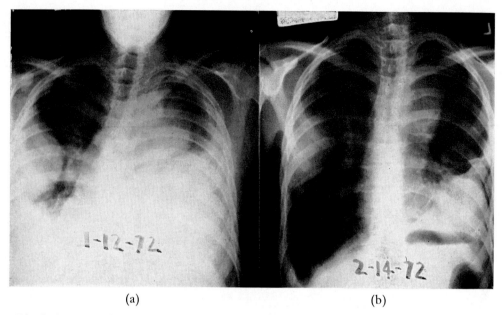

(a)   (b)

Fig. 7. (a) Chest film of Case 9 where tumor progressed after a low dose of Adriamycin. (b) chest x-ray more than a month later after 2 courses of Adriamycin at a higher dose.

occur. Pneumonectomy was therefore performed 9 months after the initial Adriamycin treatment. The lung specimen revealed a residual solitary spherical mass 3 cm in diameter. The two smaller lesions seen on initial chest X-ray were not found. Another course of Adriamycin was given. Three and one half months after pneumonectomy, he had sudden onset of right hemiparesis and dysphasia. He died 2 weeks after admission. Autopsy revealed a dilated heart weighing 450 gms with a ventricular mural thrombus. Light microscopy of the myocardial muscle revealed interstitial edema. Brain sections showed left cerebral emboli. No evidence of tumor was found. He received a total cumulative dose of 1125 mg/m² of Adriamycin in a 12·5 months period.

Case 15. P.W., a 21-year-old man, had a mid-thigh amputation in August 1967 because of osteosarcoma of the left tibia. Thirty-three months later bilateral pulmonary metastases were noted (Fig. 10(a)). Adriamycin at 35 mg/m²/day × 3 was started in August 1970 resulting in tumor liquefaction 2 weeks later. Severe anemia, leukopenia, and stomatitis occurred after each 3-day course of Adriamycin on four occasions, so the dose was decreased to 30 mg/m²/day × 3 on the fifth course. (Fig. 10(b).) A month later tumor progression was noted. A clinical trial of Guanazole was begun, but the tumor continued to grow. Resumption of Adriamycin at 35 mg/m²/day × 3, 3½ months after the last Adriamycin was given failed to slow the rapidly growing tumor and he died 12 months after the initiation of chemotherapy.

Case 16. A 37-year-old woman, had a shoulder disarticulation in November 1968 for osteosarcoma of the humerus. After the first course of Adriamycin, she had at least 25% regression of her multiple pulmonary nodules with some clinical improvement. She did not return for follow-up and died 4 months after the initial treatment.

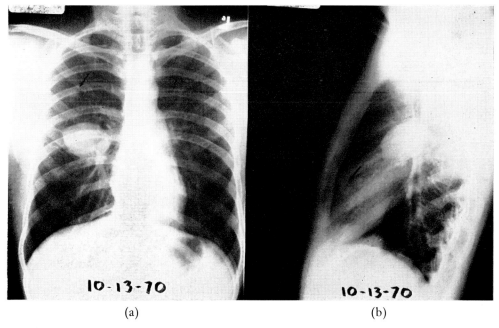

(a)   (b)

Fig. 8. Chest films of Case 14 before Adriamycin therapy. (a) posteroanterior view. (b) lateral view.

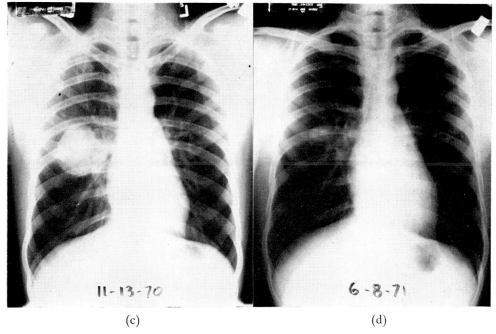

(c)   (d)

Fig. 8. (c) shows further increase of tumor mass after a course of therapy. (d) repeated courses of Adriamycin resulted in further tumor regression.

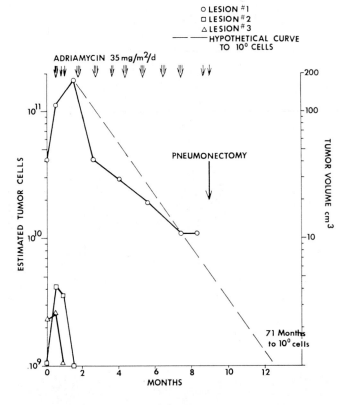

Fig. 9. Tumor volume of three unilateral pulmonary metastases of osteosarcoma measured by serial x-ray examination during Adriamycin treatment. The volumes are transformed to cell numbers by assuming 10^9 cells/cm³. The hypothetical regression line is shown. See text (Case 14).

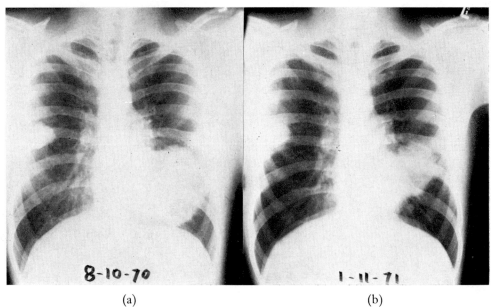

(a)   (b)

Fig. 10. Chest x-rays of Case 15 (a) before and (b) after Adriamycin therapy.

DISCUSSION

Sweetnam *et al.*[11] noted that for any treatment regimen for osteosarcoma (surgery, radiation or both), the median time to metastatic disease was 10 months. McKenna *et al.*[12] reported that at least 95% of the autopsied osteogenic sarcoma patients had demonstrable lung metastases. The average period between the discovery of pulmonary metastases and death was 6 months.[11]

Based on a meager history of chemotherapeutic effects in disseminated osteosarcoma, it is encouraging to see objective regressions in 41% of patients with this refractory disease when treated with Adriamycin (Fig. 11). The regression consisted of a shrinkage of more than 50% volume reduction in five patients and disappearance of a lesion in the lung in one patient. These results are provocative since osteosarcoma has such a poor prognosis even when initially considered operable. The nature of the remissions left no doubt that the growth of the tumor in these responding patients was dramatically altered. In some responding patients, prolongation of survival after the onset of pulmonary metastases seems real. Objective response ($>50\%$) occurred in four of four patients whose pulmonary lesions appeared 10 months and more after the initial diagnosis but in only two of 13 cases whose metastatic lesions appeared in less than 10 months. Although our series is small, this seems to correlate with the findings of McKenna *et al.*[12] They found that those patients with a longer average interval from onset of symptoms to initiation of treatment had a better prognosis than those with short duration of symptoms (7·3 months vs. 3·7 months). They also noted that 90% of the therapeutic failures (surgical ablation) were treated within 6 months of the onset of their symptoms, whereas 55% of cures were not treated until a longer interval had elapsed. These observations reflect a more malignant course manifest by shorter interval from onset of symptoms to primary treatment and earlier onset of pulmonary metastases from initial primary diagnosis,

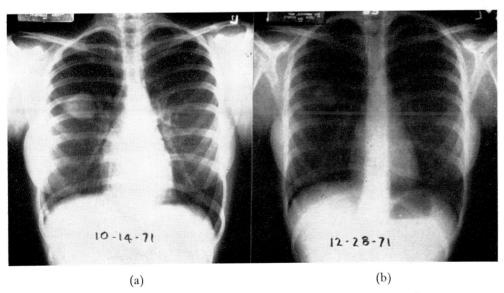

(a)   (b)

Fig. 11. Chest films of Case 8 (a) before and (b) after Adriamycin therapy.

whereas a lingering indolent prodrome may suggest a less aggressive tumor, greater host immunity or other factors at work.

Of the 17 patients, only two had metastases localized to one lung and these patients (Case 2 and 14) are our best responders. This suggests that Adriamycin therapy at an earlier stage of the disease before serious compromise of the host by extensive metastases may be a factor of importance.

The onset of the observed regressions was apparent within one month of the initial course of Adriamycin, except in two cases who required at least two courses before regression of the tumor took place. The regressions were maintained by multiple courses of Adriamycin at regular intervals. A suitable interval appears to be approximately 3 to 4 weeks as soon as the hematological toxicity has cleared.

The dosage of Adriamycin employed in the present study that produced the most frequent antitumor effects seemed to be the one that produced the most frequent leukopenia, i.e., 30 to 35 mg/m^2/day for 3 days. As with many chemotherapeutic agents the therapeutic index is small.

The manifestations of Adriamycin toxicity in this series consisted of alopecia, pancytopenia, stomatitis, nausea and vomiting and abnormal liver function tests. The occurrence of fatal cardiomyopathy in two cases with an accumulating dose of Adriamycin requires close cardiac monitoring by means of frequent EKG and may limit the total cumulative dose of Adriamycin.

Despite of the known toxic manifestations of Adriamycin, these do not preclude the practical application of this drug in the treatment of osteogenic sarcoma, a usually fatal neoplasm. The activity of Adriamycin in this refractory advanced tumor supports its exploration as a short-term adjuvant therapy with treatment of localized primary tumor because of the probability of subclinical micrometastases, a program which we are pursuing at present.

ACKNOWLEDGMENTS

This investigation was supported by U.S. Public Health Service Grants Nos. CA–5834, CA–2599 and CA–07918 from the National Cancer Institute.

From the Department of Medicine A, and Department of Pediatrics, Roswell Park Memorial Institute, Buffalo, New York.

REFERENCES

1. Cade, S., Osteogenic Sarcoma, A Study based on 133 patients. *J. roy. Coll. Surg., Edinb.*, **1**, 79–111, 1955.
2. Weinfeld, M. S. & Dudley, H. R. Osteogenic Sarcoma. *J. Bone Jt. Surg.*, **44–A**, 269–277, 1962.
3. Copeland, M. M. Primary Malignant Tumors of Bone. Evaluation of Current Diagnosis and Treatment. *Cancer*, **20**, 738–746, 1967.
4. Marcove, R. C., Miké, V., Hajek, J. V., Levin, A. G. & Hutter, R. V. P. Osteogenic Sarcoma in Childhood. *N.Y. St. J. Med.*, **7**, 855–859, 1971.
5. Phelan, J. T. & Cabrera, A. Osteosarcoma of Bone. *Surg., Gynec. Obstet.*, **118**, 330–336, 1964.
6. Lindbom, A., Soderberg, G. & Spjut, H. J. Osteosarcoma, A Review of 96 cases. *Acta. Radiol. (Stockholm)*, **56**, 1–19, 1961.

7. Hayles, A. B., Dahlin, D. C. & Coventry, M. B. Osteogenic Sarcoma in Children. *J. Amer. Med. Ass.*, **174**, 1174–1177, 1960.
8. Tudway, R. C. Radiotherapy for Osteogenic Sarcoma. *J. Bone Jt. Surg.*, **43–B**, 61–67, 1961.
9. Dahlin, D. C. & Coventry, M. B., Osteogenic Sarcoma, A Study of Six Hundred Cases. *J. Bone Jt. Surg.*, **49–A**, 101–110, 1967.
10. Coventry, M. B. & Dahlin, D. C. Osteogenic Sarcoma, A Critical Analysis of 430 Cases. *J. Bone Jt. Surg.*, **39–A**, 741–758, 1957.
11. Sweetnam, D. R., Knowelden, J. & Seddon, H. Bone Sarcoma: Treatment by Irradiation, Amputation or a Combination of the Two. *Brit. Med. J.* **2**, 363–367, 1971.
12. McKenna, R. J., Schwinn, C. P., Soong, K. Y. & Higinbotham, N. L. Sarcoma of the Osteogenic Series (Osteosarcoma, Fibrosarcoma, Chondrosarcoma, Parosteal Osteogenic Sarcoma, and Sarcomata Arising in Abnormal Bone). *J. Bone Jt. Surg.*, **48–A**, 1–26, 1966.
13. Sutow, W. W., Vietti, T. J., Fernbach, D. J., Lane, D. H., Donaldson, M. & Lonsdale, D. Evaluation of Chemotherapy with Metastatic Ewing's Sarcoma and Osteogenic Sarcoma. *Cancer Chem. Rep.*, **55**, 67–78, 1971.
14. Pinkel, D. Cyclophosphamide in Children with Cancer. *Cancer*, **15**, 42–49, 1962.
15. Haggard, M. E. Cyclophosphamide (NSC–26271) in the Treatment of Children with Malignant Neoplasms. *Cancer Chem. Rep.*, **51**, 403–405, 1967.
16. Sullivan, M. P., Sutow, W. W. & Taylor, G. L–Phenylalanine Mustard as a Treatment for Metastatic Osteogenic Sarcoma in Children. *J. Pediat.*, **63**, 227–237, 1963.
17. Sutow, W. W. Vincristine (NSC–67574) Therapy for Malignant Solid Tumors in Children (except Wilms' Tumor). *Cancer Chem. Rep.*, **52**, 485–487, 1968.
18. Selawry, O., Holland, J. & Wolman, I. J. Effect of Vincristine (NSC–67574) on Malignant Solid Tumors in Children. *Cancer Chem. Rep.*, **52**, 497–500, 1968.
19. Groesbeck, H. P. & Cudmore, J. T. Evaluation of 5–Fluorouracil (5–FU) in Surgical Practice. *American Surgeon*, **29**, 683–691, 1963.
20. Jaffe, N. Recent Advances in the Chemotherapy of Metastatic Osteogenic Sarcoma. *Cancer* **30**, 1627–1631. 1972.
21. Evans, A. E. Mitomycin C. *Cancer Chem. Rep.*, **14**, 1–9, 1961.
22. Evans, A. E. Heyn, R. M., Nesbit, M. E. & Hartmann, J. R. Evaluation of Mitomycin C (NSC–26980) in the Treatment of Metastatic Osteogenic Sarcoma. *Cancer Chem. Rep.*, **53**, 297–298, 1969.
23. Sutow, W. W., Wilbur, J. R., Vietti, T. J., Vuthibhagdee, P., Fujimoto, T. & Watanabe, A. Evaluation of Dosage Schedules of Mitomycin C (NSC–26980) in Children. *Cancer Chem. Rep.*, **55**, 285–289, 1971.
24. D'Angio, G. J., Maddock, Charlotte, L., Farber, S. & Brown, Barbara B. The Enhanced Response of the Ridgway Osteogenic Sarcoma to Roentgen Radiation Combined with Actinomycin D. *Cancer Res.*, **25**, 1002–1007, 1965.
25. Schwartz, H. S., Sodergren, J. E., Sternberg, S. S. & Philips, F. S. Actomycin D: Effect on Ridgway Osteogenic Sarcoma in Mice. *Cancer Res.*, **26**, 1873–1879, 1966.
26. Arcamone, F., Cassinelli, G., Fantini, G., Grein, A., Crezzi, P., Spalla, C. & Pol, C. Adriamycin from S. Peucetius var. Caesius. *Biotech. and Bioeng.* **XI**, 1101–1110, 1969.
27. Bonadonna, G., Monfardini, S., De Lena, M., Fossati-Bellani, F. & Beretta, G. Phase I and Preliminary Phase II Evaluation of Adriamycin, (NSC–123127). *Cancer Res.*, **30**, 2572–2582, 1970.
28. Tan, C., Wollner, N., King, O. & Ilano, D. Adriamycin, A New Antibiotic in Treatment of Childhood Leukemia and Other Malignant Neoplasms. *Proc. Amer. Ass. Cancer Res.*, **11**, 79, 1970.
29. Wang, J. J., Cortes, E. P., Sinks, L. F. & Holland, J. F. Therapeutic Effect and Toxicity of Adriamycin in Patients with Neoplastic Disease. *Cancer*, **28**, 837–843, 1971.
30. Middleman, E., Luce, L. & Frei, E. III. Clinical Trials with Adriamycin. *Cancer* **28**, 844–850, 1971.
31. Mathé, G., Amiel, J-L., Hayat, M., De Vassal, F., Schwarzenberg, L., Schneider, M., Jasmin, C. & Rosenfeld, C. Essai de L'Adriamycin dans le Traitment des Leucemies Aiques. *La Press Médicale*, **78**, 1997–1999, 1970.

32. Cortes, E. P., Ellison, R. R. & Yates, J. Adriamycin in the Treatment of Adult Acute Myelocytic Leukemia. *Cancer Chem. Rep.* In press, 1972.
33. Cortes, E. P., Holland, J. F., Wang, J. J. & Sinks, L. F. Adriamycin in Disseminated Osteosarcoma. *J. Amer. Ass. Med.* In press, 1972.

Discussion

Dr. Hale (Chairman)   I would like to ask Dr. Cortes, does he consider the presence of liver metastases a contraindication to the use of Adriamycin? Or was it in one case because of evidence of gross liver failure that he had to stop treatment?

Dr. Cortes   The presence of liver metastases does not contraindicate the use of Adriamycin. However if the liver function tests are moderately impaired, like elevation of liver enzymes and bilirubin, then one can cut down the dose of Adriamycin because of a possible delay or impaired metabolism of the drug thus resulting in more pronounced toxicity. We stopped the treatment in the particular case in question because we were really not sure about the cause of deranged liver function. But while in the process of investigating it his pulmonary metastases increased in size, so we had to discontinue Adriamycin definitely.

Dr. Brenner   I've had occasion to use Adriamycin in osteosarcoma, and I must admit that the low doses that we used, after discussion with Dr. Cortes, appear to have been inadequate. We certainly didn't see any response. We have used Adriamycin in combination with Cytoxan and Vincristine for fibrosarcoma and have been quite astonished to see partial responses that are still proceeding at the moment. From Dr. Bonadonna's symposium in Italy some time ago, he came to the conclusion that Adriamycin on its own was not an effective drug. He suggests that in fact one should use it in combination with other drugs. I would like to ask Dr. Cortes whether they have considered combined usage of other drugs with Adriamycin for the resistant cases?

Dr. Cortes   No we have not, but recently some exciting results with high-dose Methotrexate with citrovorum rescue in metastatic osteosarcoma was reported by a group from Boston. Because of their results and our Adriamycin effect a co-operative study group for osteosarcoma was formed by the National Cancer Institute. The group is proposing a combination of Adriamycin and/or Methotrexate and 5-Fluorouracil.

Dr. Jeffree   I'm sorry Dr. Cortes I didn't understand your dosage.

Dr. Cortes   Our most effective schedule ranged from 30 to 35 mg per square metre daily for 3 days, repeated every 4 weeks as soon as the blood counts are back to normal. The square metre of course refers to body surface area.

Mr. McCormack   How do you measure that?

Dr. Cortes   There is a nomograph for calculating body surface area. This consists of three vertical scales of height, surface area, and weight. A straight edge is placed on the

281

nomograph so that it goes through the points of height of the patient in inches or centi-metres and weight in pounds or kilograms. The body surface area is read at the inter-section of the straight edge with the surface area scale.

Dr. Perry I think that with the report from Buffalo and also that from the Children's Hospital, Boston, which Dr. Cortes referred to about the usage of massive doses of Methotrexate, a good deal is being done now in the States about the treatment of osteogenic sarcoma. I think this has given rise to co-operative group studies that Dr. Cortes mentioned. At the Children's Hospital, the reports that I've heard they have had 12 or 15 cases, four of which showed complete or partial remissions, two complete remissions being in those patients with pulmonary metastases. As a consequence at the Cancer Institute we formed a working party to pool the representatives from these various institutions, also to include Dr. D. L. Morton from the West Coast who has done a lot of studies on the immunological aspects of osteogenic sarcoma. One other point concerning the Adriamycin cardiac toxicity, I think Dr. Cortes that you had two cases of failure—is that correct?

Dr. Cortes Yes.

Dr. Perry I thought you said 12.

Dr. Cortes No, 12%: two out of 17.

Dr. Perry The cause of this has really been quite obscure. There was a report several years ago from this country by Dr. Barbara Smith at St. Batholomew's Hospital in the *British Heart Journal*, so it has escaped the oncologists all this time. She suggested on the basis of her experimental studies that the cardiac neurones showed some degenerative changes. We are currently pursuing this to see if that in fact is the case. Since ,as Dr. Cortes has indicated Adriamycin appears to be one of the most widely active compounds in the solid tumours that we have ever seen, this is a very critical problem.

Dr. Cortes We recently analysed the cardiotoxicity in 115 adult patients with various cancers treated with Adriamycin. Of the 100 evaluable patients with serial electro-cardiogram studies, 14 patients received a total Adriamycin dose of over 600 mg per square metre and seven of these 14 developed congestive heart failure. None of the 86 patients who had Adriamycin less than 600 mg per square metre had heart failure. We conclude, therefore, that though a valuable anti-tumour agent, administration beyond the cumulative cardiotoxic threshold of 600 mg per square metre must be approached with caution.

Dr. Makley I should just like to ask Dr Cortes about the relationship of the responders and the leucocyte count and what were the reasons for this response?

Dr. Cortes It seems that in order for Adriamycin to have its anti-tumour effect in osteosarcoma, a moderate drop of the leucocyte count is necessary. The leukopenia-antitumour effect of Adriamycin fortunately does not hold true in other types of malig-nancy like lymphomas for example. The tumour response and the leukopenia induced were demonstrated clearly in one case reported whose leucocyte count stayed within normal limits with concomitant increase in tumour size after receiving Adriamycin at 20 mg per square metre daily for 3 days. But with the induction of leukopenia at a higher dose of 30 mg per square metre daily for 3 days dramatic tumour regression was noted.

Professor Bonfiglio   If you have to induce leukopenia with Adriamycin before you can get a response, why is it that a leukopenia induced by other drugs doesn't do the same thing?

Dr. Cortes   No two drugs are the same. One drug demonstrates a different therapeutic index from another. Some could produce a response without inducing leukopenia, but most cytotoxic agents have to induce toxicity before a response is attained. In osteosarcoma it is true that many chemotherapeutic agents could produce lowering of the leucocyte count without any tumour response, but then just like an infectious disease, each micro-organism and tumour has its own drug sensitivity.

Dr. Burwood   I should like to ask Dr. Cortes about the complication rate in his case with complete remission. Were the side effects worse than in the other cases or not?

Dr. Cortes   The patient who attained a complete remission had undergone much toxicity from Adriamycin such as much moderate stomatitis and pancytopenia. During the nadir of leukopenia after her first course of therapy she developed pneumonia and had to be supported vigorously with intravenous antibiotics. She tolerated well the following course of Adriamycin at a lower dose and now she is enjoying a normal life, off therapy and free from disease for over a year.

Dr. Jeffree   What is the point in measuring drug dosage on body surface area rather than weight?

Dr. Cortes   Experience has shown that the dosage of many drugs is proportional to body weight to the 0·7 power.[1] Body surface area has also been found to be approximately proportional to body weight to the 0·7 power; thus drug dosage is directly proportional to body surface area. The relationship between drug dosage and body surface area is purely empirical and has no medical significance; however its use has been suggested as a convenient means of estimating dosages.[2]

Dr. Hale   This has recently been the tendency in paediatrics, although the pendulum is perhaps swinging back a little the other way now.

REFERENCES

1. Dreyer, G. & Walker, E. W. A. Dosage of Drugs, Toxins and Antitoxins. *Proc. R. Soc. Med., Therap. Pharmacol.* Sect. 7, 51, 1914.
2. Talbot, N. B., Richie, R. H. & Crawford, J. D. *Metabolic Homeostasis. A Syllabus for Those Concerned with the Care of Patients.* Cambridge, Harvard University Press, 1959.

Bone scanning

by

V. R. McCREADY

SUMMARY

Bone scans play a valuable part in the diagnosis and treatment of primary and secondary bone tumours. Short-lived isotopes have greatly speeded up the process, although it is still time consuming and, therefore, due attention should be paid to the correct selection of patients for investigation. Whole body scanning is still being evaluated as a method of screening for early metastases. The present techniques could still be greatly improved by reducing the time involved and improving the localization of abnormalities. It would seem that the next stage will be the development of rectilinear scanners specifically for scanning the skeleton with high sensitivity, full or minified displays, and a means of accurately correlating the X-ray and scan. A short-lived bone seeking radiopharmaceutical using $^{99}Tc^m$ as the radioisotope would be a valuable contribution to the technique. This would ensure maximum availability and economy.

INTRODUCTION

BONE SCANNING TECHNIQUES now occupy a secure place in the detection and evaluation of primary and secondary bone tumours as well as a variety of benign bone lesions. The initial enthusiasm for bone scanning, following the discovery that lesions could be detected prior to X-ray techniques,[1] has given way to a more careful evaluation of the isotope methods in relation to other diagnostic methods, particularly in surveying the whole skeleton for early metastatic involvement. There is a feeling now that lesions which were missed on routine X-rays and detected on bone scanning would be considered completely negative on review. Thus bone scanning should be considered as a complementary test and scans and X-rays should be examined together at all times.

A brief consideration of the physiology of bone can help explain many of the apparently anomalous findings between the X-rays and scans. Bone consists of inorganic and organic constituents. The organic part consists of osteoid, cells and ground substance. Radioisotopes known to concentrate in this part include cerium, and gallium in the osteoid tissue, while radiosulphur concentrates in the ground substance and selenium has been shown to label cartilage.[2] In the organic fraction radioisotopes which are known to concentrate include those of calcium, radium, strontium and barium. These isotopes probably replace calcium in the hydroxyapatite crystal while fluorine probably replaces hydroxyl or bicarbonate ions.[3] Recently there has been some evidence to show that isotopes of Indium may also concentrate in bone if enough can be displaced from the plasma proteins.[4]

The concentration of these radioisotopes in bone lesions and normal bone has been studied *in vivo, in vitro* and by biopsy or postmortem specimens.[5] Measurements on the blood following intravenous injection show a rapid clearance from the blood of both strontium and fluorine.[6] The latter clears more quickly, probably due to renal excretion and by one hour the plasma concentration of fluorine is approximately one quarter that of strontium. Gallium citrate is cleared from the blood more slowly due to protein binding.[7] Strontium is excreted through the kidneys and also through the gut. The faecal content of strontium can be seen clearly by 24 hours. The uptake of bone seeking isotopes in normal bone is rapid and in abnormal areas even more so. A clear differential between normal and abnormal bone can be seen by 20 minutes and the tumour : normal ratio increases as time proceeds (Fig. 1). Biopsy studies suggest that most of the uptake

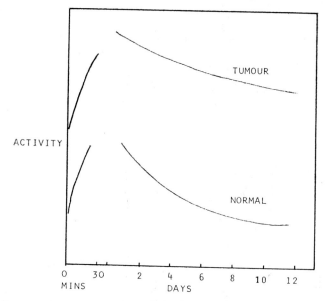

Fig. 1. A diagramatic representation of the initial and subsequent uptake of bone seeking isotopes in tumours and normal bone.

of the isotopes is in the new reactive bone which results from tumour proliferation.[5] Thus dense areas on X-rays where the reaction is complete may show little concentration and, similarly, fast-growing tumours with little reaction may show poor isotope concentration. The latter situation may be seen when there are large osteolytic areas seen on X-rays. Any area of bone formation such as is seen in fractures, joint diseases and degenerative conditions may produce bone seeking radioisotope concentration.

TECHNIQUES

The list of potential bone scanning agents continues to grow. Of these the most widely used are $^{85}Sr\ Cl_2$, ^{18}F, and $^{87}Sr^m\ Cl_2$ (Table 1). Calcium radioisotopes are not used for scanning studies due to dosimetric and instrumental reasons. Strontium-85 is probably the most widely used radioisotope because it has a convenient shelf life.[8] However, as a consequence of its long physical half life, dosimetry considerations limit the maximum activity permitted for injection to 100 μCi. The resulting scans are time consuming but can produce very clear pictures, especially if scanning is delayed. Faecal concentration of strontium may be overcome by bowel washouts or by delaying the scan for up to one week.[9] The alternative $^{87}Sr^m Cl_2$ is generator produced and is thus convenient[10] but expensive unless there is a considerable, and, more important, a regular demand for bone scans. It is possible to inject much higher activities with an improvement in image quality, but since it has a short half life the necessity for early scans results in a higher blood background level. This can produce complications in interpreting the thoracic region.[11]

TABLE 1

BONE SEEKING ISOTOPES

Isotope	Half life	Gamma energy MeV	Production	Whole body radiation dose
^{47}Ca	4·7 days	1·31	Reactor	0·7 R/100 μCi
^{85}Sr	64 days	0·513	Reactor or cyclotron	0·7 R/100 μCi
$^{87}Sr^m$	168 mins.	0·338	^{87}Y Generator	0·02 mR/mCi
^{18}F	112 mins.	0·511	Cyclotron	0·07 R/mCi

Fluorine-18 is cyclotron produced with a very short half life. The rapid blood clearance gives better scans than $^{87}Sr^m$ but also results in high bladder concentrations which tend to mar pictures of the pelvis. It too can be administered safely in millicurie activities.[12]

Bone scanning poses several particular technical problems. The distance between the area of interest and any scanning plane varies widely making setting up procedures difficult. Isosensitive scans of areas other than the thorax are possible by using dual opposed detectors. Alternatively two simultaneous but separate scans may be taken and the variation in detector-bone distance taken into account when interpreting the scans. Some rectilinear scanners have the facility for scanning the whole body during one examination.[8] The resulting picture may be minified to facilitate recording and (some people believe) interpretation. With a large detector the whole skeleton may be surveyed in approximately 40–60 minutes.

The gamma camera may also be used for localized and whole body skeletal examinations.[13] The display is poor but new systems of computer analysis may help piece the pictures together and help improve the contrast between normal and abnormal areas. The anatomical localizing system now available could help to pinpoint lesions.[14]

The localization of lesions found on scans is possible by taking long focal-skin distance X-rays with opaque markers. Transmission scanning has also been used to help localize lesions without distortion.[15]

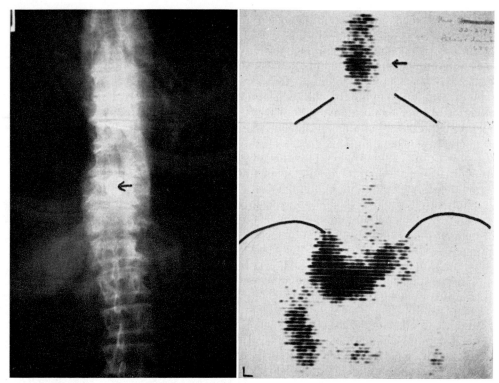

Fig. 2. This female patient, aged 67, had a carcinoma of the breast. Subsequently she complained of back pain. X-rays of the spine showed widespread degenerative changes but the bone scan (with ^{18}F) shows well defined areas of increased uptake suggesting the presence of metastases in the lower dorsal spine←and sacro-iliac joint and the left ischium (posterior view).

RESULTS

The normal skeleton as seen on bone scanning shows increased uptake at several points, particularly at the end of long bones.[16] It is usual to diagnose bone by asymmetry of uptake or by comparison with surrounding, presumably normal, bone; thus, difficulties may arise in older patients where there is osteoporosis or degenerative changes. Figure 2 shows how bone scans may be of value even in these situations. In this patient, although there were widespread degenerative changes, the area involved by metastases can be clearly seen. The region of the shoulder joints is difficult to interpret due to the inability of most scanners to cover both shoulders in one scan. Examinations of the whole spine are complicated by the wide variations in activity due both to the size of the vertebrae and its curvature. To some extent this can be reduced by scanning the patient supine with an under couch detector.

Abnormal areas of bone show as regions of localized increased uptake. The uptake is non-specific and may be due to any disease which results in new bone formation.[16] Even in cases where bone reaction is minimal lesions may still be seen (Figs. 3 and 4). Thus

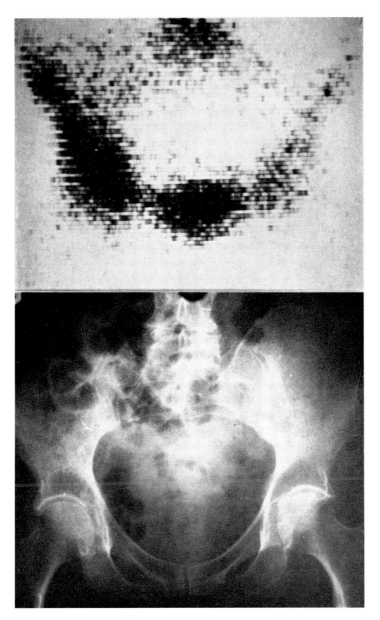

Fig. 3. The bone scan and X-ray of a pelvis in a patient with multiple myeloma. Areas of involvement can be seen in the right side of the pelvis on the bone scan. The bone scan can be of particular value in the evaluation of lesions around the acetabular fossa.

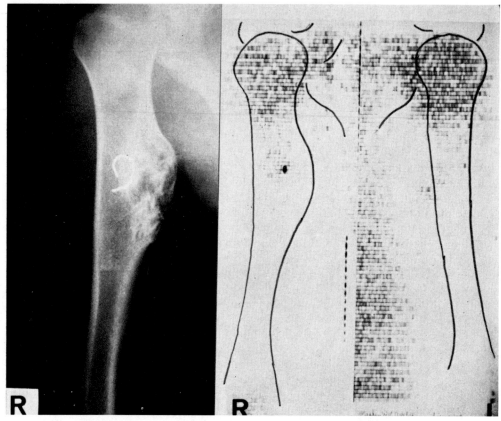

Fig. 4. In contrast to Fig. 3, this benign lesion, a chondroma, shows virtually no uptake in the region of the lesion. Note the normal increase in uptake in the head of the humerus.

both benign and malignant lesions may be seen provided they are active. The frequency with which such lesions are visualized depends greatly upon the type of patients referred and figures indicating the rate of pick up of lesions often mean little. Most lesions which eventually turn out to be positive either on X-ray or at post mortem can be detected by scanning. Rapidly growing lesions with little reaction may be missed[5] but obviously, provided both X-rays and scans are examined together, few tumours will be overlooked. Bone scans are useful in indicating where a review of the plain X-ray could be undertaken or where tomography or further views might be valuable. They are also particularly useful in deciding where or not a dense or lytic area represents an active lesion.

Whole body surveys using radioisotopes are a valuable adjunct to skeletal X-ray surveys.[13] On average at any particular point in time they will correctly diagnose more lesions than can be seen on the skeletal survey and this will, of course, change the approach to treatment of several diseases, including carcinoma of the breast. False positives do occur and the possibility must always be taken into consideration. Faecal excretion of strontium has already been mentioned. With short lived isotopes, vascular areas and renal excretion can pose problems. Hold up of radioactivity may occur at the sacro-iliac joint, simulating disease in an area which often is difficult on X-rays.[17]

REFERENCES

1. Sklaroff, D. M. & Charkes, N. D. Diagnosis of Bone Metastases by Photoscanning with Strontium 85. *J. Amer. Med. Ass.*, **188**, 1–4, 1964.
2. Moon, N. F. *The Skeleton in Principles of Nuclear Medicine*. Ed. H. W. Wagner, Chapter 15, pp. 703–719. W. B. Saunders Company, Philadelphia, 1968.
3. Neuman, W. F. & Neuman, M. W. *The Chemical Dynamics of Bone Mineral*. University of Chicago Press, 1958.
4. Mishkin, F. S. Reese, I. C. Chua, G. T. & Huddleston, J. E. Indium 113m for scanning Bone and Kidney. *Radiology*, **91**, 161–162, 1968.
5. Charkes, N. D., Young, I. & Sklaroff, D. M. The Pathologic Basis of the Strontium Bone Scan. *J. Amer. Med. Ass.*, **206**, pp. 2482–2488, 1968.
6. French, R. J. & McCready, V. R. The Use of ^{18}F for Bone Scanning. *Brit. J. Radiol.*, **40**, 655–661, 1967.
7. Popham, M. G., Taylor, D. M. & Trott, N. G. Evaluation of the Dosimetry of Intravenously Administered [67]Ga Citrate for Measurements of the Distribution in Male August–Marshall Hybrid Rats. *Brit. J. Radiol.*, **43**, 807–810, 1970.
8. Braunstein, P., Hernberg, J. G. & Chandra, R. A Practical Compromise in Bone Scanning. *J. Nuclear Medicine*, **12**, 639–640, 1971.
9. Taskinen, P. J. & Vahatalo, S. [85]Sr Profile Counting and Scanning in Early Diagnosis of Bone Metastases. *Nuclear Medizin (Stuttgart)*, **X**, 265–275, 1971.
10. Charkes, N. D., Sklaroff, D. M. & Bierly, J. Detection of Metastatic Cancer to Bone by Scintiscanning with Strontium 87m. *Amer. J. Roentgenol.*, **91**, 1121–1127, 1964.
11. Alexander, J. L. & Gillespie, P. F. The Optimum Injection-to-scan Interval for Spinal Scans using [87]Sr[m]. *Brit. J. Radiol.* **44**, 878–881, 1971.
12. McCready, V. R., French, R. J. & Gwyther, M. M. The Use of Short-lived Isotopes in Bone Scanning. *Radiosotope in der Lokalisation diagnostik.*, 407–414, 1967.
13. Galasko, C. S. B. Axial Skeletal Scintigraphy in Cancer of the Breast. *Medical Radioisotope Scintigraphy, I.A.E.A. Vienna*, Vol. II, pp. 365–377, 1969.
14. McCready, V. R. & Newbery, S. P. Co-ordinate Transfer system for the Pho Gamma III Nuclear Chicago Gamma Camera. *Brit. J. Radiol.*, **42**, 470–473, 1969.
15. Briggs, R. C., Wilson, E. B. & Sorenson, J. A. Combined Emission-Transmission Scanning of the Skeleton. *Radiology*, **90**, 348–350, 1968.
16. McCready, V. R. Skeletal Scintigraphy. In *Diagnostic Uses of Radioisotopes in Medicine*, pp. 93–100. Hospital Medicine Publication Ltd., 1969.
17. Spencer, R., Herbert, R. Rich, M. W. & Little, W. A. Bone Scanning with [85]Sr [87]Sr[m] [18]F Physical and Radiopharmaceutical Considerations and Clinical Experience in 50 cases. *Brit. J. Radiol.*, **40**, 641–654, 1967.

Discussion

Dr. Patton   I hope this is not too much of a diversion, but I was interested in the comment you made about femoral head necrosis. To what extent are these techniques likely to help one in the diagnosis of bone necrosis into double stages?

Dr. McCready   I haven't got an example myself, but in the literature you get a ring of activity on the proximal end of the necrosis. You would expect that if there is bone being turned over there it should show up and it would be an index of activity. I haven't had a case myself, but I would have thought it was very valuable in showing necrosis of the femoral head. To date most of the work has been done on the malignant situation partly because Sr^{85} is mainly used. Most of the work has been done in America and has been confined to malignant disease. With short-lived isotopes you get the same radiation dose at sea level for 2 years, I think it is, as you would from a bone scan, or if you wore a watch for 10 years with a luminescent dial. I think in the future it will spread to non-malignant conditions now that we have short-lived isotopes.

Prof. Ackerman   If you have a patient with cancer of the breast and you do a bone scan, and you find an area of increased uptake, do you then reject that patient for surgery? If you have such areas, and they can be caused by other things of course which you indicated, but you have an area which you suspect, have you proven the presence of tumour in such areas other than by follow-up?

Dr. McCready   If one takes an X-ray to ensure that you haven't got degenerative disease there, or any other cause for bone uptake, if you do that, you can be fairly confident that is a metastasis. I personally haven't proved it but other people have. They have done both biopsy and follow-up studies. We haven't done the biopsies, but we have numerous cases where it goes X-ray negative to X-ray positive. This is a standard thing.

Dr. Jacobs   I find this extremely clear except for one tiny point. That was this example of multiple chondromas that had considerable uptake, and I think you said they were still benign—those lesion hadn't become malignant. Obviously this is important if one is faced with the situation of enchondroma where the X-rays may suggest early malignancy. From that I would infer that this method isn't of use in that differential if benign ones may occasionally cause isotope uptake?

Dr. McCready   I've fallen into the trap of producing anecdotes. That happened about 3 weeks ago and of course it is the forefront of one's mind. One shouldn't show that sort of slide, one should wait for several years and see if the patient does turn out to have a malignant disease. I think possibly what is happening there is you are getting re-moulding of bones. It's very gross and the patient is quite young. I am wondering if you are getting remoulding of bones, but I can't give you an answer. In answer to the previous question; you said, "Would I change the treatment?" It depends upon the individual surgeon as to what he will do. Some surgeons are definitely changing the treatment if the bone scan is positive and the X-ray is negative. That is spreading like wild-fire through the London area.

Prof. Schajowicz I am answering Professor Ackernam's question about if you have actual proof of the presence of tumour. We had some cases in the Italian Hospital at Buenos Aires in whom we found positive scanning in several cases of slight compression fracture. Before we gave any treatment therefore we made always one or two aspiration biopsies, and in three cases we found positive scans with negative biopsies. So we rejected the tumour. It is fairly easy to find out in many cases where you suspect a malignant metastasis by doing a biopsy previous to treatment. We have seen several cases of multiple chondromatosis in Ollier's Disease. You can say very easily why you find cartilage with positive reaction and other areas with no reaction. If you have an enchondroma in Ollier's Disease it is very common to find zones of enchondral ossification with reactive bone formation which does not signify malignancy. Other tumours of the same lesion without any deposition of bone are negative in the scans.

Dr. McCready I think this is rather like Barry's question—there is no solution. The same argument is applied to liver scanning where I have found something positive, and you put a needle in and it turns out to be negative. Sometimes that would be true: on other occasions you just miss the crucial spot don't you think? I think that the proof of the pudding's in the eating. The patients where you have had positive scans and negative X-rays have a poorer survival in carcinoma of the breast than those in the other situation. There are, however, exceptions right through I think.

Mr. Wilson We have been using this scanning technique to isolate infective lesions in the spine. Could you tell us whether there would be any difference between the scans, because it seems to me that it won't help you very much if you can get the same sort of appearance in the vertebrae from the diagnostic point of view?

Dr. McCready Yes, the scans look exactly the same. We've got several of syphilis and similar lesions. You just get increased uptake. I think one has to work on probabilities. If the patient presents with an infective lesion, you assume that he hasn't got a primary tumour also; but you cannot give a definite answer. There is no way that I can see that this will ever be solved. The only answer we worked out about 5 weeks ago with this gallium story. We felt we might get uptake of gallium in the tumour, because we have lots of cases of gallium concentration, and the uptake in the bone as well. We gave them iron to unload the gallium out of the blood into the bone. We thought we might get it both ways and that this would help in that situation. But it's not to be I'm afraid.

Dr. Friedman Doesn't gallium exchange with sulphur, and if so would it be of any value in cartilagenous tumours?

Dr. McCready Cartilagenous tumours have been shown better with selenides by people in Spain. They have shown it up quite clearly. The trouble is it gives a rather high radiation dose, so you have to be sure that it is a malignant condition before you can go ahead with it. The uptake of gallium in bone I am not sure where it goes to. In ordinary tumours nobody knows where it goes to. Some people have done a lot of work on this, and they finish up as taking up in gallium or gallium-attaching particles, which is a nice way of saying you don't know. They have done ultra-centrifugation. Last week's work showed that gallium uptake goes along very carefully with DNA synthesis. If that was true we would have an *in vivo* measure of DNA synthesis, but I'm sure this won't be. Next week we will show something different.

Prof. Enneking   We have made a fairly serious effort to correlate scans, arteriograms and tomograms of primary tumours as to which technique localized best the anatomic distribution of the lesions. The radio-scan has finished a very poor third. The picture you showed of the scan of the distal femur perhaps was one way of implying that you can measure the proximal extent in the medullary canal of a primary bone tumour by scanning. We have multiple examples where they made the error of as much as 8 or 10 cm in terms of estimating where to do a local resection or an amputation. I would ask for your comments or your experience on correlating the pathology findings after amputation with scanning.

Dr. McCready   Well, having said that, in fact what the radiotherapist does is to move up to the next local joint, so it's of little practical value in giving the exact demarcation of tumour to normal. We haven't had many correlations with post-mortem specimens, because of the peculiar nature of our hospital and the way we get the patients. I can't answer that. I'm surprised it comes off a poor third. Again you see, if you met a real enthusiast he would say, "Oh, you're not scanning slowly enough", or "You're not using fluorine", or, if you were using fluorine, "You're not using strontium". Its one of these things which will take a good few years to come to absolute finite conclusions.

Mr. Sweetnam   I wonder if Dr. McCready could tell us something about the safety of administering these radioactive substances to patients. He did mention one patient with multiple exostoses who he said was rather young, and I would like to know if he was a lower age limit below which he does not give these drugs?

Dr. McCready   The official policy is that they shouldn't be given to anybody who has non-malignant disease and is under 18 years of age. In fact, if you go into it very carefully—say, take bone scanning. The figure I quote is true, the whole body dose is the same as wearing a wrist watch for 10 years or it's living at 10,000 feet in Denver, Colorado. I've forgotten the exact string of analogies, but the actual dose is not very much. One has to use one's clinical judgement. It is certainly much less that the average X-ray dose. A D.M.R.D. trainee doing a barium meal gives the patient 50 rads skin dose, and we are talking here about millirads. The whole body dose as opposed to local dose is the important thing and is what matters. That could occupy a whole conference.

Dr. Hale   May I ask if you have noticed any unusual changes when you have been doing a liver scan for instance in a patient who might have had radiotherapy to the para-aortic gland areas for seminoma of testis?

Dr. McCready   In liver scans of course, you get a standard appearance. Its quite good for checking the treatment fields actually. If you have done a mantle field and an inverted one you can see where they both meet on the liver scan with a line thin of normal tissue between. It will affect the bone marrow uptake of the colloid, but we've seen no uptake to date on the bone scans. We keep meaning to try to follow a patient right through to see if we can demonstrate any increase in blood flow during the repair process, etc., but we haven't managed this yet. The answer is—we haven't seen anything so far.

Surgical aspects of metastatic and residual sarcoma

by

D. R. SWEETNAM

SUMMARY

In Britain most patients with osteosarcoma are now treated by preliminary irradiation which can, itself, only cure a small proportion. Nice judgement is, therefore, required in deciding the correct timing of subsequent amputation, balancing the dangers of leaving possible viable tumour in the body against the fruitless mutilation by early amputation just before metastases appear. A waiting period of 6 to 8 months is supported by the author. Even with obvious metastases, palliative amputation may be required. The importance is emphasized of the judicious management of the unfortunate 80% of patients who will eventually succumb in spite of treatment.

Isolated "skip" deposits of intramedullary tumour may occur, hence disarticulation is advised for lower femoral tumours rather than ablation through the femur after which recurrence in the stump may occur in nearly 20%. Prolonged survival, produced perhaps by improved adjuvant chemotherapy, should render disarticulation even more essential if, as the author suspects, the incidence of stump recurrence might thereby increase.

Although such cases are rare, eight out of 12 patients operated upon for excision of a solitary pulmonary metastasis were alive at follow-up on average some $6\frac{1}{2}$ years later. This measure should always be considered when a lung metastasis remains solitary and when the primary tumour has been completely eradicated.

MY BRIEF THIS MORNING is two-fold, first to discuss the surgeon's approach to metastatic sarcoma—which in practice means the treatment of pulmonary metastases. Next I have to consider my views on the problem of residual sarcoma, which is a larger field and covers not only the obvious local recurrence after a full course of irradiation but also stump recurrence after inadequate amputation. Finally, and the most difficult of all, the question of when or indeed whether to amputate after irradiation when there is no clinical or radiological hint of recurrent tumour activity. In such a patient, we just do not know whether or not the whole tumour has been killed.

The basis for many of my observations this morning comes from a survey of osteosarcoma carried out for the Medical Research Council's Working Party on Bone Sarcoma,[1] and it is a pleasure to acknowledge at this stage my debt to the chairman, Sir Herbert Seddon, and members of this Working Party of which I was secretary, and particularly also to the Bone Tumour Panel of the Cancer Research Campaign who reviewed the histological material of all 469 patients studied. The members of this Panel were the

L   297

late Prof. Scarff, Dr. Ball, Dr. Byers, Dr. Mary Catto, the late Dr. Goldie, Dr. Price and Prof. Sissons, in whose Department at the Institute of Orthopaedics in London so much of the work was done. Surgeons and radiologists throughout the United Kingdom allowed me to study their patients. I know it is invidious to single out centres for acknowledgement but I cannot help but mention the Bristol Bone Tumour Registry and Westminster Hospital, both of whom provided so many patients for the survey.

Residual tumour activity apart from stump recurrence is only as old as radiotherapy, before this amputation took care of the tumour mass. In the United Kingdom to-day less than one-third of these patients are treated by primary amputation and thus the problem is a common one. Elsewhere, particularly in the United States of America, radiotherapy is much less popular, so that local recurrence except in the stump cannot be a problem. It has, as you know, been shown that even after a full course of irradiation histological examination of the amputated limb may reveal apparently viable tumour cells in one-third of the patients, and only in another third can it be said with any degree of certainty that the whole tumour is dead—the remainder may or may not harbour living tumour. We have no means as yet of telling which is which before advising completion of the programme of treatment by amputation. I agree that one must assume activity and amputate after an interval following radiotherapy—say 6 to 8 months— provided of course no metastases show themselves in the meantime. In short, I support Cade's view that this interval before amputation distinguishes those likely to survive from those doomed to early death. Surely only the former should be subjected to amputation (Fig. 1). At 7 months from the beginning of treatment 70% of those who will die of their disease already show evidence of lung metastases and as about 20% of patients survive, very few will with this regime have limbs amputated unnecessarily. I am bound to say though that in terms of survival alone there is very little if any significant difference between patients treated by primary amputation and those by intended combination of radiotherapy to be followed later by amputation—by the latter method though very many children have been spared loss of a limb in the last months of their life.

This last statement "the sparing from unnecessary amputation" is really the linch-pin of the argument in favour of Cade's combined method of treatment. Maybe the immunologists in time will give us another but they have not done so yet.

I am worried though by recurrence of the primary growth *after* lung metastases have developed, and thus after amputation has been rejected. May we have spared the child from amputation only to subject it to the horrors of massive growth, pathological fracture or even fungation before death? This is a fallacy of the available statistics. This sort of human tragedy usually occurs at home and not in hospital and *therefore does not appear in the records that we study*. May I therefore make a plea for this sort of detail to be sought out and recorded, for without it we do not really know for certain that the avoidance of amputation is necessarily best. Although I am strongly in favour of avoiding amputation in the presence of lung metastases, I am sure that the surgeon must be prepared to carry out a palliative amputation later should the need arise. In other words, the decision not to amputate should never be irrevocable.

The presence of residual tumour is not, however, a phenomenon confined to those treated initially by radiotherapy. This would imply that by amputation the whole tumour was always removed. Unfortunately this is not always the case. This example taken from the Hunterian Collection of the Royal College of Surgeons shows that skip

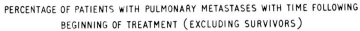

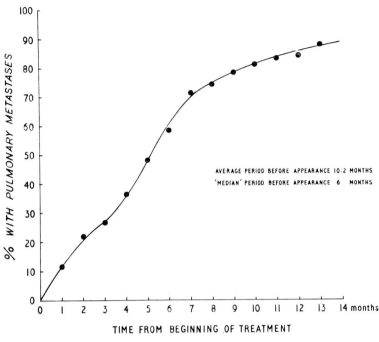

Fig. 1.

lesions can occur within the medullary cavity of a bone, and thus amputation at any level through that bone may leave behind part of the tumour (Fig. 2). Here is another example of the same sort of thing. Higher invisible such lesions if left behind will inevitably produce this sort of thing if the child lives long enough (Fig. 3).

Here then we highlight the other main field of controversy in the treatment of osteo-sarcoma. I refer, of course, to the level of amputation, and in this discussion we are not concerned whether or not amputation has been preceded by radiotherapy.

In our series of patients 83% of these tumours of the leg occurred at the knee, with twice as many in the lower femur as in the upper tibia. Thus this question of amputation level is primarily one that concerns the femur. Those who advocate leaving a femoral stump point to the advantages for limb fitting and believe local stump recurrence to be rare. The rest of us, and I number myself among this group, feel that the dangers of local recurrence outweigh the obvious advantages of retaining a thigh stump however small. We advocate disarticulation through the hip. I believe total ablation of the bone involved is necessary simply because of the high incidence of stump recurrence. Almost one out of every five patients develop such a recurrence after through-femur amputation, whether or not there has been preliminary irradiation, and one wonders how many more might also do so if they survived long enough. With a median survival time of no more than 16 months after starting treatment, and with four-fifths of all patients dying within 2 years, it seems possible at least that even this relatively high figure of recurrence

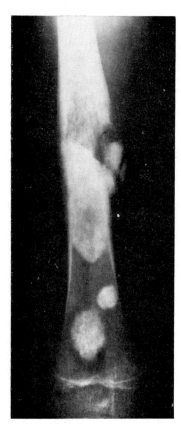

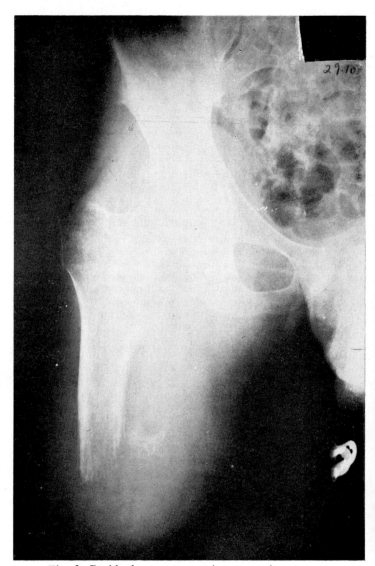

Fig. 2. Osteosarcoma of femur showing "skip" lesions in the medulla.

Fig. 3. Residual osteosarcoma in amputation stump.

might be still higher if patients had lived longer. Certainly, I feel sure that the figure is lower than the true incidence because, as I have already mentioned, details of the last months at home before death are but scant.

I cannot accept that a negative histological examination of the medullary cavity at the site of bone section indicates freedom from higher intra-medullary tumour spread with the sort of skip lesion I showed earlier. This technique is often advocated by those who claim that through-femur amputation is safe. One usually searches the literature in vain for any reference to stump recurrence. Authors seem obsessed with survival figures, forgetting that we all know that almost whatever we do to these unfortunate patients four out of five will die within 2 years. We must give more thought to the secondary aim of our treatment—the palliation of those who will die. Statistics can never do justice to this aspect of our management, even though regrettably it will prove to be the most important result of our efforts for all but the 20% or so who will survive.

I now turn to a quite different aspect of surgical management, that of the treatment of metastases. Unfortunately our efforts here by the very nature of things make up at best a minute part of the whole. We are not concerned with multiple metastases neither with lymphatic spread, which though uncommon certainly occurs.

The first account of the resection of solitary lung metastases in bone tumours was published in 1947.[2] There have been a number of resections, mainly for epithelial tumour metastases. Sarcomata we know usually produce multiple lung deposits, nevertheless there remain a very few patients in whom a single deposit remains solitary and in whom we should at least consider the possibility of resection. Five years ago Ross and I[3] collected together information on as many such patients as we could find in this country. All had primary bone tumours and all had a metastasis in the lung removed. Our search was by no means exhaustive and we found twelve. Seven osteosarcoma, two each of

OSTEOSARCOMA

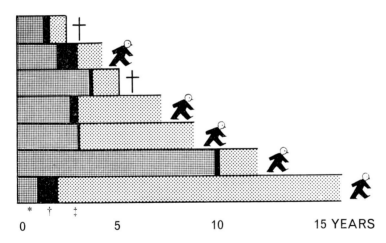

Fig. 4. Pulmonary resection for metastases showing graphically the three phases: the period after initial treatment before the metastasis was seen *: the "waiting period" †
before resection, the duration of life thereafter ‡. (The walking figure indicates that the patient remains well.)

chondrosarcoma and fibrosarcoma, and a metastasizing chondroblastoma. The first had been operated upon at the Middlesex Hospital in 1951, probably the first such operation of its kind in the United Kingdom. The patient, who had previously had a fore-quarter amputation for a chondrosarcoma of the humerus, died of an unrelated cause 15 years after lung resection. This diagram (Fig. 4) shows that of the other seven patients, five were alive at follow-up which averaged 6½ years after lung resection. These figures though in such a totally unselected series mean no more than that lung resection can work. Obviously the number of occasions when suitably solitary lung deposits present themselves must be extremely rare. Nevertheless, however rare, the fact that lives can be saved cannot be ignored. There are differing opinions concerning the indications and timing of lung resection, but at this stage when the reported number of patients is small dogmatic criteria for either cannot be stated. It is possible though to draw certain conclusions which at present appear reasonable, though which may in the light of further experience require modification. Clearly three conditions must pertain before resection is even considered. The primary growth must have been entirely eradicated, there must be no other detectable metastases, and the lung lesion must appear solitary.

The most difficult decision is the timing of resection. It must be wise to advise a period of observation after the lung lesion is first discovered. Three months has been suggested, the argument being that in favourable cases nothing is lost and an unnecessary operation avoided if the early lesion proves to be just the first of many to appear in quick succession. Although there is obvious wisdom in this council, human nature in the absence of radiological evidence of other deposits may tend to lead one to earlier lung resection. Indeed, apart from one's natural desire to rid the patient of his second lesion as soon as possible, there is the obvious alternative argument that even solitary metastases often grow quite quickly and the smaller they are the easier it is to obtain a wide clearance. It is in the judgement of this "waiting period" that most difficulty lies. The unfortunate patients, the majority of whom are children, must not be subjected to unnecessary further suffering, nor on the other hand must potentially suitable patients be denied adequate secondary surgery without too much delay. In the present state of our knowledge I believe that a waiting period of 3 months is reasonable. During the period no further metastases should have developed and just before resection a thorough search for occult deposits in the lung and elsewhere must be undertaken by all modern means.

The appearance of a solitary lung metastasis must no longer be regarded as the inevitable harbinger of death, but rather the signal for an intensive period of observation and if necessary investigation. Only in this way will suitable patients be given the benefit of further treatment. It is likely that such close surveillance will disclose an even higher proportion of suitable pulmonary lesions; for, if untreated, all must multiply and later mask the fact that at first a solitary metastasis remained uncomplicated by others for several months, the discovery and treatment of which might have prevented further spread of the disease.

REFERENCES

1. Sweetnam, R. D., Knowelden, J. & Seddon, H. Bone Sarcoma: Treatment by Irradiation, Amputation or a Combination of the Two. *Brit. Med. J.*, **2**, 363, 1971.
2. Alexander, J. & Haight, C. Pulmonary Resection for Solitary Metastatic Sarcomas and Carcinomas. *Surg. Gynec., Obstet.*, **85**, 129, 1947.
3. Sweetnam, D. R. & Ross, K. Surgical Treatment of Pulmonary Metastases from Primary Tumours of Bone. *J. Bone Jt. Surg.*, **49–B**, 74, 1967.

Discussion

Dr. Vermeij In connection with these skip lesions mentioned by Mr. Sweetnam I want to ask the following question: Do you know if thorough radiographic screening and bone scanning was performed before treatment was initiated for osteosarcoma?

Mr. Sweetnam I confess that the answer is I don't. But in view of what we heard from Dr. Enneking the other day it would seem that some of these higher lesions may be outside as well as inside the bone after biopsy. I think that it is important that we should scan them beforehand.

Dr. Vermeij I mean to search for these skip lesions inside the skeleton.

Mr. Sweetnam It sounds a good idea, but it hasn't been done to my knowledge.

Dr. Vermeij Because in the treatment of mammary carcinoma metastases if you like, at any change of your treatment you can do those things.

Dr. McCready I'm not aware that anybody has been really carrying out screening for metastases except possibly for breast carcinoma so far. We've tried it, but you must have bone deposition for it to show up and the chest ones that we have been able to see quite clearly in the X-ray didn't show up in the scan. Marrow scanning gives a high radiation dose which is probably relevant in this discussion. Very few people do bone-marrow scanning. That would probably be the answer to show up this sort of lesion. Maybe, after this conference people will approach this subject with more enthusiasm. But you know the problem—one person treats only two or three a year. There are social factors and there is some reason why you dont see the patient.

Dr. Dahlin I am interested in the high rate of recurrence in the stump—one in five, because our surgeons normally do the trans-femoral amputation for osteogenic sarcoma of the lower femur. We very rarely have recurrences in the stump. Perhaps it is because they amputate a little bit higher. Nevertheless, I looked at all the osteogenic sarcomas— several hundred cases of osteogenic sarcoma of the lower femur and I find skip areas are extremely rare in our experience. I would like to suggest that the evidence in that macerated specimen from the Hunterian Collection and also the one X-ray does not preclude the possibility, or even the likelihood, that there was unossified spread between those zones of dense bone.

Mr. Sweetnam Could I say that I absolutely agree with that. Those were just illustrative slides and in no sense were they meant to be a proof. The fact is that about 20% of this series did have evidence of stump recurrence after femoral amputation. The majority of the amputations were higher than those two slides that I showed. They were very high some of them, but still stump recurrences occured in 20%.

Prof. van Rijssel Do you know in the cases of the high amputations how far was the amputation from the upper border of the tumour? When the amputation level is close to the upper border of the tumour then trans-femoral amputation was contra-indicated and disarticulation had become essential. Do you know this?

Mr. Sweetnam Well there were a number of patients and I can't tell you the level of each one. There was nothing in the figures to suggest that the tumours—all of which were in the lower femur of course—were particularly large. There were different levels of amputation—some were very high and some apparently low.

Prof. van Rijssel But one patient in five did show stump recurrence. In these cases what was the distance between the upper edge of the tumour and the amputation level— that is the question?

Mr. Sweetnam How do you measure this distance—radiographically or by palpation?

Prof. van Rijssel I would say on the amputation specimen after the operation.

Mr. Sweetnam Even in our own cases we can only say that there were tumours of the lower femur and the amputations were performed high—in the sub-trochanteric region. I cannot tell you the distance in centimetres I'm afraid.

Mr. Eyre-Brook Our experience in Bristol from our records is not quite the same and I would like to call in one of my colleagues to give briefly our view.

Mr. Peter Hill We were obviously concerned in Bristol by the high figures Mr. Sweetnam reported in M.R.C. report (1971). I reviewed the evidence that we had here for this I found 33 cases of lower femoral osteosarcoma treated by primary amputation without any known metastases at the time of presentation. Two cases were from overseas and were omitted leaving 31 altogether that could be followed reasonably accurately.

Two of these had bony recurrences in the stump. I think of even greater interest was that there were four other patients who had evidence of tumour masses at higher levels almost always described as "ilio-inguinal". In three of them there was radiographic evidence that there was no bony involvement locally. These then were presumably due to lymphatic spread rather than intra-osseous extension. Of the two cases which did have stump recurrences one appeared about 3 months after the amputation, the other about a few months later. I'm sure that the one that recurred earlier had also other metastases apparent when the stump recurrence was first noted. This patient died fairly rapidly and obviously in a certain amount of misery in general and not particularly referred to the stump. The other patient admittedly survived rather longer with radio-therapy and local cytotoxic agents to the stump. There is no doubt that in this case the fungating mass which never really settled down did add to the terminal misery of this patient. Those are the figures I was able to find in the Bristol records.

Prof. Schajowicz I want to ask if any of you tried to find the correct amputation level by tetracycline fluorescence? It is easier and cheaper than doing bone scanning. Some people have done this successfully. It is not specific but it can help like bone scanning.

Mr. Sweetnam   The cases I am quoting were considered retrospectively. This is the sort of thing that we must all now be doing because the argument this morning about the level for amputation highlights a very deep division of opinion amongst orthopaedic surgeons. There are those who amputate through the femur and those who do not—its about 50 : 50 in this country. This controversy ought to be resolved one way or the other, but I don't think, though, that it can be decided on the sort of retrospective survey that I have reported. I think that the sort of comment you have made is very important.

Prof. Bonfiglio   Our experience in the treatment of osteosarcoma by amputation parallels that of Bristol exactly. We had two out of 32 patients who had stump recurrences and only one with lymphatic involvement. Out of 50 patients 32 had primary amputation for their treatment.

Dr. Cortes   I want to mention a really important critical observation of Dr. Martin who analysed 25 patients with osteogenic sarcoma with lung metastasis. He was measuring the doubling time of the tumour by serial X-ray examinations. Among the 25 cases he found that the doubling time was 11 to 360 days. When a patient had a doubling time of less than 20 days 50% of these cases died in about 7 months and 100% of his cases died in 15 months. When a patient had a doubling time of 21–40 days, 50% of these cases died in 12 months. Those patients who had a doubling time of 40 days or over had a median survival of 18 months and all were dead in 24 months. So that if the patient had a doubling time of 20 days or less I think that surgery has no role for resection of the tumour.

Dr. Campbell   I would like to ask Mr. Sweetnam two questions. The first is—Has he seen any survivals and any amputation specimens where there has been a hip disarticulation for osteosarcoma and there have been skip metastases present? Secondly, has he seen any survivals in cases where there have been recurrences in the stump?

Mr. Sweetnam   The answer to the second question is yes. I think that the presence of a stump recurrence does not appear to preclude the possibility of survival. I certainly know one patient who had a vicious stump recurrence with subsequent disarticulation and he survived. The answer to the other question I am not quite so certain about. I don't think I can answer that, I'm sorry.

Dr. Makley   I had the opportunity to travel around the United States looking at cases of chest metastases in osteosarcoma. We were interested in measuring from an X-ray standpoint exactly how fast these metastases grow, but not exactly the doubling time. I was impressed by the fact that we were able to follow one metastases along and made it stay the same size for some weeks whereas other metastases in the same area grew rapidly. It may then appear vice-versa—one may stop growing and the other begin to grow. I am most concerned about the usage of the doubling time from a prognostic standpoint or deciding whether you should resect the lesion or not.

Mr. Fitton   One point we haven't really touched on this morning is—if you do an amputation on a child for a sarcoma and on a child whom you expect to die, you remove the

L*

limb and hope to get better function. The quality of the function which results after disarticulation or after removal of only part of a limb leaving a stump we haven't really evaluated. The child wants to be able to walk—wants to be able to run. He wants to be able to put on his appliance fairly easily each morning—this sort of thing. Its the quality of the life that you give to the child whilst he survives that is very important. The point has been made—we don't see these children in their homes very much. I am sure that this is a criticism of our judgement. I would like to ask Mr. Sweetnam what he thinks about the quality of function in the child after high or mid-thigh amputation by comparison with disarticulation?

Mr. Sweetnam I think there is absolutely no doubt that to disarticulate through a hip is a vicious thing, and to amputate through the thigh and allow the child to walk around with a stump is obviously very much better. But this is not the only consideration. We're not talking now about survival. I cannot tell you if the figures for survival are any better with disarticulation or not. We are talking about the quality of life also for the unfortunate 80% who will die—this is what you mentioned. The figures that I have indicate that on going into this in great detail and finding out what happens to the children as far as one can after they leave the surveillance of the hospital and go home to die— about 20% develop a stump recurrence. This was a retrospective study. Now, if that is the case and if confirmed elsewhere by other series and with other methods of treatment, I would submit that it is probably better to disarticulate and avoid this horror of stump recurrence before death than to amputate through the femur with this risk. But this is a question—this is something to discuss.

Prophylactic irradiation of the lung in bone sarcoma

by

K. A. NEWTON

SUMMARY

A preliminary report of 13 patients with osteosarcoma of limb bones who received prophylactic radiotherapy to the lungs shows only four with metastases so far. Even if the other nine develop metastases forthwith then the 80% metastatic level is manifest at 18 months as compared with 8 months for the control series. Continuation of the present trend is anticipated to show a more beneficial result of this treatment.

BETWEEN 70 AND 80% OF ALL CASES of osteosarcoma succumb from pulmonary metastases.

In a proportion of patients it is possible to control the primary tumour by megavoltage irradiation. In Lee and Mackenzie's series,[1] of those ablated limbs which were examined histologically, approximately one third were found on microscopy to be tumour free, in one third viable cells persisted and in the remaining third there were cells with possible growth potential. Radiotherapy to the primary tumour is then part of a treatment policy where limb ablation is only carried out in those patients who remain metastasis free as demonstrated by whole lung tomography after a period of 6 to 9 months from the original radiotherapy treatment to the limb.

My colleague, Mr. E. Stanley Lee,[2] has demonstrated the time at which lung metastases can be seen radiographically and I am indebted to him for this information.

Using this treatment policy, 5-year survival figures are achieved which compare favourably with those obtained in other centres. I would like at this point, to acknowledge our indebtedness to Sir Stanford Cade, who, at Westminster Hospital, started this clinical trial.

In view of the high lung metastases rate from osteosarcoma, it seemed reasonable to irradiate the lungs prophylactically. Because of the intolerance of lungs to high dosage radiotherapy it is essential that the dosage be limited to a figure that can be accepted without clinical damage. The technique itself is simple, an opposing field method using megavoltage apparatus is employed and the field is fashioned by lead bricks.

Some years ago an attempt was made to irradiate metastatic disease in the lungs from radio-sensitive primary tumours. 3,000 rads was given to both lungs and in two patients severe radiation pneumonitis followed which I feel certain, contributed to their death. The pathological picture was characteristic and showed degeneration and fragmentation of elastica and ballooning of the alveolar spaces.

These severe damaging effects to the lung tissue necessitated a drastic reduction in dose and in fact, now the usual dose aimed at is 1,950 rads given at the rate of 150 rads daily—the overall time being $2\frac{1}{2}$ weeks. At this dosage level no clinical or radiological damage has been observed even on a long-term basis.

The question then arose as to whether a low dosage, in the range of 2,000 rads is likely to be at all helpful in what is tradiationally categorized as a radiation resistant tumour, i.e. osteosarcoma. As far as radiobiological evidence goes this dose would be lethal to slightly in excess of 99% of mammalian cells in a well oxygenated tissue culture medium and is equivalent to NSD of approximately 760 rets.

It is known that circulating malignant cells in the venous blood are compatible with long survival and that only a minute fraction of these circulating cells set up metastatic clones—it is possibly naive to conceive of a situation where it is doubtful as to whether a cell or small clump of cells will successfully colonize or simply fail to thrive and die. It is perhaps at this stage that radiotherapy even at low dosage may help to prevent successful growth of cells in the lung.

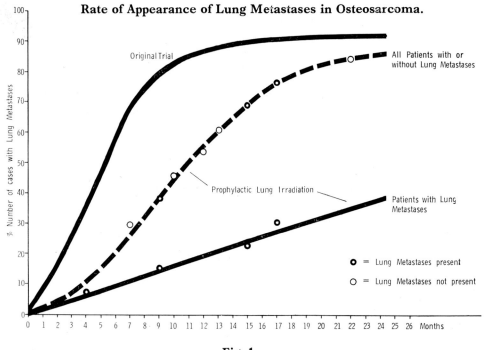

Fig. 1.

With this aim in view, during the last $2\frac{1}{2}$ weeks of radiotherapy to the limb affected by the primary sarcoma, we have somewhat tentatively given prophylactic lung radiotherapy to a small group of cases.

These 13 cases are, of course, far too small a number on which to base firm conclusions, but nevertheless I think it right to give our results even though the conclusions may be misleading and the results not substantiated by a more prolonged trial.

In this illustration (Fig. 1) relating to Mr. Lee's work on the rate of appearance of pulmonary metastases in osteosarcoma, you will observe two readings of note:

1. That 80% of patients develop metastases in 8 to 9 months.

2. Fifty per cent of patients are observed to have pulmonary metastases at 6 months.

Only four of the 13 patients given prophylactic irradiation have so far developed metastases and on this graph they are marked in the lower line. If one is to assume that the remaining nine patients remain metastasis free, then clearly the prophylactic treatment will have been remarkably beneficial but almost certainly this is an unreal conclusion. However, assuming that each of the 13 patients followed-up so far develop pulmonary metastases the day after their follow-up attendance time, then the central curve is obtained. This then must represent the worst that can happen to these patients. Even so, in this pessimistic situation, 80% will not have developed metastases until 18 months, and 50% at 11 months. If the present trend continues based on this small number of cases, then the true answer must lie somewhere between the lower curve and the central curve which does represent a very considerable delay in the appearance of pulmonary metastases. At first sight this could be interpreted as a most satisfactory result of prophylactic lung irradiation, but it could be argued that the surgeon's task is now made more difficult, in that instead of being able to advise limb ablation at 6 to 9 months with a reasonable chance that the patient is going to survive, he would no longer be in this position.

One can only hope that this prophylactic irradiation to the lungs will result in a larger proportion of patients remaining permanently metastasis free. In spite of this uncertainty it is proposed to continue with our clinical trial of prophylactic lung irradiation.

REFERENCES

1. Lee, E. Stanley & Mackenzie, D. H. Osteosarcoma. A Study of the Value of Preoperative Megavoltage Radiotherapy. *Brit. J. Surg.*, **51**, 252, 1964.
2. Lee, E. Stanley. Treatment of Bone Sarcoma. *Proc. roy. Soc. Med.*, **64**, 1179 (Sect. Radiol. p. 41), 1971.

Discussion

Dr. Suit I think this is a most interesting set of figures. I would like to ask Dr. Newton if in these patients there has been any assay of pulmonary function before and at any time following this dose of radiation?

Dr. Newton Not in this particular series but I have previously published a series of 40 patients treated by whole lung irradiation in which for the first few patients this was done at regular intervals, in one patient for as long as 12 months. There was no alteration in pulmonary function studies, not at 1950 rads in $2\frac{1}{2}$ weeks.

Dr. Suit These patients received no concomitant chemotherapy?

Dr. Newton No. These are not very recent figures. But during the last few months we have been adding concomitant chemotherapy and I am not sure what this is going to do.

Dr. Suit Which drugs?

Dr. Newton We are using a drug, the chemical name of which I do not know, but it is called ICRF 159. It was elaborated by Dr. Kurt Hellmann at the Imperial Cancer Research Fund institute. It is quite an interesting drug which it is possible does have a radiation-potentiating effect.

Prof. Duthie Irradiation of lungs must have taken place in the treatment of cases of breast carcinoma and maybe there is rather a good control from the point of view of the right to left lung fields. Has there been any study comparing the two lung fields from the point of view of follow-up after irradiation for breast carcinoma? We would like to think of the lung metastases not occurring in the irradiated lung field rather than in the unirradiated lung?

Dr. Newton I find that a rather difficult question to answer because in our particular centre we don't take in more than $3\frac{1}{2}$ cm of lung in tangential glancing fields. That is the greatest depth of lung that is irradiated, that is, $3\frac{1}{2}$ cm.

Prof. Duthie But in the older series of cases of course you were doing much more extensive irradiation. Not particularly you I mean but in other centres—like Edinburgh and so on?

Dr. Newton Yes. We have always been rather careful ourselves to avoid as much lung tissue as possible, because to give 6,000 rads to large volume lung tissue is unthinkable. I wouldn't like to do that.

Prof. Duthie   Is there any difference between the two lung fields in your series?

Dr. Newton   No.

Dr. Tudway   I should just like to take the opportunity to emphasize that so far as I know radiotherapists universally make a point of avoiding lung, and I don't think comparisons based upon breast technique would be at all helpful. And while I am on my feet could I ask Dr. Newton if there is any significance in the fact that he drew a straight line as the lower curve in his diagram?

Dr. Newton   There were just four patients and they just happened to fall in a straight line.

Autogenous lysed cell vaccine in the treatment of osteogenic sarcoma—a preliminary report on fifteen cases

by

RALPH C. MARCOVE, VALERIE MIKÉ, ANDREW G. HUVOS,
CHESTER M. SOUTHAM and ARTHUR G. LEVIN

SUMMARY

Twenty-one patients with osteogenic sarcoma of long bones treated by a lysed cell vaccine in addition to routine amputation appear to have an encouraging response to treatment, compared with both the whole cell vaccine and the control series. In view of the infrequency of follow-up chest films in the control group, an inherent bias is present in our data, making the time to metastasis for control patients appear longer thus adding more weight to the vaccine therapy. In addition, all patients in the control group have been followed well over two years, whereas only four of the six disease-free patients in the lysed cell series have had a full 5-year follow-up.

INTRODUCTION

A RECENT ATTEMPT at modern immunotherapy for a patient with osteogenic sarcoma was made by the senior author in June 1963. A lyophilized homogenous vaccine prepared from the primary tumor tissue was given to a child who had pulmonary metastases already present. During the 15 days of injections the child gained 7 lb, but after this treatment period he returned to a downhill course and subsequently died. However, his temporary improvement suggested that tumor growth may have been inhibited. and this encouraged a controlled trial of immunotherapy in less advanced disease.

A formal trial was begun in April 1966. Included in the study were patients under the age of 25 with osteogenic sarcoma of the long bones but no evidence of spread beyond the primary site who were treated by amputation. The autogenous whole or lysed cell vaccine was given in the post-operative period following amputation. With the appearance of metastases (usually pulmonary) the vaccine was judged a failure. If there was subsequent pulmonary resection, any observed beneficial effect was credited to this pulmonary surgical treatment. Our experience with multiple pulmonary resections in the treatment of osteogenic sarcoma has been reported by Martini et al.[10]

This paper is a preliminary report on the patients who received vaccine treatment through March 1972.

TABLE 1

FOURTEEN PATIENTS WHO RECEIVED WHOLE CELL VACCINE

No.	Initials	Age	Sex	Site of Tumor	Date of surgery	Date of last negative X-ray	Date of Metastases	Pre-Operative symptoms
1	N.H(L).	16	F	Humerus L.	19/12/67	29/4/68	25/7/69	5 months duration
2	P.M.	15	F	Tibia R.	1/5/68	June '69	Jan. '70	November 1967, Mid-thigh amputation
3	J.S.	10	F	Femur L.	16/5/68	1/7/69	18/9/69	Early April 1968
4	C.P.	16	F	Humerus L.	22/7/68	—	D17/7/69	2 months before admission
5	E.M.	11	M	Tibia	16/8/68	—	11/12/68	1½ months
6	K.G.	12	F	Femur R.	3/9/68	3/12/68	4/2/69	—
7	S.G.	10	F	Tibia L.	2/10/68	5/8/69	9/9/69	2 weeks before admission
8	K.K.	11	F	Tibia L.	4/10/48	Dec. 1972	—	1 month before admission
9	R.B.	14	F	Fibula L.	7/10/68	18/3/69	22/4/69	6 weeks before admission
10	D.S.	16	M	Tibia L.	30/10/68	27/2/68	D 27/3/69	3 months before admission
11	A.R.	15	M	Femur R.	10/12/69	6/3/69	17/4/69	6 weeks before admission
12	E.W.	19	M	Femur L.	24/1/69	20/3/69	2/5/69	January 1969
13	G.P.	14	M	Femur R.	22/9/69	29/11/69	30/12/69	Pain in thigh August 1969
14	M.B.	20	F	Femur R.	23/9/69	—	6/3/70	—..

Note—one patient well to December 1972.

MATERIALS AND METHODS

The clinical presentation of osteogenic sarcoma is most often that of several months of dull, low-grade pain and gradual swelling. If the pain is too intense or the swelling is too sudden and the radiologic demonstration of the bone lesion equivocal, one must be alerted to the possibility of another disease process, for instance osteomyelitis, eosinophilic granuloma or aneurysmal bone cyst.

The roentgenogram usually presents either a lytic, a blastic or mixed picture permeating the bone and often an adjacent soft tissue mass can be identified with productive radiologic densities consistent with ossification, calcification, or both. Skipped areas of tumor up and down the involved bone shaft are most often so small that they are not demonstrated by the initial roentgenogram, even if they are grossly identifiable. The medullary extension of the lesion is usually distant to the soft tissue mass.

On microscopic examination this lesion exhibits a markedly variegated pattern, but the essential finding is that of malignant spindle cell stroma forming osteoid or immature bone which is neither reactive nor periosteal in nature. As the bone production becomes more dense, the osteocytes become more mature (Phemister's normalization process).[11,12] Large areas of spindle cells or cartilage formation may be present including bone formation by the process of endochondral ossification.[7] This latter mechanism of bone formation can also be seen in chondrosarcoma and therefore is not in itself diagnostic for osteogenic sarcoma.[1,3,6] A small biopsy specimen, especially a needle aspiration, may display only a few spindle cells which also can be seen in a reticulum cell sarcoma or a fibrosarcoma, making a false diagnosis a real possibility. Likewise a limited area may

TABLE 2

FIFTEEN PATIENTS TREATED WITH LYSED CELL VACCINE

No.	Initials	Age	Sex	Site	Date of surgery	Date of last negative X-ray	Date of metastases	Pre-operative symptoms
1	J.R.	15	F	Femur L.	1/4/66	21/11/71	5/3/68*	9 months tenderness
2	K.P.	4	F	Tibia R.	16/5/66	Dec. 1972	—	4 weeks pain and swelling
3	C.N.	18	F	Tibia L.	3/6/66	Dec. 1972	—	—
4†	J.R.	17	M	Fibula R.	1/7/66	31/10/66	22/2/67	1 month before admission
5	G.K.	15	M	Tibia R.	10/10/66	—	4/1/67	4 months before admission
6	K.W.	8	M	Femur L.	9/2/67	5/5/67	20/6/69	December 1966
7	L.J.	12	F	Humerus R.	23/2/67	24/10/67	2/1/68	January 1967
8	P.D.	7	M	Humerus L.	21/7/67	Dec. 1972	—	Fracture May 1967
9	R.F.	16	M	Tibia	9/8/67	24/1/69	8/4/69	—
10	J.R.	16	M	Tibia R.	10/9/67	Dec. 1972	—	November 1966
11	C.C.	14	F	Humerus R.	21/9/67	1/11/67	Feb. 1968 D 24/11/68	Several months before admission
12	M.C.	11	M	Femur L.	13/12/67	—	D 28/5/69	—
13‡	W.M.	24	M	Hip L.	14/2/69	Dec. 1972	—	6 weeks before admission
14‡	J.C.	20	M	Femur L.	3/3/69	Dec. 1972	—	Several weeks before admission
15‡	R.S.	12	M	Humerus	5/9/69	—	20/1/70	1 month before admission

* Metastasis removed from lung.
† Tumour irradiated before vaccine prepared.
‡ Water-lysed vaccine.
Six of 15 (40%) patients have no metastases to December 1972 when all survivors had recent normal chest X-ray films.

show only cartilaginous tissue, hence a diagnosis of a chondrosarcoma could be entertained. Other limited tissue samples may exhibit giant cells, large angiomatous formations mimicking a giant cell tumor or an angiosarcoma.[4] This study therefore emphasizes the importance of large, adequate, open biopsy specimens for diagnostic purposes.

The Memorial Hospital experience with osteogenic sarcoma under the age of 21 has been reviewed by Marcove *et al.*[8,9] This series included 145 consecutive cases treated between January 1949 and December 1965. Nine additional cases, patients between the ages 21 to 25, seen during the same time period, have been added to this series to provide a control group for the vaccine study (154 patients).

Tables 1 and 2 give a summary of the basic data on the patients who received vaccine treatment.

The trial began with the administration of a UV-irradiated lysed cell vaccine. The tumor specimen and about four times its weight of saline were put into a Viritis homogenizer in an ice water bath, which was operated at maximum speed for 15 minutes. This ruptures virtually all of the cells and a large proportion of the nuclei. The resulting suspension was then centrifuged for 15 minutes at 8,000 G, which sediments intact cells and nuclei but leaves the cell sap, microsomes, mitochondria, and membranes in the supernatant which was harvested. Transmission of 253·7 mμ ultraviolet light through this supernatant was measured in a Beckman DU Photometer and the specimen was diluted in sufficient isotonic saline to allow at least 50% transmission through a depth of 2 mm. If the preparation contained large amounts of hemoglobin a considerable dilution was necessary to accomplish this objective. The preparation was then placed in open Petri dishes to a depth of 2 mm and irradiated from a "germicidal" UV lamp (General Electric Co.) to provide a dose of 50,000 ergs/mm^2 at the bottom of the fluid layer. The material was ampouled aseptically in volumes of from 1 to 5 ml. Concentrations of these extracts and the total dosage given to the patients varied widely. We have no data on actual concentration, or the actual amount of tissue solids which were administered, but the supernatants which were irradiated represented the yield from as much as 200 mg of tumor tissue per ml to as little as 31 mg per ml, and the total dosage administered per patient was the yield from as much as 14 gm of tumor tissue to as little as 1·8 gm. Vials were stored in a "Revco" freezer at approximately −60°C until use.

A gamma irradiated whole cell suspension, described below, was given during 1968 and 1969 and was abandoned as being ineffective. Three patients in 1969 received a water lysed cell preparation and are included in the lysed cell series. The trial with the lysed cell vaccine was resumed in 1971. Nine patients of the total of 21 in the lysed cell series have not developed pulmonary metastases at the time of writing.

To prepare the whole cell suspension, the tumor was minced with scissors and scalpels. Fragments were eliminated by sedimentation or by filtration through surgical gauze. The resulting suspension, which consisted predominantly of single cells, was centrifuged and the cells were suspended in Solution A (15) at a concentration of 10 million cells/ml. The suspensions were irradiated from a ^{60}Co source to a dose of 10,000 rads, ampouled in 1 ml aliquots, and stored at −60°C. Immediately before administration, a vial of vaccine was allowed to thaw at room temperature. The contents were mixed by drawing in and out of a syringe twice, and were administered by subcutaneous or intra-muscular injection into the gluteal or deltoid region.

The 14 patients who received the whole cell preparation are listed in Table 1. Only one of these is still free of disease at this time.

The injections were usually started between 7 and 10 days after surgery (never later than 28 days) and continued at approximately bi-weekly intervals for as many doses as were available. Patients who lived outside the commuting area for Memorial Hospital received at least the first dose of vaccine while hospitalized, and thereafter therapy continued through the cooperation of their local doctors. For shipment, the vaccine was packed in dry ice, and was stored frozen thereafter, usually in a household type deep freezer at temperatures around −10°C.

RESULTS

The data recorded for each patient in the control and vaccine groups included race, sex, age, site of tumor, pre-operative duration of symptoms and/or signs, and the date of amputation. For patients with no evidence of disease the date of latest follow-up was noted, and for patients with pulmonary metastasis the time from amputation to last negative and first positive chest X-ray (Tables 1 and 2).

It was necessary to employ a historical control, as the scarcity of cases of osteogenic sarcoma did not permit randomization. But the control group consisted of a consecutive series from Memorial Hospital, and all slides were reviewed by the same pathologist.

Examination of the control and the vaccine series showed the distribution of patients by race, sex, age, site, and pre-operative duration to be similar in the three groups. A few of the patients in the control and lysed cell series had received pre-operative radiation therapy, and none in the whole cell series (the practice has been discontinued at Memorial Hospital in the last few years), but the analysis of the control series had revealed no evidence of an effect of radiation therapy on the course of the disease.[9]

It was felt that the most suitable criterion for evaluating the effect of the vaccine was the length of the disease-free interval from surgery to the onset of pulmonary metastasis, as estimated by the date of the first positive X-ray (Fig. 1). It is important to note here, however, that X-rays were not taken on a regular basis in the control series since no treatment was available for pulmonary metastases. This meant that metastases would tend to be diagnosed at a later date, making the disease-free interval appear longer. The median interval from the last negative to the first positive chest film was 7 months for the

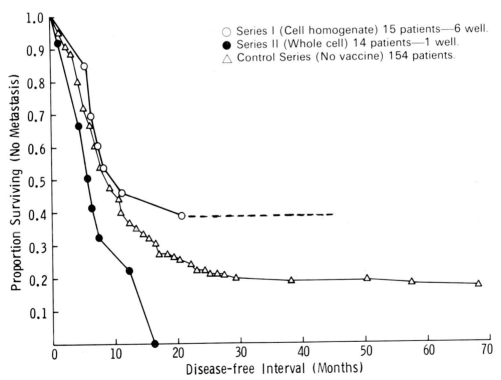

Fig. 1. Comparison of the lysed cell and whole cell vaccine series with control group in terms of the disease-free interval from amputation to detection of pulmonary metastases.

control series. For 28 patients in the control series the closest available date for the onset of pulmonary metastasis was the date of death, because of complete lack of follow-up X-ray examination.[9]

The curve for patients treated with the lysed cell vaccine (Fig. 1) may show some actual benefit. Statistical analysis of the difference between the results of the two vaccine treated groups when computed by the life table method[2] and evaluated by the Wilcoxon–Gehan two sided test[5] yields $P < 0.02$. In view of the restricted nature of the data presented however caution must be used in accepting this estimate as evidence of anything beyond a trend in favour of the lysed cell vaccine therapy. Nevertheless, it is sufficient to encourage continuation of the trial.

ACKNOWLEDGEMENT

The authors are grateful to Pat Middleman for technical assistance in the preparation of the paper.

REFERENCES

1. Copeland, M. & Geschickter, C. F. Malignant Bone Tumors, Primary and Metastatic. A Monograph. *Amer. Cancer Soc., Inc.*, **13**, 4–6, 1963.
2. Cutler, S. J. & Ederer, F. Maximum Utilization of the Life Table Method in Analyzing Survival. *J. Chron. Dis.*, **8**, 699–712, 1958.
3. Dahlin, D. C. & Coventry, M. B. Osteogenic Sarcoma. A Study of Six Hundred Cases. *J. Bone Jt. Surg.*, **49–A**, 101–110, 1967.
4. Farr, G. H., Huvos, A. G., Marcove, R. C., Higinbotham, N. L. & Foote, F. W., Jr. *Telangiectatic Osteogenic Sarcoma*. In preparation.
5. Gehan, E. A. A Generalized Wilcoxon Test for Comparing Arbitrarily Singly-Censored Samples. *Biometrika*, **52**, 203–223, 1965.
6. McKenna, R. J., Schwinn, C. P., Soong, K. Y. & Higinbotham, N. L. Sarcomata of the Osteogenic Series (Osteosarcoma, Fibrosarcoma, Chondrosarcoma, Parosteal Osteogenic Sarcoma, and Sarcomata Arising in Abnormal Bone). An Analysis of 552 Cases. *J. Bone Jt. Surg.*, **48–A**, 1–26, 1966.
7. Marcove, R. C. & Huvos, A. G. Cartilaginous Tumors of the Ribs. *Cancer*, **27**, 794–801, 1971.
8 Marcove, R. C., Miké, V., Hajek, J. V., Levin, A. G. & Hutter, R. V. P. Osteogenic Sarcoma in Childhood. *N.Y. St. J. Med.*, **71**, 855–859, 1971.
9. Marcove, R. C., Miké, V., Hajek, J. V., Levin, A. G. & Hutter, R. V. P. Osteogenic Sarcoma under the Age of Twenty-One. A Review of One Hundred and Forty-Five Operative Cases. *J. Bone Jt. Surg.*, **52–A**, 411–423, 1970.
10. Martini, N., Huvos, A. G., Miké, V., Marcove, R. C. & Beattie, E. J., Jr. Multiple Pulmonary Resections in the Treatment of Osteogenic Sarcoma. *Ann. Thoracic Surg.*, **12**, 271–280, 1971.
11. Phemister, D. B., A Study of the Ossification in Bone Sarcoma. *Radiology*, 17–23, 1926.
12. Phemister, D. B. Chondrosarcoma of Bone. *Surg. Gynec. Obstet.*, **50**. 216–233 1930.

Discussion

Prof. Middlemiss   May I ask a question which is really not directed to Dr. Marcove, but at pathologists here. Dr. Marcove is the first person to have mentioned osteoid tissue in this Symposium up to date, and I would like to know whether you all accept this as being essential to the diagnosis of osteosarcoma?

Professor McKenzie   Of course it does depend to some extent upon how much tissue you have available for study. If a biopsy is done in a child or young adolescent, and it shows malignant spindle celled tissue and maybe a focus of malignant cartilage as well, then in a very small biopsy I don't think that the absence of osteoid or tumour bone formation prevents one from making the diagnosis of osteogenic sarcoma; any more than I think that the absence of cross striations stops one making the diagnosis of rhabdomyosarcoma in cases which are otherwise typical.

Dr. Price   I think that perhaps you can get a little closer than that by combining cytological, cytochemical and histological methods. It is my experience that if you can demonstrate the tumour consists predominantly of cells which are either functional or morphological malignant osteoblasts you are home and dry with the diagnosis. That one can usually do on cytological smear or imprint preparations and the alkaline phosphatase preparation. By and large there are very few exceptions here, and the only things I can recall which could be easily confused have been smears from very florid callus. So you don't need osteoid necessarily.

Dr. Ball   I would like to go on record as saying that my practice is like that of Memorial Hospital, I would not like to diagnose osteosarcoma unless I could be convinced that tumour bone had been produced, or tumour osteoid or calcified osteoid. I would like to mention that I have another difficulty, that whilst everyone is agreed that this is a common definition of osteosarcoma—i.e. the presence of tumour osteoid, it's very rare to find the following sentence telling you how to recognize osteoid. It is as though a tacit compliment is being paid to everybody—that they will know it when they see it. I am not so sure that this is always the case—at least in the British Bone Tumour Panel we can argue sometimes about what is or is not osteoid. So the question is not quite so easy as some pathologists might perhaps think.

Dr. Marcove   When I was working with Jaffe in pathology we routinely would take an amputated specimen and slice it and X-ray every slice. And if in one slice you saw a little suspicious area of calcification that is where we made our sections from and then you found osteogenic sarcoma. Of course, not all osteoid is calcified to bone, but that was his criterion and whether other people agree with him or not. . . .

Dr. Price   Dr. Marcove, that is all very well, but just as Dr. Ball has hinted not all osteoid belongs to the tumour—some of it may be residual—some of it may be reactive. And to a large extent that is the crunch.

Dr. Marcove Yes, that is so. Also I have long discussions as to what is reactive bone in a Ewing's sarcoma, you can find plenty of bone there, and plenty of bone in a chondrosarcoma too.

Professor Bonfiglio I would like to ask, a question of the pathologists. My old friend Dr. Dahlin and I have discussed this at great length. How much osteoid or tumour bone will they accept to call a lesion an osteosarcoma? I have tried to differentiate between osteosarcoma and other types of tumours forming in bone which are in the "blanket" title of "osteogenic sarcoma", which is I think where one of our real world difficulties lies in coming to grips with the terminology. identification and classification of lesions. And how much will one accept? Is a small focus of tumour bone sufficient to call it an osteosarcoma, as compared with fibrosarcoma, when 99.9% of the lesion is fibrosarcomatous in nature, or chondrosarcomatous in nature?

Professor Ackerman This has sufficiently stimulated me to suggest that if we have a lesion which is a malignant bone tumour—then if its a cartilaginous tumour we have to take into consideration that we will look at the X-rays too. If it is a chondrosarcoma that has some metaplastic bone, that can be easily identified by just looking at it. Now the second point is that there are cases that you put in the text-book, anybody can look at them a mile away and say—"that's osteoid". Then I hate to hear these confessions of our inadequacies here in public. I admit that I can't identify osteoid with confidence—I don't know any way you can do that by looking at an H & E slide with absolute confidence. However, the problem may arise when you have a tumour which is a fibrosarcoma, but the surgeon says "Are you sure that it isn't an osteosarcoma?". And so the question is—"Is this an osteosarcoma just sort of masquerading as a fibrosarcoma?" I think that Dr. Price has rendered a great service by showing that we don't just have to look at the slides—we can see what the tissue can do and what it can produce. As he has indicated, when you have a fibrosarcoma which is really fibrosarcoma it doesn't make alkaline phosphatase, and you can find that out. Now a Ewing's tumour is all the same so you don't have any problems. When you have a highly pleomorphic tumour and it has the characteristics radiographically and clinically of an osteosarcoma, such as those that are sometimes. telangectatic, you may have to hunt a long time for osteoid and probably wouldn't find it But still if you give it a little time and do some of the other things that Dr. Price has said, I think it can be identified with confidence as osteosarcoma. So I think that this is not such a big problem. We have our inadequacies—but they are not that big !

Dr. Jeffree The following point has really been made for me, but it is this point of alkaline phosphatase in an apparent fibrosarcoma. Dr. Price will remember a case where the first specimen we had was a typical fibrosarcoma histologically and it was choc-a-block with alkaline phosphatase and I had never seen anything like it. Well, the medullary tumour was typical osteosarcoma. It was the bit outside the bone that we looked at first and the content of alkaline phosphate definitely pointed to osteosarcoma, but you could not see this in the initial sections.

Dr. Suit I would like to go back to Dr. Marcove's paper. I think that the implications of the data if we can accept them at their face value are quite important. I wish to know if you have performed any investigations of the patient's reactivity to his own tumour cells? Have you made any assay to see if there is any recognition by the patient of the antigens of his own osteosarcoma cells? If so, was there any correlation between that kind of reactivity and the patients who remained metastasis-free?

Dr. Marcove   We are trying to do it. There are three immunologists working at Sloan–Kettering on this. Also our sera are being sent to the Kleins in Sweden and we're all trying to show increased cytotoxic effect of serum. We have demonstrated it, but not in titres yet. I'm not sure that the antibody–antigen reaction that we are showing really is important in survival of the patient. There are many different types of antibody–antigen reactions. We have published a fractionation of urinary S1 antigen into S1 and S2 antigens. I suspect that there are many antigens and reactions; and whether they are important for the patient's survival or not I do not think is known. The only way to do it is to try it on patients and study the cases.

Professor Barnes   One of the most remarkable things which has come out of this Symposium, and nobody has really commented about it today, is the extraordinary variation in 5-year survival results for osteosarcoma from the various centres. In Israel none; in Canada—5%; in Great Britain—somewhere between 15 and 21%. If we assume that we are all talking about the same tumour then these differences really are quite remarkable. Does it in fact mean that a different type of technique of irradiation is being employed in these various centres? For example, in Israel is the whole length of the femur being irradiated—or only part of it?

   Dr. Enneking yesterday did point out the dangers of wide spread or spillage of the tumour after biopsy. One wonders if in some of these instances only a part of the affected bone was being irradiated and not the whole. Does this in some way influence the long-term results? It would really be fascinating to hear the opinions of the people from these three centres: Westminster Hospital, Toronto General and Israel as to what is their opinion about this extraordinary difference in the 5-year survival rates.

Dr. Hale (Chairman)   May I call upon anyone who is willing to contribute to this. Before we start I am not so sure that the radiotherapy to the primary lesion is the key to this problem—I think it may be surgery.

Professor Van Rijssel   It also depends upon the number of cases I think. As far as I have understood, the number of cases that people from Israel referred to was 40 cases. The number of cases treated in Holland with a result of 20% survival for 5 years were about 300.

Professor Barnes   But a survival rate of nil amongst 40 patients must surely be significant, and I don't think you can ignore that.

Professor Van Rijssel   But I think that they were not the same patients!

Dr. Brenner   I think that is a very good point because we heard now that the number of cases seen in individual centres and from particular pathology registries has varied enormously—from 300 down to our 40 and 30 in Toronto. I think that this is probably the real indication of what is going on. Our cases for the most part were rather late when they were seen at our Institution. They were referred cases, and I think Dr. Spira will bear me out that they were for the most part almost inoperable *ab initio*. Nevertheless, it's a very small series, and although we have no survivors amongst 40 cases, one patient who had extra-corporeal irradiation lasted $4\frac{1}{2}$ years. Small numbers don't mean a thing in percentages. When you have a large series of cases—e.g. over 300, you may still get between 5 and 15%. I think it is significant that the cure rate is very low whatever the method has been. In Israel I was the radiotherapist for most of these cases, but I do know that at that time the technique was to irradiate mainly the tumour and not the whole bone. I don't believe myself that whole bone irradiation is going to make any difference whatsoever. I think that the main trouble here is that we have disseminated disease: I don't think that the local disease itself is a big problem. If it were then the disarticulations would get far better results than the difference of only 5 or 10%. Now I think that this is a generalized disease and should be treated as such. The only reason that we proposed our extra-corporeal irradiation was that this enables the child to go back to school fairly rapidly with his own leg. We don't ever claim that this is a curative procedure.

Dr. Newton   My experience of patients treated in Israel totals one. This patient was referred to us and it was quite clear that the irradiation didn't cover the entire extent of the tumour. As demonstrated by bone scanning about 5 or 6 cm was involved above the irradiation field. Perhaps this one case is deceiving. Usually our own technique embraces a minimum field length of 32 cm and a minimum dose of 6,000 rads. Part of the treatment is given pre-operatively: most of the cases have it done before biopsy, as 1,000 rads given in one treatment, and a biopsy is then performed on that day or the following day. Then the main 5,000 rads follow after an interval of 1 week. The area treated is always very generous, but even so I am inclined to agree that the secret does not lie in the technique of the radiotherapy.

Professor Dahlin   It is probably superfluous to mention this but I think that we should have a statistician here. It is obvious that small numbers of cases are not important as far as determining exact percentages is concerned. I also think from our own experience I can say safely that unless one follows up a very high percentage of the cases, and knows exactly what happens to them, one is apt to find that it is the long survivors who get lost. In our country the surgeons know what happens to those that get into trouble because they come back to them. But they forget about the survivors because literally many of them move to California. So I think that as exact statistics as we can get are vital to this whole subject.

Mr. Lee   Could I just go back to this question of the survivals for a moment, because I think it is important. Nobody of course has done a really controlled trial of different methods of treatment; perhaps Dr. Marcove comes nearest to it. Much depends upon the kind of material that is referred to a particular institution and I think this must vary a great deal. We had 187 cases when we drew up this 21% survival rate and this included every single case that came to the hospital, even some who developed metastases when they were having their radiotherapy. I think this is another question which must be asked: How do you calculate your percentages? From every case that was seen in the hospital, or from every case that was accepted for treatment, or from every case that completed treatment—and so on? I think that the differences between one institution and another are so great that we cannot very closely compare the figures. This is why anything between 10 to 14 or 20% is perhaps as near as we can get.

Professor Enneking I would like to make one comment in regard to that. We have recently tried to go through the world literature and find out what the natural curve of survival in the *disease-free interval* is for osteosarcoma treated only by surgery. We would use that curve to compare other forms of treatment. As Prof. Barnes has pointed out the crude survival rates are very variable. The thing that falls within the confidence levels that Dr. Marcove showed is the disease-free interval from the time of operation, to the time of first appearance of pulmonary metastases. Every published curve falls within this confidence level of 95% with the exception of one which presented in Holland the other day. From the point of 2 years onwards to 5 years there are varying declines in crude survival rates. So I think in terms of using a yardstick by which to measure the effectiveness of treatment the disease-free interval following the removal of the primary is probably the closest for everyone to count, because there are very few cases now not treated with something else other than pure surgery.

About a year and a half ago we gathered over 400 cases in which we wanted to try and demonstrate not only the survival rate, and the growth rate of pulmonary metastases but also the metastases to other organs. We wanted to have children before the age of 21. From all these cases all over the United States only 6% had three or more chest X-rays and accurate documentation of the date of death, and an autopsy. Only 22 cases, and this was from about 14 different centres: so that the opportunity I think of documenting accurately the natural history and follow-up course of osteosarcoma after primary removal and treatment is probably past us. All that we can do is to try to accumulate the world literature and draw up a reasonably confident curve of the disease-free interval to compare with other forms of treatment.

Experimental studies

Transplantation of canine osteosarcoma

by

L. N. OWEN

SUMMARY

Canine foetuses *in utero* were inoculated with living spleen cells from a dog bearing a spontaneous osteosarcoma. At birth osteosarcoma from the donor was inoculated into puppies and a successful transplantation occurred. Using the inoculation of trypsinized tumour cells into foetuses *in utero* or into dogs immunosuppressed with A.L.S. serial transplantation has been carried out.

From the fourth *in vivo* transplantation the tumour was successfully grown in tissue culture and is now in its 280th passage. Fatal malignant sarcomas occur when foetal dogs are injected with these tumour cells or when the cells are injected into new-born immunosuppressed dogs. If osteosarcoma tissue culture cells are injected intra-arterially into immunosuppressed puppies tumours develop in the bones of the injected limb.

Following intravenous injection tumours develop in the lungs and this tumour growth can be reduced by X-irradiation of the thorax. Trials are in progress in clinical cases in dogs using a linear accellerator to X-irradiate only one lung. Some effects of anti-tumour drugs on canine osteosarcoma cells in tissue culture are given.

INTRODUCTION

OSTEOSARCOMA IS THE MOST common primary sarcoma of bone in man and dog (Owen, 1969a). Most tumours arise in the metaphysis of a long bone, common sites being the distal femur and proximal tibia in man and the proximal humerus and distal radius in the dog. The radiographical and histological features are similar in both species but age incidence of tumour onset differs in that the condition occurs mainly in middle age in the dog, whereas in man most cases occur in the first three decades of life. The natural history of the condition is similar in both species, lung metastases, however, developing earlier in the dog as would be expected in an animal of shorter life span.

Because of its larger size the dog is better suited for research on surgical, irradiation and perfusion techniques than other smaller laboratory animals. Many studies have been made on the spontaneous tumour in the dog but large numbers of cases are difficult to obtain and much of value can be learned from a transplantable osteosarcoma in the dog.

METHODS OF TRANSPLANTATION

The methods of transplantation have previously been described (Owen and Nielsen 1968, Owen 1969b, Bostock and Owen 1970).

INTRA-FOETAL INJECTION

In the original transplantation 10^8 spleen cells from an Alsatian cross-bred male dog bearing a spontaneous osteosarcoma were injected intraperitoneally into canine foetuses on the 54th day of gestation. At birth the puppies were injected subcutaneously with tumour from the same donor. In one animal the tumour grew progressively and from this tumour, which was more cellular and less calcified than the original, a cell suspension was made and injected again into canine foetuses. Serial transplants were made by this technique on six occasions.

ANTI-LYMPHOCYTE SERUM

Anti-lymphocyte serum (A.L.S.) made by standard techniques in rabbits, pigs, cows or horses from thymus and mesenteric lymph nodes of 3-month-old puppies has proved to be a highly successful method for immunosuppression and tumour transplantation in the dog. An initial dose of 3 ml/kg subcutaneously followed by 1·5 ml/kg s/c three times weekly has been used. Suspensions of tumour cells usually 10^6–10^8 have been injected subcutaneously, intravenously or intra-arterially into puppies the day following the first injection of A.L.S. Tumours are frequently palpable or radiographically visible within 3 weeks and in many animals injected intravenously the advanced state of tumour growth necessitates euthanasia after 5–6 weeks. Animals injected subcutaneously with tumour live longer.

TISSUE CULTURE

Subcutaneous tumour from the fourth (intra-foetal) passage in a Retriever puppy was removed surgically, diced in Hanks' solution and trypsinized at 38°C for 20 minutes. Centrifuged cells at a concentration of $1·25 \times 10^6$ cells/ml were re-suspended in TC199 containing 20% foetal calf serum. These cells grew well and later *in vitro* passages grew in TC199 with only 10% calf serum. This canine osteosarcoma cell line has been maintained for 3 years and is now in its 280th passage. The tumour is of fibroblastic appearance and 10^6 tissue culture cells or more injected intraperitoneally into foetuses at about the seventh week of gestation or injected into newborn puppies immunosuppressed with A.L.S. produce fatal sarcomas in nearly all instances.

ANATOMICAL DISTRIBUTION OF TUMOURS

(a) Puppies injected intraperitoneally as foetuses developed sarcomas in many sites including peritoneum, pleura, pericardium, heart, lungs, kidneys, meninges and bones. In four puppies osteosarcoma of the gums occurred at about 3 weeks of age coinciding with the time of milk tooth eruption (Fig. 1). In one of these animals this was the only site of tumour occurrence found at post-mortem examination.

(b) Following intravenous injection of A.L.S.-treated dogs with *in vivo* transplanted cells or cells grown in tissue culture there was rapid development of tumours in the lungs. In some instances tumours were widespread in the bones, both limb bones and skull bones being affected.

(c) Intra-arterial injection. Following injection of 10^6–10^7 tumour cells into the femoral artery of new-born puppies treated with A.L.S., sarcomas developed in the bones

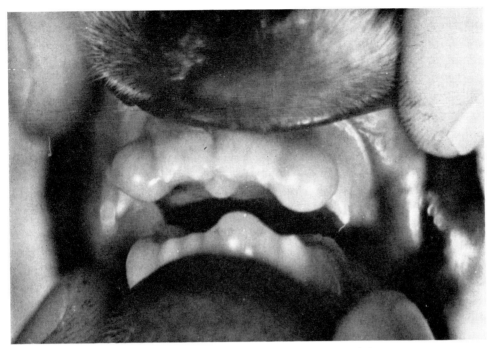

Fig. 1. Three-week-old puppy with osteosarcomas of the gums.

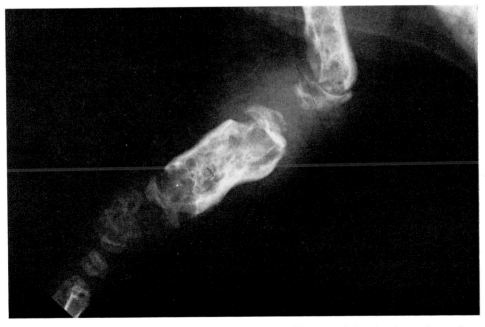

Fig. 2. Sarcomas of hind limb bones in a 6-week old puppy following intra-femoral arterial injection of osteosarcoma cells at birth.

of the affected limb (Fig. 2) and smaller tumours occurred in the lungs and elsewhere in the body. In some new-born animals it has been possible to produce limb bone tumours which progressed in non-immunosuppressed animals but the number of "takes" in normal animals is very variable.

HISTOLOGY AND HISTOCHEMISTRY

In tumours serially transplanted *in vivo* the appearance of the transplanted tumour was essentially similar to the spontaneous original tumour. Osteoid or new bone was present in all transplants and cells showed the characteristically high alkaline phosphatase content of an osteosarcoma; lactic acid dehydrogenase and β-glucuronidase activities were also positive.

Chromosome studies made from tumour in a female animal showed the tumour to be male, the same as the original donor, and the normal 78 chromosomes were present.

Histological examination of tumours grown from tissue culture cells has shown in most areas closely packed cells with little intercellular matrix. In other areas the appearance was of a fibrospindle cell sarcoma, well collagenized. Alkaline phosphatase was absent in these tumours except in those tumours developing in bone. The reactive bone cells around the tumour were positive for this enzyme.

TUMOUR GROWTH RATE

The original donor dog with an osteosarcoma of the proximal humerus had multiple metastases in the lungs. Under standard reproducible conditions a series of chest radiographs was made weekly over a period of 46 days and seven metastases of clear definition were measured. One hour before euthanasia 6 mCi of tritiated thymidine was injected intravenously. Autoradiographs were made from metastatic lung tumours of similar size to those which had been measured radiographically. Growth measurements were also made on transplanted tumours in A.L.S.-treated dogs. The results are as follows (Owen and Steel 1969):

Terminal volume doubling times of lung metastases of the spontaneous original tumour: 11, 12, 20, 25, 26, 37, 40 days—mean 24 days.

Labelling index: 9·7%

Potential doubling time: 2·6 days.

Cell loss factor: 89%.

Transplanted tumour terminal volume doubling times: small tumours 2–3 days; larger tumours approximately 5 days.

It will be seen that actual doubling times become much shorter as has also been found to occur with transplanted tumours in rodents.

X-IRRADIATION OF LUNGS

Osteosarcoma in man kills in nearly all cases because of lung metastases. It is likely that in the early stages of the condition the microscopic metastases in the lungs are the only metastases present in the body. Methods may eventually be developed which will destroy these relatively few tumour cells by radiotherapy, chemotherapy, immuno-therapy or a combination of these methods. The canine osteosarcoma model developed can be used to study some possible methods of achieving this object.

New-born puppies have been immunosuppressed with A.L.S., and injected into the jugular vein with a well-dispersed suspension of osteosarcoma cells grown in tissue culture. Twenty-four hours later in some of these dogs one or both sides of the thorax have been irradiated with 600 r X-irradiation from a 230 kV radiotherapy machine. In some animals repeat doses of irradiation have been given. The experiments are still in progress but some early results are shown in Tables 1, 2 and 3 (heavy weights given in grammes.)

TABLE 1

X-IRRADIATION OF RIGHT LUNG

600 r given one day after injection of cells and lungs
examined 32–35 days later

Dog No.		No. of cells	Weight left lung	Weight right lung
1		10^8	28	17
2		5×10^7	37·2	20·8
3		5×10^7	22	12·0
4		5×10^7	11·8	11·0
5	Control. No irradiation	10^8	33	29·4
6	Control. No irradiation	5×10^7	27	28·8

TABLE 2

X-IRRADIATION OF LEFT LUNG OR BOTH LUNGS

5×10^6 cells intravenously. 600 r X-irradiation
24 hours later, then weekly at doses at 300 r. Lungs
examined 28–35 days post-injection

Dog. No.	X-irradiation dose		Weight left lung	Weight right lung
1	Both	900	9·7	7·1
2	Both	1200	4·7	7·7
3	Both	1500	7·3	7·8
4	Left	1800	14·0	40·5
5	Nil		71	49

TABLE 3

X-IRRADIATION OF LEFT LUNG OR BOTH LUNGS

2×10^7 cells intravenously. 600 r X-irradiation 24 hours later,
then weekly at doses of 300 r

Dog No.	X-irradiation dose		Weight left lung	Weight right lung	Days post-injection
1	Left	900	15·3	23·6	16
2	Both	900	9·9	8·1	27
3	Left	1200	12·8	42·6	23
4	Both	1200	9·1	16·4	31
5	Both	1500	5·2	6·5	31
6	Nil		10·9	15·7	25
7	Nil		25·9	37·8	32

In most instances there was a considerable reduction in the amount of tumour in the irradiated lung compared with the non-irradiated. In occasional animals which have not shown marked differences growth of the tumour has been poor.

As well as measurement by weights of tumour in lungs histological studies of tumour volume on a dissecting microscope indicate impressive tumour reduction following irradiation.

CHEMOTHERAPY

To canine osteosarcoma cells growing in Leiden tubes a number of drugs have been added at concentrations shown in Table 4. The medium containing the drug was replaced with fresh medium after 24 hours. Cells were examined at 24 and 72 hours for cytopathic effects.

The most marked cytopathic effects were shown by the first five drugs in the table, viz. Actinomycin D, Vinblastine, Vincristine, Mycophenolic acid and Ethoglucid. With other drugs effects were minimal or non-apparent. It is hoped at a later stage to correlate these results *in vitro* with the effect of the drugs on tumours *in vivo*. If the Vinca alkaloids are classified as one drug the modes of action of the four effective drugs are all different and combination therapy could be of value.

X-IRRADIATION OF PRIMARY TUMOURS AND LUNGS IN CLINICAL CASES OF OSTEOSARCOMA IN DOGS

Nine dogs with a primary spontaneous osteosarcoma in a limb bone and without radiographic evidence of lung metastases have been X-irradiated using a linear accelerator. Doses of 4,000 to 5,000 r usually fractionated at 1,000 r at weekly intervals have been

TABLE 4

CANINE OSTEOSARCOMA TISSUE CULTURE CELLS

Drug	Concentration γ/ml
Actinomycin D	0·01
Vinblastine	0·2
Vincristine	0·1
Mycophenolic acid	10
Ethoglucid	10
CB1954	1·0
CB1955	5·0
Chlorambucil	1·0
Cyclophosphamide	20
5 Fluorouracil	15
Melphalan	2·5
Methotrexate	1·0
Stilboestrol diphosphate	7·5
Triaziquone (Trenimon)	0·02
Prednisolone phosphate	20 mg/ml
Thio-tepa	3 mg/ml
Neomycin	2,500 units

given to the primary tumour. Within 2 days of the first dose pain was considerably decreased and lameness improved. Except in two very advanced cases the tumours have shown regression and radiographical changes. When pain recurred or there was an increase in tumour size euthanasia was carried out. Of 6 dogs now dead the pain-free survival time varied between 1 and 7 months (Owen and Bostock 1972). On the first occasion that the primary tumour was irradiated the right thorax in these dogs was also irradiated at a dose of 600 r and this dose was repeated 1 week later. In one dog the affected limb was ablated surgically and the right chest irradiated with 600 r on two occasions with one week interval. Post-mortem examination on three dogs where the primary tumour was treated with X-irradiation and in one dog surgically has shown less tumour tissue on the irradiated side in two dogs but in the other two dogs there was no appreciable difference. It is expected that during the next year more cases will be evaluated and a conclusion reached on the effect of this clinical procedure.

In lungs which contain no tumour cells at the time of irradiation the possibility exists of causing lung damage by the irradiation which may then favour the future lodgement and growth of tumour cells shed from a primary X-irradiated tumour. This aspect is being investigated experimentally.

ACKNOWLEDGEMENTS

Much of the above work is joint work with Mr. D. E. Bostock. I wish also to acknowledge the help of Professor W. I. B. Beveridge, Professor J. S. Mitchell, F.R.S.,

Dr. C. H. G. Price, Dr. G. M. Jeffree, Dr. H. A. van Peperzeel, Dr. D. W. van Bekkum and Dr. G. S. Steel. The investigation was supported by grants from the Cancer Research Campaign and the Medical Research Council.

REFERENCES

Bostock, D. E. & Owen, L. N. Transplantation and Tissue Culture Studies of Canine Osteo-sarcoma. *European J. Cancer*, **6**, 499, 1970.

Owen, L. N. *Bone Tumours in Man and Animals*. Butterworth, London, p. 201, 1969a.

Owen, L. N. Transplantation of Canine Osteosarcoma. *European J. Cancer*, **5**, 615, 1969b.

Owen, L. N. & Nielsen, S. W. Transplantation of Canine Lymphosarcoma. *European J. Cancer*, **4**, 391, 1968.

Owen, L. N. & Steel, G. G. The Growth and Cell Population Kinetics of Spontaneous Tumours in Domestic Animals. *Brit. J. Cancer*, **23**, 493, 1969.

Owen, L. N. & Bostock, D. E. Preliminary Report on the Treatment of Canine Osteosarcoma using the Linear Accelerator. *Vet. Rec.*, in the press, 1972.

Discussion

Dr. Moore To anticipate something that Dr. Finkel might say is wrong, an obvious experiment here I think, Dr. Owen, would be the attempt to transmit osteosarcoma to the foetuses by intra-uterine injection of cell-free material from your primary osteosarcomas. Have you tried this? If not I think it should be high on the list of your priorities.

Dr. Owen Yes we have. It is an obvious thing to do and we have done it. It's difficult to get accommodation for large numbers of dogs to keep over a long period of time. We have made extracts of various types and injected them into foetuses. Some animals we have also put onto anti-lymphocyte serum for some period after birth. But we've got nothing. They are all perfectly normal at the moment. What we have also done and are continuing to do is to grow normal embryonic tibial bone and frontal bone from dogs—as we think frontal bone may be a good source of supply of pure osteoblasts. and getting a pure osteoblast culture is very difficult to prove—but its the nearest thing we could get. They grow very well in tissue culture—at least for a period of time. Then we have put frozen and thawed osteosarcoma material (Moloney extract) on these cells. Osteosarcoma cells given 10,000 rads of irradiation have also been put on these cells, and also one or two other methods to see if we can get transformation and we have grown up the query transformed cells and the normal cells and injected them into immunosuppressed animals. In two instances we have got something that looks like sarcoma, but regresses in two dogs. But in instances where this was done the control cells died out before we were able to inject them. So its not a fool-proof experiment and has never gone into print, nor will it go into print until we can repeat it. This is the approach we are making.

Dr. Suit I would like to know if in your primary sample material you are making any study of the host reaction to the individual sarcoma cells?

Dr. Owen We have only just started this. We have read with great interest D. L. Morton's work and Dr. Moore's work is here now, and others on immunofluorescence and other methods in this. As far as we have gone which isn't very far we don't get the same results. I think this is a question of technique, but there may be some other reasons. We do at the moment get some peri-nuclear fluorescence which we can't explain at all. We are pursuing this line actively and shall continue to do so. There is a W.H.O. meeting on animal tumours at Geneva in July and we hope to introduce not only classification which is now going well, but a co-operative therapy group. If anyone here has any ideas on the clinical osteosarcomas that we get I shall be very pleased to hear them. We can get collaborators in America, Holland and in Britain who will all adopt the same therapy. We would like to do something a bit different that also might pay off, and not use exactly the same things that have been described this morning.

Dr. Price I am terribly interested in these extraordinary gum tumours in your puppies. Could you give any indication about the frequency with which they have appeared in that particular situation? I believe it was an intra-peritoneal injection of a cell suspension that you gave them. Also would you have any clues as to why they appear in this extraordinary site?

Dr. Owen   We have only seen this phenomenon in four instances. This was in the early *in-vivo* transplants before we got the tumour growing in tissue culture. We've injected very large numbers of dogs with tissue culture material and not seen this phenomenon since. I must admit that we are mostly injecting now for various reasons animals that are immunosuppressed at birth rather than foetuses. Three of eight dogs were in one litter which we injected intra-peritoneally and one dog was in another litter. Their litter-mates (5) did not develop gum tumours. As to why they should develop, this is obviously a very vascular area and there is trauma here from an erupting milk tooth. One must assume that the conditions are favourable for tumour growth, but what these are it would be very nice indeed to know, or even how to find out.

Dame Janet Vaughan   I would only say in connection with these gum tumours that we found when we used ^{90}Sr in rabbits it was a very favourable site for the development of tumours. Dr Halse of Harwell when he was using neutron bombardment of the whole body in rabbits also found that the one site where tumours developed in his rabbits was also this area where there was a growing tooth. When our jaws were sectioned, Rushton who was a very well known dental pathologist did demonstrate this as a site of very active proliferating tissue. One knows that malignancy is apt to arise in very actively proliferating cells. I too was very interested to see these gum tumours. It would appear that in animals at least there is something in dogs and rabbits about this area which is very conducive to tumour growth.

Professor Sissons   In relation to this last question, can I ask whether these are tumours of the soft tissues of the gums or arising in bone?

Dr. Owen   The tumours are osteosarcomas developing in the soft tissues of the gum and can be round almost. You can dissect them away from the bone.

Professor Sissons   In this sense they are rather different from the tumours which Dame Janet was referring to which were osteosarcomas in the bone of the jaw.

Dr. Owen   No, they are in gum tissue itself, which at the time is being damaged by milk tooth eruption.

Professor Bonfiglio   Does this mean that they will also develop metaphyseal tumours in time?

Dr. Owen   In one animal of the four there were only gum tumours. The other three animals did not have tumours in the bones in this particular instance, but tumours in other sites in the body—in other soft tissues such as the kidney and pleura and so on.

Professor Duthie   In your typical trial of your clinical cases are you basing your criterion of entering into your trial on radiology alone, or are you also combining it with surgical biopsy? You might be able to run two trials there—two systems of diagnosis plus treatment without any surgical intervention.

Dr. Owen   At the moment we are doing everything on biopsy. We are doing everything in the diagnosis as in the human field to make the results comparable. But I accept your point on the question of biopsy, as to whether it is a good thing.

Professor Van Rijssel   Can you tell me is there some difference in the physiology of bone in dogs compared with humans? For instance is the replacement more rapid? I enquire because of the difference of the age group in which tumours occur, much later after epiphyseal fusion.

Dr. Owen   I don't think that there are any really fundamental differences known between dogs and man. In explanation I assume that one possibility is a virus and the latent period might be a number of years. It's not too far different if we get a 9-year-old dog and the human surgeon has a 15-year-old child. There is very little difference in years, but in the life span it is quite different in the dog. It's usually more than half the life span before the tumours develop.

M*

Investigation of a transplantable murine osteosarcoma

by

BARRY FRIEDMAN, and ALEX FINSTERBUSH†

SUMMARY

A transplantable murine osteosarcoma which arose spontaneously in a C3H mouse has retained its bone-forming capability through more than 200 generations of transplantation. It has also retained its malignancy in uniformly causing death by pulmonary metastases unless amputated one week or less following implantation. The tumor has been transplanted to other strains of mice retaining to some degree its bone-forming ability as well as its ability to metastasize to the lungs. The virus particles which are present in Dunn osteosarcoma cells may not be etiologically related to the tumor on the basis of evidence presented.

INTRODUCTION

Two PREVIOUS REPORTS, both concerned with bone induction experiments have included brief descriptions of an osteosarcoma transplantable in C3H mice.[4,6] The tumor was obtained through the courtesy of Dr. Thelma Dunn of the National Cancer Institute who discovered it in 1955 when it arose spontaneously in the tail vertebra of a 21-month-old female C3He/b mouse. The mouse had been injected with an extract of AKR spontaneous leukemia cells as a newborn, but no other mice in the group developed osteosarcoma. Dr. Dunn maintained the tumor by serial subcutaneous transfer and we in our laboratory have done likewise at approximately monthly intervals for over 4 years. The tumor has now been transplanted for over 200 transplant generations and we now report in somewhat greater detail the histological changes which have occurred through the many transplant generations, and some of the biological characteristics of the Dunn osteosarcoma.

MATERIALS AND METHODS

The experiments were performed using either C3H/HeJ (Jackson Laboratories, Bar Harbor, Maine) or CF1 (Carworth Farms, Portage, Michigan) 6-week-old female mice. The C3H is an inbred agouti, the CF1 is a random-bred albino mouse.

* Supported by PHS Grant DE-02587 from National Institute of Dental Research of NIH and the Research Fund of Mount Sinai Hospital, Cleveland, Ohio.

† From the Orthopaedic Research Laboratory of Mt. Sinai Hospital, Cleveland and the Materials Science Center of Case Western Reserve University.

Tissue taken for light microscopy was fixed in acetic acid formalin and following decalcification paraffin-embedded sections were stained with hematoxylin and eosin. Localization of alkaline phosphatase was carried out by a modification of the method described by Molbert et al.[11] Tissue for electron microscopy was fixed in 6% glutaraldehyde, post-fixed in osmium tetroxide, dehydrated and embedded in Araldite. Thin sections were contrasted with uranyl acetate and lead citrate.

TRANSPLANTATION OF TUMOR CELLS

Donor mice were killed by cervical dislocation and the skin overlying the tumor was shaved and swabbed with alcohol. Using sterile instruments and solutions the tumor was dissected out and was either cut into $2 mm^3$ fragments which were implanted subcutaneously through a 5 mm incision in the skin of recipient mice, or was finely-minced in saline in a Petri dish. Fascia and necrotic tissue were discarded and the tumor cell suspension strained through sterile gauze. Cell counts were obtained in a hemocytometer and the cell suspension was brought to the desired dilution by addition of saline. Injection of tumor cell suspensions was performed into the lower thigh muscles of the right hind leg after shaving the overlying skin. A volume of 0·1 ml containing the desired number of tumor cells was used for injection.

DETERMINATION OF THE NUMBER OF TUMOR CELLS REQUIRED TO TRANSFER THE TUMOR

Cell suspensions containing 2×10^4, 5×10^5, and 10^6 were injected into groups of 10 to 20 mice.

EFFECT OF REMOVAL OF TUMOR-BEARING EXTREMITY ON SURVIVAL

In order to determine if removal of the tumor would prevent metastatic spread, disarticulation of the tumor-bearing extremity was carried out in groups of 20 animals at 1 and 2 weeks after tumor implantation. Animals were killed and autopsied 4 weeks later. This procedure was preferable to waiting until the animals died of their tumors, because surviving C3H mice cannibalize their dead.

TRANSPLANTATION OF DUNN OSTEOSARCOMA FROM C3H MICE TO CF1 MICE

Six-week-old CF1 female mice were obtained from Carworth Farms, Portage, Michigan, average weight 16 gm. Tumor transplantation was carried out by implantation into CF1 mice of fragments of tumor, intramuscular injection of tumor cell suspension, or intraperitoneal injection of tumor cell suspension using Dunn osteosarcoma tissue from C3H mice. In some experiments CF1 mouse tumor tissue which had been successfully transplanted from C3H mice was removed and either implanted as tumor fragments or injected as cell suspensions into other CF1 mice or were transplanted back into C3H mice.

ATTEMPTS TO INDUCE TUMORS WITH CELL-FREE EXTRACTS OF TUMORS

Because virus particles had been observed in cells of the Dunn osteosarcoma by electron microscopy,[4] attempts were made to induce the tumor into C3H mice by injection of cell-free extracts of the tumor. Tumor extracts were prepared by homogenizing freshly excised tumor tissue in 10 times its volume of minimal essential medium (Eagle)

with 10% bovine serum, glutamine, penicillin and streptomycin added. Further preparation of extract was accomplished in two ways: (a) centrifuging homogenized tissue
twice at 5,000 rpm at 0°C and filtering the last supernatant through 0.45μ millipore
filters; (b) freeze-thawing three times in liquid N_2, centrifuging between each freeze-
thaw cycle. Cell-free extracts were injected subcutaneously into groups of six mice in
each of three separate experiments. In addition, in order to "mature" immature viruses
before injection, extracts prepared as in (a) above, were diluted 1, 2, 4, and 8 times with
culture medium and incubated at 37°C with cultures of hamster kidney cells or with
cultures of whole C3H mouse embryo cells (Microbiological Assoc., Bethesda, Maryland)
for 72 hours. Cultures were then trypsinized, centrifuged and the supernatant injected
into groups of newborn and 6-week-old C3H mice.

OBSERVATIONS AND RESULTS

Tissue sections obtained from the original tail vertebra osteosarcoma, the first generation and 111th generation transplanted tumors, as well as their pulmonary metastases,
were kindly furnished by Dr. Dunn. As shown in Fig. 1, the tumor is a well-differentiated bone-forming tumor which has eroded the cortex of the vertebral body and grown
subperiosteally. Except for the increased cellularity and the invasiveness of the tumor,
the osteoblasts appear similar to active osteoblasts in normal bone-producing tissue.
Hyperchromicity, mitotic figures and pleomorphism are not prominent and only occasional bizarre cell forms are seen. The malignant character of the tumor, however, is
proved by the presence of pulmonary metastases (Fig. 2). The tumor tissue present in
the lung of the original animal has the same well-differentiated appearance as does that
of the primary site.

The tumor tissue from the first generation transplant of the tumor shows more pleomorphism, mitoses and increased cellularity than the original, but is still producing
fairly well-differentiated tumor bone (Fig. 3).

The tumor has undergone de-differentiation with subsequent transplantations. The
amount of trabecular bone is considerably less than the original tumor and the trabeculae
are now thin and strand-like in contrast to the thicker woven bone of the original tumor
(Fig. 4).

Bone formation, at present, is confined to the central portions of the tumor. Cells
undergoing mitotic division are numerous, especially close to the tumor periphery. After
3 weeks following implantation the center of the tumor undergoes necrosis and this
becomes more extensive as the tumor grows peripherally (Fig. 5 and 6).

The Dunn osteosarcoma metastasizes to the lungs by the ninth or tenth day resulting
in death of the animals by about 6 weeks following tumor implantation (Fig. 7). Tumor
tissue in the lung appears similar to that of the primary tumor at the transplant site,
usually contains osteoid and, in larger tumor nodules, the osteoid becomes calcified.
Most metastatic nodules in the lungs are demarcated from the surrounding alveoli by
one or more circumscribed zones of flattened fibrous tissue cells, but acute or chronic
inflammatory cells are not seen unless there is an associated pneumonitis which is
occasionally present.

Metastasis to organs other than lung occurs in less than 5% of the mice autopsied.
The kidneys and the adrenals are the most frequent extra-pulmonary sites of metastasis.

342

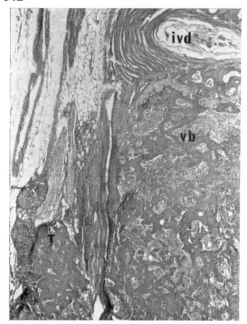

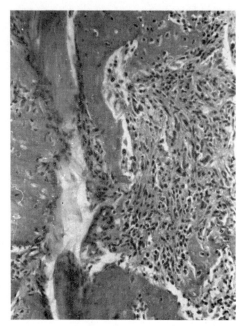

Fig. 1-A.　(H & E ×31.) Low magnification photomicrograph of original Dunn osteosarcoma in a tail vertebra of a C3H mouse. Intervertebral disc (ivd) is seen above. Below it is the vertebral body (vb). Increased cellularity and tumor bone formation is seen in lower half of vertebral body. Some tumor bone has perforated cortex (T) and is seen in extra-vertebral tissues.

Fig. 1-B.　(H & E × 236.) Higher magnification showing tumor at right breaking through cortex and at left tumor bone which appears mature.

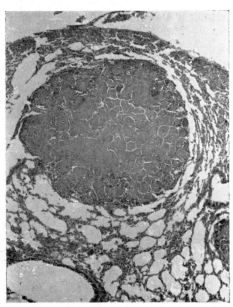

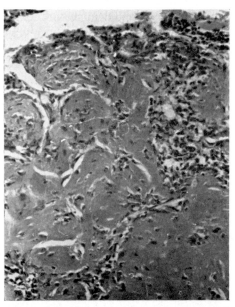

Fig. 2-A.　(H & E × 31.) Pulmonary metastasis from original Dunn osteosarcoma. Tumor nodule consists of dense bone trabeculae.

Fig. 2-B.　(H & E × 283.) Higher magnification of metastatic nodule in lung showing masses of mature bone surrounded by tumor osteoblasts.

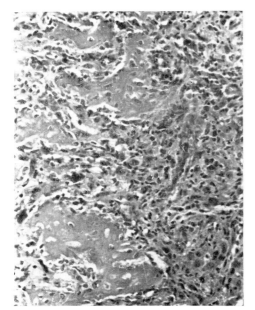

Fig. 3. (H & E × 236.) Photomicrograph of first generation transplant of Dunn osteosarcoma. There is more pleomorphism and mitoses. Bone trabeculae are still quite thick, although less numerous than in primary tumor and there is increased cellularity.

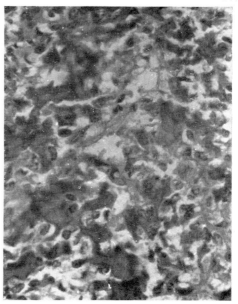

Fig. 4. (H & E × 393.) Photomicrograph from tumor of 111th generation transplant. The bone trabeculae are now slender, smaller in size and considerably more irregular. Tumor cells are more numerous and pleomorphic.

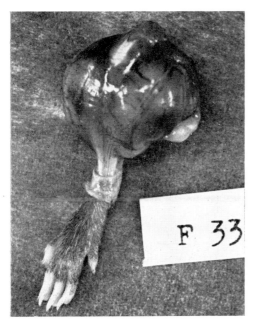

Fig. 5. Gross specimen of tumor 4 weeks following injection of tumor cell suspension.

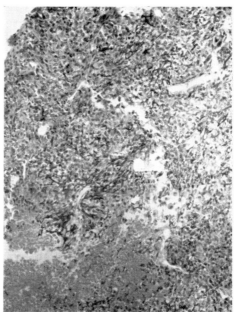

Fig. 6. (H & E × 31.) Low magnification photomicrograph of tumor showing peripheral portion at upper left. The cells here are less differentiated than those in the more central portions of the tumor where a number of lacy bone trabeculae can be seen. Central portion of the tumor at the bottom of the figure shows necrosis.

The spine has been involved in several instances, however, in each case spread to the spine and subsequently to the dura occurred in animals in whom the tumor had been transplanted subcutaneously into the flank. Spinal involvement in these cases may well have resulted from extension of the tumor rather than from metastatic seeding.

Tumor tissue has not been found in regional lymph nodes, spleen or thymus. We have not attempted to culture tumor cells from the blood stream.

The tumor cells are rich in alkaline phosphatase as determined by histochemical determination for this enzyme. Alkaline phosphatase is present in tumor cells of metastatic foci as well as in the primary tumor.

Electron microscopy reveals that the cytoplasm of the tumor cells contain an abundance of endoplasmic reticulum cisternae and a variable number of mitochondria, Golgi complexes, and free ribosomes (Figs. 8 and 9). Virus particles measuring 75 to 90 millimicrons in diameter are present within the endoplasmic reticulum of all tumor cells and can be seen budding from the membranes of the endoplasmic reticulum. Mature viruses consisting of a dense nucleoid enclosed within three electron dense concentric shells are seen in the extracellular spaces.

Where tumor bone is present it consists of masses of electron dense crystals which have the appearance of confluent, roughly spherical clumps. The bone mineral is always found in relation to collagen fibrils and at higher magnifications a mineral-organic matrix relationship similar to that present in normal bone can be identified. The major ultrastructural difference between the tumor bone trabeculae and normal bone is the relative disorientation of the former in contrast to the orderly pattern of normal bone trabeculae.

Electron microscopic examination of tumor in the pulmonary metastases shows cells which in no way differ from the primary tumor and, like them, contain virus particles. Adjacent lung tissue, however, appears relatively normal and cells of the adjacent alveoli are free of virus particles.

Subcutaneous implantation of tumor fragments into C3H mice was successful in transplanting the tumor in all but a few animals. The few transplant failures were probably technical errors since second transplant attempts in the same animals were uniformly successful. Injection of 10^6 tumor cells in suspension was likewise 100% successful in producing tumors, although some tumors were induced with injections of 2×10^4 cells.

When the tumor-bearing legs of C3H mice were amputated 1 week after implantation of tumor, most of the mice survived. Death from pulmonary metastasis in these animals could usually be attributed to a local recurrence of the tumor due to incomplete amputation. Even following disarticulation or hemipelvectomy local recurrence of the tumor in the skin occasionally occurred. When amputation was delayed for 2 weeks following tumor cell implantation, fatal pulmonary metastases occurred in all animals. These animals remained healthy for 4 to 6 weeks longer and had survival times that were comparably longer than animals whose primary tumor was not removed.

Of 52 CF1 mice in whom the Dunn osteosarcoma was transplanted from C3H mice, 12 developed tumors at the site of implantation as well as pulmonary metastases. In addition, three CF1 mice developed tumors which spontaneously regressed and disappeared. Two of these were abdominal masses following intraperitoneal injections of tumor cells. In these animals the abdominal masses were first noted 2 weeks after the intraperitoneal injection of 3×10^5 Dunn sarcoma cells in saline suspension. Although

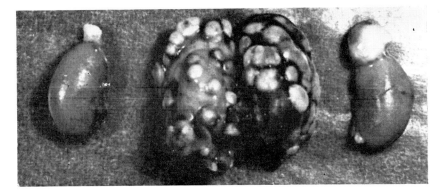

Fig. 7. Lungs and kidneys of C3H mouse 6 weeks following tumor cell suspension injection into leg. Massive metastatic nodules in lungs are evident. Kidney to the right of the lungs shows a large adrenal metastasis and a small metastatic nodule at its lower pole.

the tumor masses were not biopsied, the 2 week interval between injection and appearance of the masses is more consistent with the development of a tumor than an abscess due to infection, although the latter possibility cannot be discounted. Regression occurred gradually over the subsequent 2 weeks. In the third instance a tumor cell suspension was injected subcutaneously into the left leg and 3 weeks later a tumor cell suspension was injected into the right leg. Tumors developed in both legs, the right leg was amputated and histological sections confirmed the presence of the tumor. Four weeks later the tumor in the remaining left hind leg was noted to be regressing and by 8 weeks following the implantation of tumor cells, had completely regressed. Unfortunately, this was an isolated occurrence and attempts to reproduce it have failed.

Histologically the tumors in the CF1 mice differed from those of the C3H mice in that the tumor cells appeared to be larger with respect to both nucleus and cytoplasm. Osteoid, some of which was calcified, was present in a lattice-work pattern between the tumor cells in about half of the CF1 mice that developed tumors (Fig. 10). In the other tumor-bearing CF1 mice a collagenous intercellular matrix was frequently seen (Fig. 11).

Attempts to induce the tumor by injecting cell-free extracts of the Dunn osteosarcoma prepared as described in the Methods section, have been unsuccessful. Even extracts which were prepared by incubation of tumor extracts with embryo cells in culture and injected into newborn mice whose cell-mediated immunity was presumably undeveloped failed to produce the tumor.

DISCUSSION

A number of transferable murine osteosarcomas have been previously reported.[1,2,3,9,12] The major difference between the Dunn osteosarcoma of the present report and most of those previously described in the literature is that it has retained to at least a minor degree its capability of forming bone while remaining a malignant metastasizing tumor. The osteogenic sarcoma described by Hilberg[9] also arose in a C3H mouse and was transplantable, but eventually lost its ability to form bone in sub-

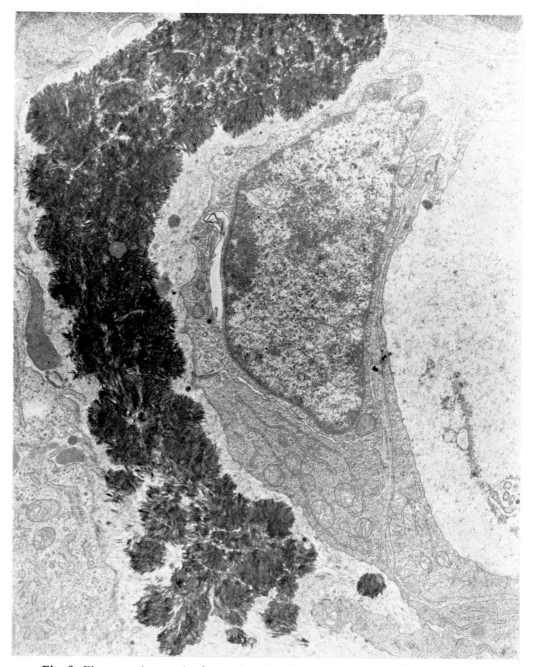

Fig. 8. Electron micrograph of a portion of a Dunn osteosarcoma. The dark boomerang-shaped mass in the center is a portion of a bone trabeculum composed of clumps of bone mineral crystals superimposed on collagen fibrils. The needle-like crystals can be identified at periphery of the trabeculum. Cells to the right of the trabeculum are surrounding a small blood capillary space while those to the left are tumor osteoblasts. Mitochondria and endoplasmic reticulum cisternae may be seen in cytoplasm. (×5,100).

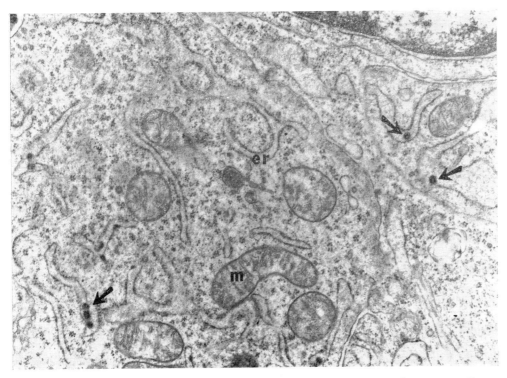

Fig. 9. Higher magnification electron micrograph of cytoplasm of a tumor cell. Mitochondria (m), endoplasmic reticulum (er) cisternae are seen in cytoplasm which also contains many small clumps of free ribosomes. Virus particles are seen in several endoplasmic reticulum cisternae (arrows). (× 30,000.)

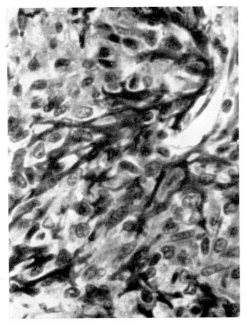

Fig. 10. (H & E × 370.) Tumor cells and lattice-work of bone trabeculae from osteosarcoma which had been transplanted to CF1 mouse. Nuclei and cytoplasm of these cells is somewhat larger than those of the tumors in C3H mice.

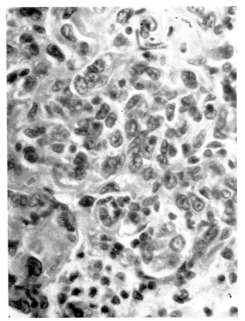

Fig. 11. (H & E × 400.) Tumor in CF1 mouse showing tumor cells surrounded by a collagenous matrix.

cutaneous transplantations. Albala and Esparza[1] have described a transplantable osteogenic sarcoma in AKR mice which has retained its bone forming ability through 44 generations, but did not metastasize.

The ability of the Dunn osteosarcoma to retain its bone forming capability when transplanted to another strain of mouse (CF1) is a further indication that its cells can produce an ossifiable collagen. Finally, its ability to stimulate host tissues to form bone in proximity to the tumor even when the tumor tissue was sealed within a millipore diffusion chamber as previously reported,[6] is additional evidence of its bone inducing capability.

The virus seen in electron microscopy of this tumor tissue is similar in appearance to murine viruses previously described.[13,15] Its abundance in tumor cells both at the primary site and in metastases, as well as its absence in normal tissues adjacent to the tumor, leaves little doubt that the virus grows and lives in the tumor cells. Whether the virus is related to the causation of the tumor is another matter. The virus discovered by Finkel, Biskis and Jinkins[3] appears to be etiologically related to an osteosarcoma in CF1/Anl mice since cell-free extracts of this tumor were found capable of inducing osteosarcomas in other CF1/Anl mice. We have attempted to induce the Dunn osteosarcoma by the injection of cell-free extracts without success. Nor were we able to induce the tumor by injection of the cell-free supernatant of embryo C3H mouse cells which had been cultured with the cell-free tumor extract in an effort to mature immature viruses before attempting tumor induction. Furthermore, as we have previously reported, the failure of tumors to develop in proximity to millipore diffusion chambers containing Dunn osteosarcoma tissue which were implanted subcutaneously into isogeneic mice, is further evidence against an etiological relationship between the virus and the tumor. It seems likely, on the basis of these facts, that the virus in the Dunn osteosarcoma cells is merely a passenger in the transfer of tumor cells from animal to animal.

Transplantation of tumors from one strain of mice to another as was done in the present study can sometimes be accomplished after the tumor has been carried through a number of transplants within the original strain.[10] Although the reasons are not well understood the ability to grow successfully what amounts to an allograft has been attributed by some investigators to a weakening or simplification of the antigenicity of rapidly growing tumor cells due to a genetic alteration in the cells. Others believe that some tumor cells containing tumor specific transplantation antigens evoke a response in the susceptible host which actually enhances the growth of the tumor.[7] Support for the latter concept may be found in several recent experimental and clinical reports by the Hellströms and associates.[8] They have shown that the sera of tumor-bearing animals and individuals contain factors which block the cytotoxic immune mechanisms that would normally protect the animal or individual from growth of the tumor.

Histocompatibility testing was not carried out between the C3H and CF1 mice in the present study and since the latter are a random bred strain the individual histocompatibility genotypes for each of the mice used cannot be assessed. Finkel (personal communication) has successfully transplanted the Dunn osteosarcoma into CBA mice, a strain that like the C3H/HeJ mouse has its strong histocompatibility gene at the H-2^k locus[14] but differs at other H loci. The ability to cross genetic lines with the tumor has given us a valuable tool for studies of tumor immunity.

ACKNOWLEDGEMENTS

We wish gratefully to acknowledge the contributions to this study made by Dr. Hideya Hanaoka and Miss Patricia Shaffer.

REFERENCES

1. Albala, M. M. & Esparza, A. R. Transplantable Osteogenic Sarcoma in Inbred AKR Mice. *Cancer Res.*, **29**, 1519–1522, 1969.
2. Barrett, M. K., Dalton, A. J., Edwards, J. E., Greenstein, J. P. & Briggs, V. C. A Transplantable Osteogenic Sarcoma Originating in a C3H Mouse, *J. nat. Cancer Inst.*, **4**, 389–402, 1944.
3. Finkel, M. P., Biskis, B. O. & Jinkins, P. B. Virus Induction of Osteosarcomas in Mice *Science*, **151**, 698–701, 1966.
4. Friedman, B., Heiple, K. G., Vessely, J. C. & Hanaoka, H. Ultrastructural Investigation of Bone Induction by an Osteosarcoma using diffusion Chambers. *Clin. Orthop.*, **59**, 39–57, 1968.
5. Hauschka, T. S. The Chromosomes in Ontogeny and Oncogeny. *Cancer Res.*, **21**, 957–974, 1961.
6. Heiple, K. G., Herndon, C. H., Chase, S. W. & Wattleworth, A. Osteogenic Induction by Osteosarcoma and Normal Bone in Mice. *J. Bone Jt. Surg.*, **50–A**, 311–325, 1968.
7. Hellström, I. & Hellström, K. E. Colony Inhibition Studies on Blocking and Non-Blocking Serum Effects on Cellular Immunity to Moloney Sarcomas. *Int. J. Cancer*, **5**, 195–201, 1970.
8. Hellström, I., Sjögren, H. O., Warner, G. A. & Hellström, K. E. Blocking of Cell-mediated Tumor Immunity by Sera from Patients with Growing neoplasms. *Int. J. Cancer*, **7**, 226–237, 1971.
9. Hilberg, A. W. Morphologic Variations in an Osteogenic Sarcoma of the Mouse when Transplanted to the Kidney. *J. nat. Cancer Inst.* **16**, 951–959, 1956.
10. Liebelt, A. G. & Liebelt, R. A. Transplantation of Tumours. In *Methods in Cancer Research*, **Vol. 1**, pp. 143–242, Harris Busch, ed., Academic Press, N.Y., 1967.
11. Molbert, E. R. G., Duspiva, F., & Von Deimling, O. H. The Demonstration of Alkaline Phosphatase in the Electron Microscope. *J. Biophys. Biochem. Cytol.*, **7**, 387–391, 1960.
12. Pybus, F. C. & Miller, E. W. The Gross Pathology of Spontaneous Bone Tumors in Mice. *Amer. J. Cancer*, **40**, 54–61, 1940.
13. Smith, K. O. Identification of Viruses by Electron Microscopy. In *Methods in Cancer Research*, **Vol, 1**, pp. 545–572, Harris Busch, ed., Academic Press, N.Y., 1967.
14. Snell, G. D. & Stimpfling, J. H. Genetics of Tissue Transplantation. In *Biology of the Laboratory Mouse*, Earl L. Green, ed. 2nd Ed., McGraw-Hill Co., New York, pp. 457–491, 1966.
15. Wivel, N. A. & Smith, G. H. Distribution of Intracisternal A-particles in a Variety of Normal and Neoplastic Mouse Tissues. *Int. J. Cancer*, **7**, 167–175, 1971.

Discussion

Dr. Moore I would like to sound a cautionary note about the value of this experimental model in relation to primary osteosarcoma in other animal systems and certainly in relation to human disease for this reason. Dr. Friedman's best results were obtained when he transplanted a C3H tumour into a CF1 mouse, in other words across a histocompatibility barrier. Therefore the regressions that had been noted I would probably wager were due to isoantigenic differences betwixt the tumour and the host, and not due to any antigens that the tumour itself possessed in relation to its original host. The other cautionary note I would sound is that this tumour was induced in 1955 and is therefore 17 years old. It was induced with an extract from a spontaneous leukaemia that arose in an AKR mouse, I think that all these features, the introduction of many variables here make this a considerably less than ideal model for the study of the various immunological parameters in osteosarcoma. Also (if I may ask him) I am very much unclear as to what was the point of the experiment in which he passaged the C3H tumour in the CF1 mouse which is known to have indigenous FBJ virus, with the object of inducing tumours back into C3H mice. I couldn't quite see the rationale behind that particular experiment. I would have thought that there was the possibility that the virus which was noted by electronmicroscopy was almost certainly a passenger, particularly in view of the very varied history of this tumour's life?

Dr. Friedman I couldn't agree with you more. I have to keep telling myself that this is not a human osteosarcoma and that this does not probably bear any relationship to human osteosarcoma. It does provide a good tool for applying some methods which possibly may have some use in human tumours. Much of the information that we have got in cancer research has stemmed from animal experimentation. Whether this does or does not develop into anything that is of value, I think is almost secondary. We have got something here at least that we can work with which does at least, if nothing else, give us a little food for thought. On one thing I must correct you. You said that this tumour was produced by injection of spontaneous leukaemia cells from AKR mice, this is not entirely so. These mice had received spontaneous AKR leukaemia cells as newborns. This was the only mouse of a large number, I can't tell you how many, but Dr. Dunn I am sure could. This was the only mouse that did develop a spontaneous osteosarcoma, and I think it more likely that this is a spontaneously arising osteosarcoma—rather than one which is associated with the leukaemia cells. With respect to the virus particles I have tried every way that I know, and the ways that other people have advised me to induce the tumour by cell-free extracts or by the virus alone and have not been successful. I am assuming this is a passenger virus—unless it is a helper virus, or one of these other strange things. Not being a virologist I can't answer the question any more fully than that. The rationale was to try to see whether or not we could pass the H2 histocompatibility barrier of these mice. Actually, these C3H mice of this particular strain have the strong histocompatibility gene at the locus $H-2^k$. The CF1 mice that we use were random bred and we did not do histocompatibility testing, so that I really can't tell you whether or not the mice that accepted the tumour were crossing the H2 barrier. That was one of the things we have on our schedule, but the reason for doing it was to see if it were possible to pass the H2 histocompatibility barrier.

Dr. Price   In your transmission experiments with this tumour to other mice did any of the recipient animals ever turn up with leukaemia?

Dr. Friedman   None of the animals that I have been working with have developed leukaemia. I would like to make one further comment and that is with respect to the CBA mice. I gave some of these cells to Dr. Miriam Finkel and she first transplanted them in CBA mice and subsequently we were able to do the same. I think you have done these into other strains Dr. Finkel?

Dr. Finkel   It takes very well in CBA's. I can guarantee it.

Bone tumor viruses

by

MIRIAM P. FINKEL, CHRISTOPHER A. REILLY, Jr., BIRUTE O. BISKIS,
and ISABEL L. GRECO

SUMMARY

The following three viruses, which induce bone tumors when injected into newborn mice, have been isolated from murine bone tumors: (1) FBJ-osteosarcoma virus, originally from a spontaneous CF1 osteosarcoma, is a C type RNA virus. FBJ-tumors contain many virus particles. (2) RFB-osteoma virus, originally from spontaneous CF1 osteomas and radiation-induced osteosarcomas, resembles intracisternal type A particles in some respects. RFB-tumors are very rich in virus. (3) FBR-osteosarcoma virus, originally from a radiation-induced X/Gf osteosarcoma, probably is a C type particle morphologically similar to FBJ virus. Although extracts of FBR-osteosarcomas produce many tumors very quickly following injection into newborn mice, very few particles appear in the tumors.

Evidences for a human bone tumor virus are the appearance of bone tumors and fibrosarcomas in Syrian hamsters inoculated soon after birth with cell-free extracts of human osteosarcomas, the presence of human sarcoma-specific antigen in some of the experimentally induced hamster tumors, and the presence of C type particles in both the human and hamster tumors.

WHEN EVIDENCE WAS FIRST presented that chicken sarcomas,[36] rabbit fibromas and papillomas,[38,39] mouse mammary tumors,[2] mouse leukemia,[24] and mouse parotid gland tumors[25] could be passed by cell-free extracts of these tissues, it seemed most unlikely that bone tumors could have a similar etiology. However, Rous, Murphy and Tytler reported cell-free passage of a chicken osteochondrosarcoma,[37] and in 1960 Stewart reported the appearance of bone tumors in 22% of Swiss mice inoculated at birth with SE polyoma virus,[41] the parotid gland agent originally reported by Gross. These demonstrations of tumor induction by viruses prompted us in 1961 to embark on a search for a similar causative agent in spontaneous and radiation-induced osteogenic sarcomas of mice. Our endeavors resulted in the discovery of FBJ-osteosarcoma virus[6] and the extension of our search to canine and human bone tumors. We now have isolated two different murine bone-tumor viruses and accumulated substantial evidence for a human osteosarcoma virus.

Whereas 20 years ago strong opposition greeted proponents of viruses as etiologic agents for even a few neoplasms, it is now readily accepted that many tumors are caused by viruses or virus-associated inherited information. Indeed, the fact that we could isolate three viruses from bone tumors of mice favors the view that most tumors have a viral agent.

In the present communication we summarize our work with FBJ-osteosarcoma virus, describe the new murine RFB-osteoma and FBR-osteosarcoma viruses. and review the current evidence obtained in our laboratory for a human osteosarcoma virus.

FBJ-OSTEOSARCOMA VIRUS

In the original search for virus in murine osteogenic sarcomas we examined seven radiation-induced and four spontaneous bone tumors of CFl/Anl mice.[6] FBJ virus was derived from one of the spontaneous tumors, a parosteal sarcoma. Two of the mice that had received a cell-free extract of that tumor soon after birth died with bone tumors 280 and 337 days later, respectively. In the second passage a parosteal sarcoma was detected in 69 days, and with successive passages tumor incidence increased and latent period decreased.[7,10]

Except for X/Gf mice, all mouse strains that have been tested respond to neonatal injection of FBJ virus with the production of osteosarcomas.[29,42] Syrian hamsters also develop FBJ osteosarcomas.

Horizontal transmission from tumor-bearing animals to uninoculated cage mates has not been demonstrated, and several attempts to demonstrate vertical transmission have not been successful. Following intraperitoneal injection of extract into newborn mice, FBJ-osteosarcomas can occur anywhere in the skeleton; ribs and diaphragm are favored sites (Fig. 1). Multiple primary tumors are common, but metastases to soft tissues are rarely seen. Growth is usually rapid and moderately invasive. FBJ tumors are very firm, smooth, pale pink, and of homogeneous texture, although heavy central or diffuse focal ossification is seen occasionally. They arise on the periosteum or in muscle adjacent to bone and display considerable histologic diversity from area to area; predominant cells can be fibroblasts, giant cells, or osteoblasts, and the amount of osteoid and degree of ossification are quite variable.

FBJ virus is a C type RNA virus containing the group-specific complement-fixing antigen of the murine leukemia-sarcoma complex.[29,30] Type C virus regularly buds from the cell membrane, and both mature and immature particles appear in intercellular spaces (Fig. 4). In FBJ tumors with abundant virus, production also occurs within cisternae of the rough endoplasmic reticulum, where the particles seem to emerge together and remain connected with each other.[1]

Attempts to isolate FBJ virus from radiation-induced bone tumors of CFl mice have not been successful. Forty-three extracts have been injected into newborn animals, and recipients of six of them developed osteosarcomas. In a few cases mice given extracts of these tumors also developed osteosarcomas, but so far none of the passages has resulted in the rapid appearance of a large number of malignant bone tumors such as occurred during the original isolation of FBJ virus. Nevertheless, three lines of evidence point to the presence of FBJ virus in at least some of these tumors: ( ) The interactions between FBJ virus and ^{90}Sr on tumor induction produce complex results: FBJ virus either enhances or inhibits ^{90}Sr-tumor induction, depending upon the experimental conditions.[13,15] For example, virus given at birth decreases the latent period but also decreases the incidence of tumors induced by ^{90}Sr given at 28 days of age. (2) The plasma of some mice bearing ^{90}Sr-induced osteosarcomas neutralizes FBJ virus.[17,34] (3) Type C particles

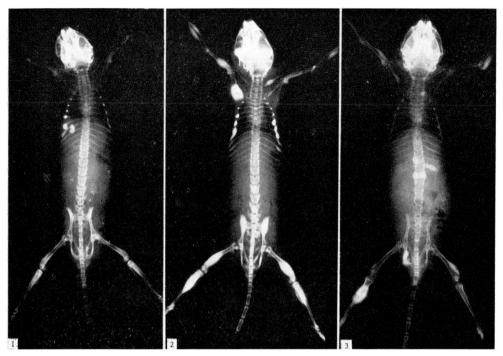

Fig. 1. Radiograph of 47-day-old CF1 mouse with FBJ-osteosarcoma of sixth, seventh, and eighth ribs; the seventh rib has two areas of ossification. The peripheral portion of the tumor mass is not calcified. The increased density of the ilia, distal femurs, and proximal tibias frequently preceeds the appearance of FBJ-tumors.

Fig. 2. Radiograph of 63-day-old CF1 mouse with RFB-osteomas in mandibles, long bones, spine, girdles, and ribs. There is no soft tissue involvement.

Fig. 3. Radiograph of 43-day-old X/Gf mouse with FBR-osteosarcomas of right humerus, left ulna, sixth and seventh cervical vertebrae, twelfth thoracic vertebra, thirteenth rib, first lumbar vertebra, right ischium, right tibia, and left femur.

morphologically similar to FBJ virus have been found in thin sections of most ^{90}Sr-induced osteosarcomas (Figs. 5 and 6).

RFB-OSTEOMA VIRUS

Old CF1 mice have a very high incidence of spontaneous osteomas; 10 to 20% of animals permitted to live until natural death possess one or more of these benign bone tumors.[5,14] The earliest lesion usually is a small area of cortical exostosis, which then may progress slowly to become a solid, bony hard, somewhat spherical, non-invasive tumor, sometimes exceeding 1 cm in diameter. We have now isolated a virus that induces these tumors a few weeks after injection into newborn CFl/Anl mice.

The first potent osteoma-virus extract was prepared from three neoplasms of one CFl mouse. This mouse had received FBJ virus soon after birth, and when it was killed 369 days later it had a 2 cm FBJ-osteosarcoma of the tibia, a 6 mm osteoma of the femur, and

356

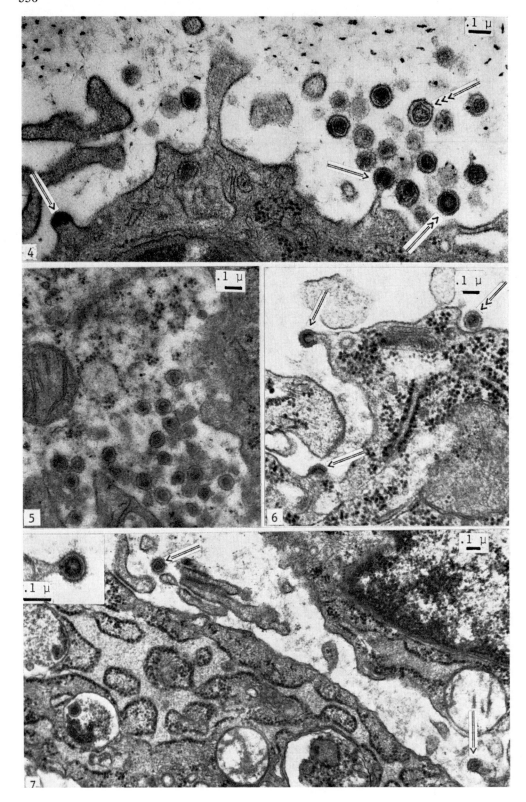

a lymphosarcoma involving thymus, spleen, and lymph nodes. Most recipients of this three-tumor extract had palpable bone tumors when they were examined 87 days after injection. The roentgenographic appearance of the tumors was similar to the usual CFl osteomas, but these were remarkable because so many were present in such young animals (Fig. 2). One mouse had 16 osteomas; the average number in the 17 mice of the group was five.

Some of these osteomas were immediately extracted for injection into another group of newborn mice. Again many osteomas quickly appeared. This procedure has been continued, and in less than 2 years this osteoma line has been passed serially eight times. The extracts have gone through 0.45μ millipore filters without loss of oncogenicity, but a modified Moloney extracting procedure[27] greatly reduced oncogenic activity. Attempts to demonstrate placental passage have failed.

Six other lines of benign bone tumors, histologically and roentgenographically identical to those described above, are being carried by cell-free passage in CFl/Anl mice. Five were derived from ^{90}Sr-induced osteosarcomas; the sixth originated from an extra-osseous osteosarcoma that arose in a mouse treated at birth with ether-inactivated FBJ virus. We have not yet established the identity of the agents in these seven lines, but we suspect that they are the same virus, tentatively named RFB-osteoma virus (Reilly–Finkel–Biskis).

The virus-induced osteomas grow very rapidly at first. Eventually growth rate slackens, and most of the tumors are not a serious threat to life. Those that occur on the mandible, a frequent location, sometimes interfere with eating, and those that impinge on the spinal cord occasionally cause paralysis.

RFB-osteomas consist of osteoblasts and osteocytes in dense, well organized, non-invasive lesions. There are few mitotic figures and no indication of malignancy, even in tumors present for a year or more.

Electron microscopy of the osteomas shows a great number of particles, 100 to 150 mμ in diameter, resembling type C virus in most respects (Figs. 8 and 9). Immature particles have a dense ring around a pale nucleoid; mature particles have a large, very dense, central nucleoid. Only rarely have budding forms been observed. In addition to the morphologic differences between RFB and FBJ viruses, there are antigenic differences as well, since plasma of mice with RFB-osteomas failed to neutralize FBJ-osteosarcoma virus.

Fig. 4. Electron micrograph of FBJ-osteosarcoma in CF1 mouse with budding (single arrow), immature (double arrow), and mature (triple arrow) C type virus particles.

Fig. 5. Electron micrograph of ^{90}Sr-induced osteogenic sarcoma in CF1 mouse with many mature C type particles.

Fig. 6. Electron micrograph of osteosarcoma in CF1 mouse that had received an extract of ^{90}Sr-induced osteogenic sarcoma soon after birth. There are two budding (single arrow) and one mature C type particles (double arrow).

Fig. 7. Electron micrograph of FBR-osteosarcoma in X/Gf mouse wth a few C type particles (arrow). The budding particle in the inset occurred in another FBR virus-induced osteosarcoma.

358

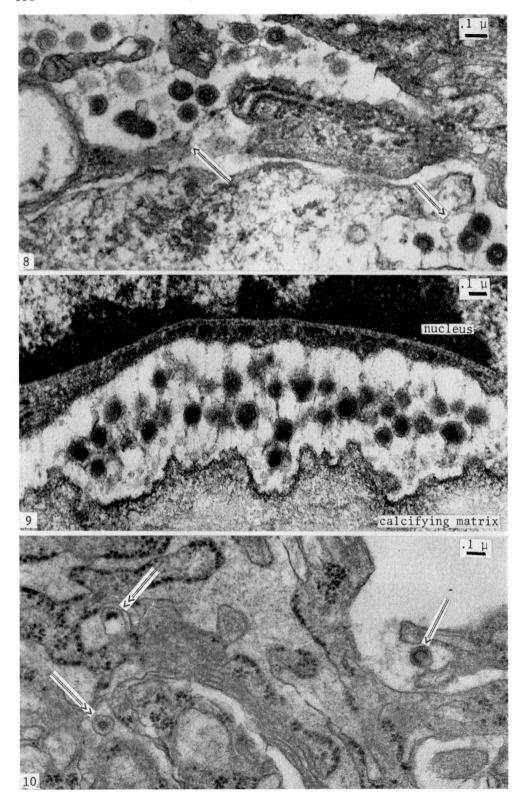

FBR-OSTEOSARCOMA VIRUS

The X/Gf mouse, developed by Dr. Anna Goldfeder and distinguished by the fact that it has a very low incidence of spontaneous tumors, is also resistant to tumor induction by external irradiation, SE polyoma virus, and FBJ virus, and it is relatively resistant to tumor induction by urethan and Friend leukemia virus.[19,22] In the course of an experiment in our laboratory to determine whether X/Gf mice are resistant to ^{90}Sr as well, many osteosarcomas were produced, and 18 extracts were prepared for injection into neonatal X/Gf mice. Four of the extracts induced one tumor each: an osteoma, a hemangiosarcoma of bone, a fibrosarcoma in the pelvic muscles, and a lymphosarcoma. A fifth extract induced two tumors: an osteosarcoma and an atypical reticular tissue tumor with blast cells and large histiocytes. Both reticular tumors gave rise to lines that are being carried by cell-free passage. In one of these lines, after two passages of cell-free extracts of leukemic spleens and lymph nodes, one animal developed both an osteosarcoma and a reticulum cell sarcoma. An extract prepared from these two tumors was injected into seven newborn mice; osteosarcomas appeared in five and both osteosarcomas and reticular tissue tumors in two. The established osteosarcoma line, now in its ninth cell-free passage, produces bone tumors in less than 4 weeks in almost all X/Gf mice inoculated at birth. Whether or not a leukemia agent is still present in the osteosarcoma extracts is not known because the animals become moribund very quickly with bone tumors. Our designation of this agent is FBR-osteosarcoma virus (Finkel–Biskis–Reilly).

FBR-osteosarcomas resemble FBJ-tumors in many respects. After intraperitoneal injection of cell-free extracts into newborn X/Gf mice, tumors arise anywhere in the skeleton, most frequently in ribs and thoracic and lumbar spine, and they often appear first as regions of periosteal proliferation (Fig. 3). FBR-osteosarcomas usually are more densely osteoblastic than FBJ-tumors, but they are very similar histologically. They show comparable diversity from area to area; primary cell types range from spindle cells to osteoblasts and osteocytes.

Electron microscopic examination of second and third passage FBR-osteosarcomas showed only occasional mature C type particles in intercellular spaces and a few immature forms budding from the cell membrane (Fig. 7). This paucity of virus-like particles is not consistent with the marked potency of the extracts, but examination of later passage tumors may show more prolific virus production.

Although the oncogenic activity of FBR virus is similar to that of FBJ virus, its counterpart in CFl mice, we suspect no close relationship between them since FBJ is not oncogenic in X/Gf mice. Whether FBR virus is oncogenic in CFl mice is under investigation.

Fig. 8. Electron micrograph of RFB-osteoma in CF1 mouse showing immature particles resembling C type particles in most respects.

Fig. 9. Mature osteoma virus particles with very large, electron-dense, central nucleoid.

Fig. 10. Electron micrograph of hamster fibrosarcoma showing a budding C type particle (single arrow) and H particles, one of which is incomplete (double arrow).

INDICATIONS FOR A HUMAN OSTEOSARCOMA VIRUS

The three lines of evidence from our studies with human osteosarcomas which imply that the human disease, like that of mice, is associated with a virus are: (1) induction of sarcomas in Syrian hamsters with cell-free extracts of human osteosarcomas, (2) demonstration of sarcoma-specific antigen in human osteosarcomas and demonstration of the same antigen in the experimentally induced hamster tumors, and (3) presence of C type particles in human osteosarcomas and in the induced hamster sarcomas.

Six years ago we prepared our first extract of a human osteogenic sarcoma and injected it into 49 newborn Syrian hamsters.[8] Nineteen died before weaning, six were used for special study, and the remaining 24 were permitted to live as long as possible. Two of these died with fibrosarcoma; one had a fibrosarcoma of the leg 581 days after injection,[11,12] and the other a fibrosarcoma of the premaxilla at 619 days. We now have inoculated hamsters with extracts of 100 human malignant tumors occurring in bone: 91 osteosarcomas, four chondrosarcomas, three fibrosarcomas, one giant-cell tumor, and one reticulum cell sarcoma. At the present time recipients of osteosarcoma extracts have had 14 osteosarcomas, four osteomas, two fibrosarcomas of bone, and eight fibrosarcomas of soft tissue.[35] More tumors are likely to appear since many of the animals are considerably younger than the youngest to have died so far with sarcoma or osteoma. In our control hamster population there has been only one sarcoma, which arose in the subcutaneous tissues of the neck. Since osteosarcomas, osteomas, and fibrosarcomas are very uncommon in this species, treatment with human osteosarcoma extracts probably was instrumental in the induction of most of these 28 tumors. Carcinomas and tumors of the reticular tissues, however, are relatively common, and the number of these tumors seems not to have been influenced by treatment with extracts of human tissues.

At last count, taken when extracts from 60 patients had been under test for at least 200 days, 12 of them had induced osteosarcomas, fibrosarcomas, and osteomas in hamsters. However, only 2% of the hamsters that received material from these 12 patients developed tumors.

Six of the hamster sarcomas have been maintained by subcutaneous transplantation. After 10 transplant generations a cell-free extract of one of them, a fibrosarcoma of the leg, induced diffuse abdominal fibrosarcoma in a hamster inoculated soon after birth, and there have been three more cell-free hamster-to-hamster passages of this tumor since that time. The tumor was re-established as a subcutaneous transplant after the first cell-free passage, and after 13 transplant generations it was established in tissue culture.

Recently we confirmed the results of Morton and Malmgren[31] and of Priori, Wilbur, and Dmochowski[32] that demonstrated cross-reactivity between sera and tumors of osteosarcoma patients. In our studies, 57 of 58 sera from osteosarcoma patients detected sarcoma-specific antigen in cryostat sections or tissue culture cells from six human osteosarcomas in an indirect immunofluorescence test.[33,35] In addition, we showed that human osteosarcoma serum also detected human sarcoma-specific antigen in five of the six hamster sarcoma transplants and in one primary experimentally induced hamster sarcoma. The sixth transplanted hamster sarcoma did not react with human osteosarcoma serum, nor did two hamster carcinomas, four reticular tissue tumors, and a number of normal tissues.

In order to rule out the possibility that the positive reactions were due to an isoantibody or globulins bound to the tissue before testing, one human osteosarcoma and five of the hamster sarcomas were retested with serum from two rabbits immunized against different human osteosarcoma extracts. The human tumor and four hamster tumors that reacted in the first test again reacted; the hamster sarcoma that had been negative was again negative. Other non-reacting tissues in this second test were a hamster reticulum cell sarcoma, two FBJ-osteosarcomas, and a number of normal hamster tissues.

Other evidence against the possibility that positive immunofluorescence results were due to non-specific reactions is that tumor cells, both human and hamster, grown for a minimum of three passages in tissue culture, reacted just as well as did cryostat sections of solid tumors. It is particularly significant that the hamster sarcoma that had been passed cell-free from hamster to hamster was subsequently shown still to contain human sarcoma-specific antigen.

Particles resembling type C virus have been found in all human osteosarcomas that have been carefully examined, both in sections of intact tumors and in sections of pelletted extracts.[8,11] Since none of the preparations have been rich in particles, we are now re-examining the tumors after they have been established in tissue culture.

All but one of the sarcomas induced in hamsters by cell-free extracts of human osteosarcomas that have been examined with the electron microscope have contained C type particles, but only a few were found after careful search (Fig. 10). The tumor lacking C type particles had an abundance of type A cytoplasmic particles;[12] this tumor also lacked human sarcoma-specific antigen.[35] All the hamster tumors regularly contain the relatively large cytoplasmic particles with small nucleoid and radial rays between nucleoid and outer membrane that have been variously called Bernhard particles, spoked virus, type H particles, and type R particles (Fig. 10).

The agent associated with human osteosarcomas does not seem to be immunologically related to FBJ-osteosarcoma virus since attempts to neutralize FBJ virus with serum of five osteosarcoma patients and hamsters bearing three sarcoma transplant lines were not successful.

DISCUSSION

When we began our search for virus in CFl osteogenic sarcomas in 1961 we had little hope of success. Now, however, we feel that probably all tumors carry inherited viral information and that it should be possible to obtain an active agent from many of them. The implication is that information for neoplastic change and virus are closely related, but every tumor does not contain an abundance of formed virus, and every virus seen in tissue sections does not indicate neoplasm. Views somewhat similar to these have been expressed in Huebner and Todaro's oncogene-virogene theory of oncogenesis.[28]

With the CFl mouse, only four spontaneous osteosarcomas were extracted before FBJ-osteosarcoma virus was isolated. On the other hand, 43 extracts of radiation-induced osteosarcomas have not yielded a potent osteosarcoma agent, although five have supplied an osteoma agent. This is a most unexpected result in view of the fact that bone-seeking radionuclides have not been shown to increase the incidence of benign bone tumors. RFB-osteoma virus was also isolated from two non-radiation-induced CFl bone tumors. It is interesting that, although the initial potent extract included an FBJ-osteosarcoma, no

N

FBJ-tumors have appeared in subsequent passages. Either RFB virus inhibits FBJ, or the latter has been diluted out during the rapid passage of RFB virus.

Contrary to the situation in CFl mice, in the tumor-resistant X/Gf strain 18 extracts of ^{90}Sr-induced osteosarcomas have provided three malignant tumor lines maintained by cell-free passage. It is curious that, although the original extracts were of osteogenic sarcomas, two of the lines induce reticular tissue tumors and the third, an osteosarcoma line, came from a second-passage reticular tumor.

Intercellular type C particles appear only occasionally in FBR-osteosarcomas of X/Gf mice. However, they are frequent in the reticular tissue tumors, where immature forms emerging in cisternae of the rough endoplasmic reticulum are also seen. Goldfeder[23] and Goldfeder and Ghosh[20,21] found A and B particles, but not C particles, in X-ray and urethan-induced thymic lymphoma and mammary tumors in this strain. C particles were noted, however, in Friend-leukemia-infected X/Gf mice.[22]

Some understanding of the tumor-inducing mechanisms should emerge from careful study of the contradictory, yet somewhat similar, experiences with CFl and X/Gf mice. The former strain ordinarily has a high incidence of a variety of spontaneous tumors;[4] the latter very rarely has tumors of any kind.[19] In CFl mice spontaneous bone tumors have provided an osteosarcoma virus and an osteoma virus; radiation-induced tumors have yielded only the osteoma virus. Contrariwise, in X/Gf mice radiation-induced bone tumors have provided both a leukemia and an osteosarcoma virus, but not an osteoma virus. Further investigations of the biologic activities and immunologic relationships of these agents should be useful in determining their roles and the role of radiation in the oncogenic process.

Harvey and Moloney viruses induce bone tumors in rats and hamsters,[18,26,40] but we are aware of no work on the isolation of a virus from either spontaneous or radiation-induced osteogenic sarcoma in these species. Our search for an agent in radionuclide-induced bone tumors in beagles has not provided an active virus,[9] but our current results with human osteosarcomas give clear evidence of a causative viral agent. Preliminary results showed that 20% of the extracts of human osteosarcomas induced tumors in hamsters, but only 2% of the hamsters inoculated with material from these patients developed tumors. Therefore, although hamsters are receptive to the oncogenic agent in human bone tumors, the number of responding animals is small.

Only one of the human tumors tested so far, an osteosarcoma in the third metacarpal of a former radium dial painter (Case 03–429),[3] was radiation-induced. Three hamsters inoculated with extract of that tumor survived to weaning; none died with tumor. Osteosarcomas arising from therapeutic radiation may be satisfactory sources of virus, but if the situation in man resembles that in CFl mice rather than X/Gf mice, virus extraction from spontaneous tumors will be more successful than from radiation-induced tumors.

The most convincing evidence of a human osteosarcoma virus has been the demonstration of human osteosarcoma-specific antigen in experimentally induced hamster sarcomas. Of particular importance is the presence of the antigen in a hamster sarcoma that had been carried as a subcutaneous transplant for 13 passages after it had gone through cell-free passage from an extract of a 10-generation subcutaneous transplant. In other words, the tumor that reacted with human osteosarcoma serum was 24 hamster-passages removed from the animal originally inoculated with human osteosarcoma extract.

ACKNOWLEDGEMENTS

We gratefully acknowledge the assistance of many past and present members of our research group, particularly R. W. Camden, D.V.M., P. J. Dale, E. W. Jackson, P. B. Jinkins, G. Rockus, and L. L. Stewart. This work was supported by the United States Atomic Energy Commission.

REFERENCES

1. Biskis, B. O. & Finkel, M. P. Electron Microscopy of the FBJ Osteosarcoma Virus. In *Proceedings Twenty-seventh Annual Meeting Electron Microscope Society of America*, C. J. Arceneaux, Ed. Claitor's Publishing Division, Baton Rouge, pp. 384–385, 1969.
2. Bittner, J. J. Some Possible Effects of Nursing on the Mammary Gland Tumor Incidence in Mice. *Science*, **84**, 162, 1936.
3. Finkel, A. J. Miller, C. E. & Hasterlik, R. J. Radiobiological Parameters in Human Cancers attributable to long-term Radium Deposition. In *Radiation-Induced Cancer*. International Atomic Energy Agency, Vienna, IAEA-SM-118/7, pp. 183–202, 1969.
4. Finkel, M. P. & Scribner, G. M. Mouse Cages and Spontaneous Tumors. *Brit. J. Cancer*, **9**, 464–472, 1955.
5. Finkel, M. P., Biskis, B. O. & Scribner, G. M. The Influence of Strontium-90 upon Life Span and Neoplasms of Mice. In *Progress in Nuclear Energy*, Series VI, Vol. 2. Pergamon Press, London, pp. 119–209, 1959.
6. Finkel, M. P., Biskis, B. O. & Jinkins, P. B. Virus Induction of Osteosarcomas in Mice. *Science*, **151**, 698–701, 1966.
7. Finkel, M. P., Jinkins, P. B., Tolle, J. & Biskis, B. O. Serial Radiography of Virus-induced Osteosarcomas in Mice. *Radiology*, **87**, 333–339, 1966.
8. Finkel, M. P., Biskis, B. O. & Farrell, C. Pathogenic Effects of Extracts of Human Osteosarcomas. *Arch. Path.*, **84**, 425–428, 1967.
9. Finkel, M. P. & Biskis, B. O. Search for Virus in Canine Osteosarcomas. *Proc. Amer. Ass. Cancer Res.*, **8**, 18, 1967.
10. Finkel, M. P. & Biskis, B. O. Experimental Induction of Osteosarcomas. In *Prog. Exp. Tumor Res.*, Karger, Basel, **Vol. 10**, pp. 72–111, 1968.
11. Finkel, M. P., Biskis, B. O. & Farrell, C. Osteosarcomas Appearing in Syrian Hamsters after Treatment with Extracts of Human Osteosarcomas. *Proc. nat. Acad. Sci. (Wash.)*, **60**, 1223–1230, 1968.
12. Finkel, M. P., Biskis, B. O. & Farrell, C. Nonmalignant and Malignant Changes in Hamsters Inoculated with Extracts of Human Osteosarcomas. *Radiology*, **92**, 1546–1552, 1969.
13. Finkel, M. P. & Biskis, B. O. Osteosarcomas induced in Mice by FBJ Virus and ^{90}Strontium. In *Delayed Effects of Bone-Seeking Radionuclides*, Ed. C. W. Mays, *et al.*, University of Utah Press, Salt Lake City, pp. 417–435, 1969.
14. Finkel, M. P., Biskis, B. O. & Jinkins, P. B. Toxicity of Radium-226 in Mice. In *Radiation-Induced Cancer*. International Atomic Energy Agency, Vienna, IAEA-SM-118/11, pp. 369–391. 1969.
15. Finkel, M. P., Biskis, B. O. & Reilly, C. A. Jr. Influence of FBJ Osteosarcoma Virus given before or after Strontium-90 upon the Induction of Bone Cancer in Mice. IVe Congrès International de Radiobiologie et de Physico-chimie des Rayonnements, Livre des Résumes, p. 72, 1970.
16. Finkel, M. P., Biskis, B. O., Reilly, C. A. Jr., Camden, R. W. & Farrell, C. Evidence for a Bone Tumor Agent in Human Osteosarcomas. *Proc. Amer. Ass. Cancer Res.*, **12**, 48, 1971.
17. Finkel, M. P., Biskis, B. O. & Reilly, C. A. Jr. Interaction of FBJ Osteosarcoma Virus with ^{90}Sr and with ^{90}Sr Osteosarcomas. In *Oncology*, **Vol. 1**, *Cellular and Molecular Mechanisms of Carcinogenesis*, Ed. R. L. Clark. Year Book Medical Publishers, Chicago, pp. 422–434, 1971.

18. Fujinaga, S., Poel, W. E. & Dmochowski, L. Light and Electron Microscope Studies of Osteosarcomas Induced in Rats and Hamsters by Harvey and Moloney Sarcoma Viruses. *Cancer Res.*, **30**, 1698–1708, 1970.

19. Goldfeder, A., Kauffman, S. L. & Ghosh, A. K. Carcinogenesis in Naturally Tumour-resistant Mice. X-irradiation versus Urethane as a Carcinogenic Agent. *Brit. J. Cancer*, **20**, 361–374. 1966.

20. Goldfeder, A. & Ghosh, A. K. Radiation Studies on Mice of an Inbred Tumor-resistant Strain. V. Possible Evidence for Activation of the Mammary Tumor Virus (MTV) by urethane as observed by Electron Microscopy. *Tex. Rep. Biol. Med.*, **25**, 396–409, 1967.

21. Goldfeder, A. & Ghosh, A. K. Unusual Ultrastructures in a Thymic Lymphoma of an X-ray- and Urethan-treated X/Gf Mouse. *Cancer Res.*, **29**, 1889–1892, 1969.

22. Goldfeder, A., De Harven, E. & Friend, C. Studies on Mice of a Tumor-resistant Strain (X/Gf). VIII. Type C Particles in Mammary Tumors of Friend Leukemia Virus-infected Mice. *Europ. J. Clin. & Biol. Res.*, **16**, 323–328, 1971.

23. Goldfeder, A. Studies on Oncogenesis in Mice of a Tumor-resistant Strain X/Gf. *Proc. Amer. Ass. Cancer Res.* **20**, 1972.

24. Gross, L. "Spontaneous" Leukemia Developing in C3H Mice following Inoculation in Infancy, with Ak-leukemic Extracts, or Ak-embryos. *Proc. Soc. exp. Biol.*, **78**, 27–32, 1951.

25. Gross, L. A Filterable Agent, recovered from Ak-leukemic Extracts, causing Salivary Gland Carcinomas in C3H Mice. *Proc. Soc. exp. Biol.*, **83**, 414–421, 1953.

26. Harvey, J. J. Replication of Murine Sarcoma Virus-Harvey (MSV-H) in Tissue Cultures of Virus-induced Sarcomas. *J. gen. Virol.*, **3**, 327–336, 1968.

27. Huebner, R. J., Hartley, J. W., Rowe, W. P., Lane, W. T. & Capps, W. I. Rescue of the Defective Genome of Moloney Sarcoma Virus from a Noninfectious Hamster Tumor and the Production of Pseudotype Sarcoma Viruses with Various Murine Leukemia Viruses. *Proc. nat. Acad. Sci. (Wash.)*, **56**, 1164–1169, 1966.

28. Huebner, R. J. & Todaro, G. J. Oncogenes of RNA Tumor Viruses as Determinants of Cancer. *Proc. nat. Acad. Sci. (Wash.)*, **64**, 1087–1094, 1969.

29. Kelloff, G. J., Lane, W. T., Turner, H. C. & Huebner, R. J. *In vivo* Studies of the FBJ Murine Osteosarcoma Virus. *Nature, (Lond.)*, **223**, 1379–1380, 1969.

30. Levy, J. A., Hartley, J. W., Rowe, W. P. & Huebner, R. J. Biologic Characteristics of the FBJ Osteosarcoma Virus. *Proc. Amer. Ass. Cancer Res.*, **10**, 50, 1969.

31. Morton, D. L. & Malmgren, R. A. Human Osteosarcomas: Immunologic Evidence Suggesting an Associated Infectious Agent. *Science*, **162**, 1279–1281, 1968.

32. Priori, E. S., Wilbur, J. R. & Dmochowski, L. Immunofluorescence Tests on Sera of Patients with Osteogenic Sarcoma. *J. nat. Cancer Inst.*, **46**, 1299–1308, 1971.

33. Pritchard, D. J., Reilly, C. A. Jr. & Finkel, M. P. Evidence for a Human Osteosarcoma Virus. *Nat. New Biol.*, **234**, 126–127, 1971.

34. Reilly, C. A. Jr. & Finkel, M. P. Evidence of FBJ Virus Antigen in ^{90}Sr-induced Osteo-sarcomas. *Radiat. Res.*, **47**, 252–253, 1971.

35. Reilly, C. A. Jr., Pritchard, D. J., Biskis, B. O. & Finkel, M. P. Immunologic Evidence Suggesting a Viral Etiology of Human Osteosarcoma. *Cancer*, **30**, 603–609, 1972.

36. Rous, P. Transmission of a malignant New Growth by Means of a Cell-free Filtrate. *J. Amer. med. Ass.*, **56**, 198, 1911.

37. Rous, P., Murphy, J. B. & Tytler, W. H. The Relation between a Chicken Sarcoma's Behavior and the Growth's Filterable Cause. *J. Amer. med. Ass.*, **59**, 1840–1841, 1912.

38. Shope, R. E. A Filterable Virus causing Tumor-like Condition in Rabbits and its Relationship to Virus Myxomatosum. *J. exp. Med.*, **56**, 803–822, 1932.

39. Shope, R. E. Infectious Papillomatosis of Rabbits. *J. exp. Med.*, **58**, 607–624, 1933.

40. Soehner, R. L. & Dmochowski, L. Induction of Bone Tumours in Rats and Hamsters with Murine Sarcoma Virus and their Cell-free Transmission. *Nature, (Lond.)*, **224**, 191–192, 1969.

41. Stewart, S. E. The Polyoma Virus. In *Advances in Virus Research*, Ed. K. M. Smith and M. A. Lauffer. Academic Press, Inc., New York, **Vol. 7**, pp. 61–90, 1960.

42. Yumoto, T., Poel, W. E., Kodama, T. & Dmochowski, L. Studies on FBJ Virus-induced Bone Tumors in Mice. *Tex. Rep. Biol. Med.*, **28**, 145–165, 1970.

Discussion

Dr. Murray   I was particularly fascinated by the second case of transmitted multiple osteomata. A lot of those lesions were in the mid-shafts of the long bones, and they bore a considerable resemblance to Englemann's disease, which we have always accepted as being one of the congenital dysplasias. I have never been quite happy about it being a congenital dysplasia because it is a condition which presents very often in adult life. It does occur in children sometimes. It is accompanied by a specific bone pain and I can't help wondering if this is a clue to this being a virus disorder. I don't know if you have thought about this?

Professor Bonfiglio   There is a similarity also to infantile cortical hyperostosis, some of those roentgenograms were quite characteristic of that process as well.

Dr. Finkel   I would say that we have been able to extract this particular virus from CF1 mice seven different times, so this is certainly something that is endemic in the CF1 strain. We have not yet had a chance to investigate other mouse strains to see if there is something similar there. Nor have we been able to test this virus in other systems. It seems most remarkable to me that it has been so simple to pull this osteoma virus out. I am sorry I don't have histologic material to show you here, but there wasn't time to prepare it.

Dr. Price   I would like to comment for a moment on what Dr. Murray mentioned. I think there is also another very interesting condition which is rare admittedly but occasionally confused with Caffey's Syndrome—that is the post-vaccinial reaction. This of course is due to a viral agent. Another thing which I think is tremendously interesting is that in the work that Dr. Moore and I have done using FBJ virus in CBA mice, I noted that additional to being an oncogenic agent it also stirs up a considerable periosteal reaction which may go on to produce a good deal of metaplastic cartilage and bone. I have one further comment to make and perhaps Dr. Owen would be able to speak on this, as well. I was struck in the radiographs of the monstrous osteomata that there was some similarity again to Marek's disease, the osteopetrosis lymphomatosum of Galla Domestica, particularly where we saw these so called osteomata in the long bones.

Dr. Owen   I would support Dr. Price on that. I would like to see the histology before you say it resembles osteopetrosis, but the radiographic appearance is similar.

Dr. Moore   An important feature of FBJ virus is the fact that it was the first sarcoma virus to be isolated from a spontaneously arising solid tumour. This contrasts with other strains of MSV (e.g. Harvey and Moloney) which were isolated from leukaemia virus preparations. The association of type C particles with human neoplasms has been the subject of considerable controversy. One series of investigations, despite extensive search, failed to identify virus in biopsies or tissue cultures derived from human sarcomas (Giraldo *et al.*, 1971)[1] However, Hall, Morton and Malmgren (1970)[2] reported the presence of particles morphologically similar to C type viruses in cultured human liposarcoma cells and more recently McAllister and his colleagues (1972)[3] identified a virus (RD114) released from human rhabdomyosarcoma cells which possessed all the characteristics of a mammalian C type virus. No definitive statements may presently be made about the oncogenicity of these particles in man.

Dr. Finkel   I think one of the important things that I would like to emphasize in the work I have presented here is that sometimes when there is an oncogenic agent you can see it. It's a type C virus and there is no question about it. Other times you can see particles in tumours and you can't do anything with them. These are particles that are there, they are apparently not oncogenic or they are defective for some reason. They are not going to induce tumours no matter what our normal procedures are. In other cases where you can see no virus you can actually get active extracts. You know you have an oncogenic agent but it just doesn't happen to have a protein coat. You can't see it with the electron microscope. Certainly with our X/Gf osteosarcoma agent, we have the agent there, but we can't see it. With Barry Freidman's Dunn osteosarcoma he can see the particles but he hasn't been able to pass that tumour cell-free. So that just the fact that you see the virus doesn't mean the agent is not there.

Professor Sissons   Dr. Finkel, I wonder if you would expand just a little on the tumour specific antigens that you told us were a feature of the induced tumours with your material?

Dr. Finkel   I really can't tell you very much about them because I don't know much about them myself. I can merely say that with using the indirect immunofluorescence technique, and using human osteosarcoma serum checked against a primary hamster osteosarcoma, and against osteosarcoma that were induced in hamsters which we have been carrying in tissue culture, and fibrosarcoma in hamsters that we have been carrying in tissue culture, and subcutaneous transplants, we get a reaction. So that I don't know what explanation we would have for this kind of reaction unless these hamsters were carrying human antigen. If they are doing this, and it is the same antigen, perhaps it is a virus.

REFERENCES

1. Giraldo, G., Beth, E., Hirshaut, Y., Aoki, T., Old, L. J., Boyse, E. A. & Chopra, H. C. Human Sarcomas in Culture. Foci of Altered Cells and a Common Antigen: Induction of Foci and Antigen in Human Fibroblast Cultures by Filtrates. *J. exp. Med.*, **133**, 454–478, 1971.
2. Hall, W. T., Morton, D. L. & Malmgren, R. A. Virus Particles in Tissue Cultures of a Human Liposarcoma. *J. nat. Cancer Inst.*, **44**, 507–513, 1970.
3. McAllister, R. M., Nicolson, M., Gardner, M. B., Rongey, R. W., Rasheed, S., Sarma, P. S., Huebner, R. J., Hatanaka, M., Oroszlan, S., Gilden, R. V., Kabigting, A. & Vernon, L. C-type Virus Released from Cultured Human Rhabdomyosarcoma Cells. *Nat. New Biol.*, **235**, 3–6, 1972.

A study of metastasizing S.E. polyoma virus-induced fibrosarcoma in the Syrian golden hamster

by

ROBERT B. DUTHIE

SUMMARY

Tumour progression was studied in a polyoma virus-induced fibrosarcoma of a golden hamster, the tumour being examined histologically and micro-autoradiographically 24 hours after "flash" labelling with tritiated thymidine. Although this rapidly growing tumour is readily grafted, no significant rise in viral (H.I.) antibody titres was found in the recipients. In a group of 100 flank grafted hamsters the tumours were repeatedly excised at a size of 2·5 cm, this regime being accompanied by increasing metastatic frequency. In a second group of 62 animals with renal sub-capsular implants early nephrectomy likewise showed a reduced incidence of lung secondaries. The radioactive marker was noted in the engrafted tumour, but not in the metastasizing cells. These results may be explained either by a time factor or by tumour progression caused by the serial excisions.

FOULDS (1949)[4] INTRODUCED the concept of tumour progression as "the development of an irreversible qualitative change in different directions to give an increase in size". It is not constant in either speed or amount but depends upon:

1. Preferential selection of certain cells to survive.
2. Adaptation of these cells to their environment.
3. Some stimulating factor being added to their normal habitat.

Clinically it is very unusual to see radiographic evidence of lung metastases when the diagnosis is first made of giant-cell tumour, chondrosarcoma, or even osteosarcoma. It is also an unusual feature of any of the old reports of untreated bone malignancies, for the lungs alone to be involved except in the terminal stages.

It is most difficult to study the features of progression in humans and therefore one has to turn to animal models.

Viruses were first implicated as causing tumours in animals by Borrell in 1903.[1] It is now commonly stated that the virus theory of cancer has become "respectable" but Dalldorf believed it was better to state that this theory had become more rational to "respectable" experts. This form of extra-chromosomal "carcinogen" has been found to produce many forms of tumour, but with accompanying uncertainty and controversy. Although many of these lesions were proliferative and hyperplastic, many regressed and did not satisfy Goodpasture's[5] definition of a cancer as being "an autonomous new growth in which there is an irreversible change so that they fail to respond to normal cell control". Viruses are regarded as producing cellular mutations which may or may not disappear. The virus aetiology of cancer has been aggravated by extending the definition of virus to include nucleic acids and other self-replicating structures (Grace 1962).[6] However, in 1958 the polyoma virus of Stewart et al.[10] and Eddy et al.[2] satisfied Goodpasture's definition and established the importance of the DNA oncogenic viruses in animals.

The S.E. polyoma virus has been shown to produce a multiplicity of tumours in the majority of the rodent family. Because their tumours can be transplanted into various sites while still retaining their original morphological and behavioural characteristics, and not arising de novo, it was decided to study the metastasizing properties of transplanted fibrosarcoma obtained from a virus-induced tumour in a golden hamster.

MATERIALS AND METHODS

Mouse embryo cultured leukaemia virus (No. 695-26B) was obtained from Dr. Bernice Eddy and after thawing and reconstituting with distilled water, 0·4 ml. was injected subcutaneously into Syrian golden hamster (Criceti aurati) neonates obtained from the Animal Research Centre, Bainbridge, N.Y., and which had never before been exposed to polyoma virus. Within a month, pleomorphic tumours of heart, kidney, spleen, liver and subcutaneous sites were found (but none of bone) and this aspect of the work has been well documented by others. It is noted that the S.E. polyoma virus will produce bone tumours in the Swiss S.K. strain of mice for example, but very rarely in hamsters or large rodents. Autopsy and microscopic examination was carried out after "flash" injection of radioactive tritiated thymidine 24 hours before sacrifice of all animals carrying the transplanted tumour for microautoradiographic study as well as staining various tissues with Toluidine Blue solution and for the Feulgen reaction.

A tumour arising in the myocardium from one of these hamsters was minced up in sterile saline and implanted, as small pieces 2–3 mm in diameter, in the dorsal subcutaneous area or under the capsule of the kidney of homologous weanling hamsters for five serial passages. No immunological conditioning by irradiation or by steroid administration was necessary for 100% "take" in these animals. These were then operated upon with excision of the growing transplanted tumours when the mass had reached a size of 2·5 cm in diameter. Polyoma hemagglutination inhibition (HI) antibody titres were determined in the blood removed by cardiac puncture in nine animals and from emulsified tumour tissues (9) according to the technique of Eddy et al. (1958)[3] by Dr. Donald Hare. All showed non-significant titre levels for the viral antibodies, i.e. less than 1/80 HI, with "normal" controls being 1/40 HI antibodies. This failure to demonstrate these antibodies appeared to show that there was not an induced antibody response by the host to the tumour tissue. But it is well established that infection by the virus does give marked elevation of the polyoma antibodies. Such low titre levels also suggested that the transplanted tumour tissue did not contain live virus material.

RESULTS

The histochemical properties, such as metachromasia, the Periodic Acid Schiff reaction, the Feulgen reaction for desoxyribonuclei acid, and the alkaline phosphatase

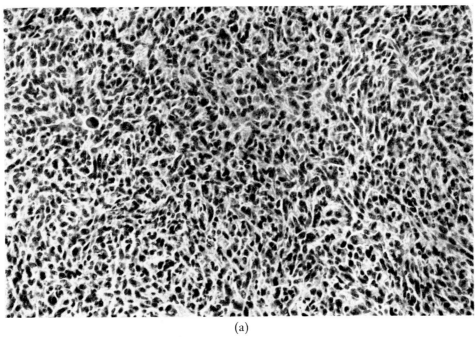

(a)

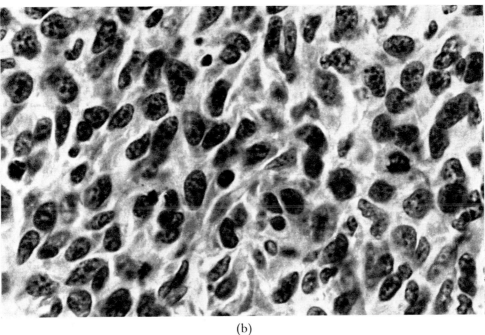

(b)

Fig. 1. (*a*) Photomicrograph (H & E ×200) to show the fibroblastic cellular content, making up the fibrosarcomatous tumour. (*b*) Photomicrograph H & E ×600) of the same field showing the large, irregularly placed nuclei containing chromatin and mitotic figures of the tumour cells.

N*

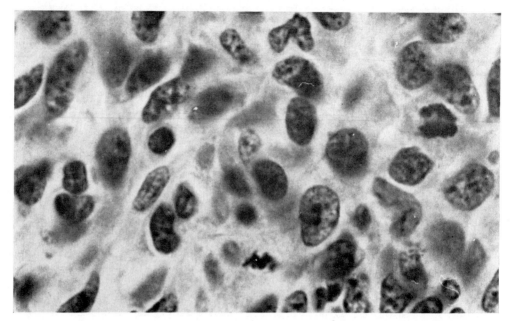

Fig. 2. Photomicrograph (Feulgen stained × 800) from similar tissue to show further definition of the characteristic nuclear structure of a virus infected cell or of a rapidly dividing tumour cell.

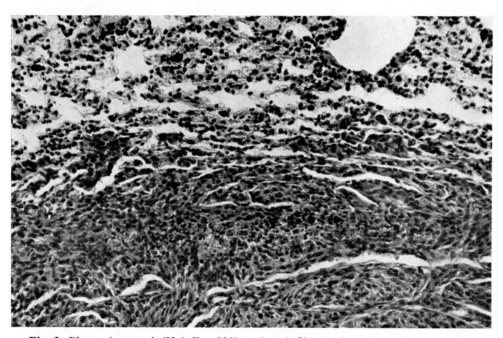

Fig. 3. Photomicrograph (H & E × 200) to show infiltrated lung tissue above and the tumour tissue below.

content were seen in all the transplanted tumours. Although the alkaline phosphatase demonstration by the Gömöri technique was an obvious feature of this tumour, its transplantation into a joint (10 animals), adjacent to fracture callus (10 animals) or under the capsule of the kidney (34 animals) failed to demonstrate any osteogenic potency. The tumour cell was fibroblastic (Fig. 1(a) and (b)) giving rise to a fibro-myxosarcoma appearance with a large eccentrically placed nucleus (Fig. 2) heavily stained with the Feulgen reaction. Thin walled vessels were plentiful. The circumscribed tumours had a pseudo-capsule. Several contained areas of cartilaginous metachromatic tissue of a "metaplastic" type but were otherwise highly differentiated and uniform in appearance. The uptake of tritiated thymidine (H^3) by the nuclear content of the tumour was clearly seen on autoradiography and grain counting was possible. These corresponded to areas of strongly positive DNA staining material and indicated either that these cells were undergoing rapid replication or were cells which had been infected by a virus.

It was found that the "untreated" transplanted tumour would kill the host within 4 weeks by local growth, invasion and ulceration without metastasizing to the lungs or elsewhere.

TABLE 1

TOTAL NUMBER OF ANIMALS USED IN THE SUBCUTANEOUS TRANSPLANTATION SERIES = 100
FIVE WERE STILL ALIVE AT END OF EXPERIMENT. TWELVE DIED BEFORE THE FIRST EXCISION
OF TUMOUR

No. of animals with tumour	Excision of tumour and day	No. of animals sacrificed and examined on day	Pulmonary Metastases	
			Present	Absent
86	1st at 17th	36 at 24th	18 (51%)	17 (one animal eaten)
47	2nd at 42nd	29 at 49th	27 (93%)	2
18	3rd at 60th	14 at 67th	14 (100%)	0
4	4th at 85th	3 at 92nd	2 (2/3)	1
1	5th at 107th	1 ——	1 (1/1)	—

A series of 100 hamsters who had successful transplantation of the muscle tumour into the dorsal subcutaneous site, received five consecutive excisions of the growing transplanted tumour (see Table 1).

The lung metastases had similar histochemical properties as the primary tumour (Fig. 3) except when the primary tumour was strongly labelled with the tritiated thymidine label, few of the tumour cells of the lung metastases had positive autoradiographs.

TABLE 2

TOTAL NUMBER OF ANIMALS USED IN THE KIDNEY TRANSPLANTATION SERIES = 62
EIGHT DIED BEFORE NEPHRECTOMY AND FIVE ANIMALS WERE NOT EXAMINED FOR
METASTASES

Nephrectomy at 20th day
Lung metastases in nine animals on sacrifice   = 39%
Normal lungs in 14 animals on sacrifice

Death of all animals by 40th day
Lung metastases in 16 animals   = 50%
Normal lungs in 16 animals

DISCUSSION

Although some S.E. Polyoma induced lung tumours—mainly adenomatous in type—have been reported, these were not found to arise in this strain of golden hamsters. The most uniform method of producing lung tumours is by the intranasal inhalation route. Stanton (1960)[9] has shown that this oncogenic effect of the polyoma virus is local rather than systemic. He has described that the stimulus for cell proliferation may be a virus-induced cellular change rather than any direct effect of the virus passing from cell to cell, i.e. these tumours do not act as a culture medium but rather that with division of the cells altered DNA content may be carried on. This may or may not produce further malignant change depending upon the host/cell response and what is happening within the host.

Another point to be considered is the uncertainty whether a continued viral insult is necessary to maintain the progression of the tumour. Habel and Silverberg (1960)[7] have shown that a C57-695 tumour transplant growing in mice did not arouse an antibody response in the host and this tumour transplant did not contain any virus. Similarly their hamster tumour transplant line—except for one—gave no consistent evidence of association between virus and continued tumour growth. Sambrook *et al.* (1968)[8] have described how the viral DNA becomes a part of the genetic material of some transplanted cells and that some of the attributes of the transformed cells may result from the expression of these viral genes.

Stewart *et al.* (1959)[10] have shown in rodents that it is rare for polyoma virus-induced tumours to metastasize, indicating any systemic aggressive behaviour—except for the angioid type of tumour.

In our series there was increasing incidence of lung metastases when the subcutaneous and kidney transplanted tumours were repeatedly excised. (Tables 1 and 2). These excisions certainly carried the host animals past the time of local invasion which usually killed the host. Therefore the important factor may simply be that of time. But it is of interest that the lung fields were the only site of metastases except in a few animals in which tissue had been involved from the implanted tumour. Here the mode of spread might well have been by direct invasion rather than by the blood stream. On the other hand excision may well have changed the aggressive character or progression of this particular tumour. This type of tissue study does not really indicate whether the physical trauma of operative excision changes the spreading properties of this tumour, or liberates tumour cells for their spread to the susceptible environment of lung fields. This is unlikely in the present series since the lung tumour did not present with any tritiated thymidine label similar to the primary subcutaneous or kidney implanted tumour.

ACKNOWLEDGEMENT

It is a pleasure to acknowledge that the majority of this work was supported by an N.I.H. research grant No. CY 4265(3) of the National Cancer Institute, Bethesda, Md., U.S.A.

REFERENCES

1. Borrell, A. Epithelioses Infectieuses et Epitheliomas. *Ann. Inst. Pasteur*, **17**, 81–122, 1903.
2. Eddy, B. E., Stewart, S. E., Young, R. & Mieler, G. B. Neoplasms in Hamsters induced by Mouse Tumour Agent Passed in Tissue Culture. *J. nat. Cancer Inst.*, **20**, 747–761, 1958.
3. Eddy, B. E., Rowe, W. P., Hartley, J. W., Stewart, S. E. & Huebner, R. J. Hemagglutination with the S.E. Polyoma Virus. *Virology*, **6**, 290–291, 1958.
4. Foulds, L. Mammary Tumours in Hybrid Mice: Growth and Progression of Spontaneous Tumours. *Brit. J. Cancer*, **3**, 345–375, 1949.
5. Goodpasture, E. W. Personal communication, 1956.
6. Grace, J. T. Neoplasia and Viruses. *Health News* (*N.Y.*), **39**, No. 4, 4–12, 1962.
7. Habel, K. & Silverberg, R. J. Relationship of Polyoma Virus in Tumour *in vivo*. *Virology*, **12**, No. 3, 463–476, 1960.
8. Sambrook, J., Westphal, H., Srinivesan, P. R. & Dulbecco, R. *Proc. nat. Acad. Sci.* (*Wash.*), **60**, 1288, 1968.
9. Stanton, M. F. The Local Oncogenic Response of Hamster Tissues to Polyoma Virus. *Cancer Res.*, **20**, 487–491, 1960.
10. Stewart, S. E., Eddy, B. E. & Stanton, M. F. Neoplasms in Rodents induced by S.E. Polyoma Virus. *Acta Un. int. Cancr.*, **25**, 842–851, 1959.

Discussion

Dame Janet Vaughan   It is very odd that the tritiated thymidine label wasn't carried in the metastasizing tumour cells. Has Professor Duthie any explanation for this?

Professor Duthie   I think that we have to look at it, whether the tumour cells that were discovered in the lung actually had arisen after the flash labelling had taken place in the transplanted tumour. The set-up was particularly designed to show whether after flash labelling of the transplanted tumour that once you excised it, those tumour cells with access spread to the lung fields—and they haven't. Well they certainly didn't carry in the label.

Professor Bonfiglio (Chairman)   Did you look at any of the vessels leading from the tumour as to whether there were tumour plugs in them at any point along the line either before or after excision?

Professor Duthie   No, because reading from the flank there would be quite a difficult anatomical exercise.

Professor Bonfiglio   No, just histologically. Meaning in the ones that you had excised before autopsy for instance?

Professor Duthie   No we haven't. Because I would imagine there would be several draining areas, or many.

Professor Bonfiglio   I just wondered if you had noticed any tumour thrombi anywhere along the line.

Dr. Price   Am I right in interpreting what you said as implying that the S.E. polyoma virus agent has been lost in the process of this experiment and is indicated by the absence of the positive auto-radiograph? If that is so, would it be worthwhile to attempt perhaps to recover it by means of differential sucrose gradient centrifugalization?

Professor Duthie   No I don't think we are labelling the virus, we are labelling purely the DNA content of these tumour cells.

Dr. Price   But that indicates DNA synthesis doesn't it?

Professor Duthie   That indicates DNA synthesis. Well, it indicates that at a particular moment really the DNA had become labelled by tritiated thymidine, but it is really no indication of the viral content.

Dr. Moore   Did you actually undertake any other experiments to determine whether this tumour was immunogenic in this strain of hamster? Did you attempt to induce resistance to the tumour by other methods such as by giving them irradiated grafts? Because presumably unless this tumour was exceptional it would carry the polyoma virus-specified antigens common to all polyoma virus-induced tumours. I would have expected some degree of immunogenicity of the tumour, and I was wondering whether in the course of time you were going to attempt to correlate this with the results you have got from repeated excision?

Professor Duthie That would be a good experiment.

Dr. Price Could I please make one further comment. Again, this is to a certain extent based on an assumption. You showed us a photomicrograph of a cellular tumour with a little area of cartilage. That to my mind was really a beautiful example of perhaps a part of our contention this morning. That to me was clearly metaplastic cartilage not tumour cartilage, that is to say it is a change taking place in a tumour matrix. Of late years having worked a little bit with experimental rodent tumours, I have now to some extent modified my concept of what constitutes an osteosarcoma. I do differentiate very carefully now a sarcoma which produces a matrix which may undergo metaplastic chondrification and ossification but this does not indicate that one should regard it as a chondrosarcoma or osteosarcoma, I think that is a beautiful example.

Professor Duthie This one I put in the rather firm diagnosis of being a fibromyxosarcoma. That was the uniformity of it.

Skeletal tumours induced by internal radiation

by

JANET M. VAUGHAN*

SUMMARY

Four variable factors are recognized which may affect the oncogenic behaviour of bone-seeking radionuclides: the type and site of cells "at risk", the physical characteristics of the isotope under study, its site of deposition in bone and the pattern of bone trabeculation for which there are known species differences. It is essential to recognize the relationship between the particle range and the size of the bone trabeculation and the marrow cavities, likewise the importance of the energy of the radiation and the half life of the radionuclide.

Thus experiments have shown that short-range radionuclides induce mainly tumours of the osteogenic tissues while those of longer range cause a wider variety with in addition neoplasms of marrow origin involving haematopoietic, reticuloendothelial and stromal elements.

THE NOMENCLATURE of skeletal tumours has long been a difficult problem, owing to the complex histological picture they often present (Jaffe 1958, Willis 1967, Sissons 1966). It appears possible that an analysis of the character of radiation induced skeletal tumours, in relation to the type of radiation that has initiated the malignant transformation, may lead to a recognition of the cell or cells from which the malignant process has originated. Before attempting this analysis it is necessary to examine, first of all the tissues at risk, secondly the relevant characteristics of the radiations involved, particularly their energy, and their range, thirdly the site of deposition of the radionuclides involved and fourthly the character of the bone trabeculation which is being irradiated.

1. SKELETAL TISSUES AT CARCINOGENIC RISK

The tissues associated with the skeleton which are at carcinogenic risk from internally deposited radionuclides are: (1) osteogenic tissue on bone surfaces which contains osteoprogenitor stem cells; (2) bone marrow which contains haemopoietic, reticuloendothelial and stromal stem cells. (The recent work of Loutit and his colleagues (Barnes, Carr, Evans and Loutit 1970) suggests that in post-foetal life of the mouse differentiated osteoprogenitor cells are probably not present in the marrow); (3) epithelium lining the cranial sinuses of the skull, outside bone, but closely adherent to it (International Commission on Radiological Protection 1968, Loutit and Vaughan 1971). The last does not

* From the Bone Research Laboratory, Churchill Hospital, Oxford.

concern the present discussion. The site of the fibroblast stem cell is at present not clear. In 1968 Barnes and Khrushchov provided good experimental evidence that it was in the marrow. More recent experimental evidence suggests that fibroblast stem cells may exist in other connective tissue (Barnes, Evans and Loutit 1971).

2. CHARACTERISTICS OF THE RADIATIONS

The bone seeking radionuclides which will be discussed are ^{228}Th, ^{226}Ra, ^{224}Ra, ^{239}Pu, ^{45}Ca and ^{90}Sr and its radioactive daughter ^{90}Y. A mention is also made of ^{89}Sr. The characteristics of these radionuclides which are particularly relevant to the present discussion are shown in Table 1. The first four are primarily alpha emitters. The beta

TABLE 1

SOME CHARACTERISTICS OF CERTAIN BONE-SEEKING RADIONUCLIDES

(*Bleaney 1971, by courtesy of author*)

Radionuclide	Half-life	Radiation	Energy MeV	Range in Soft tissue	Site
^{228}Th	1·9 years	α	5·4–8·8	39–88 μm	Surface
^{226}Ra	1,620 years	α	4·6–7·7	31–70 μm	Volume
^{224}Ra	3·69 days	α	5·4–8·8	39–88 μm	Surface
^{239}Pu	$2·4 \times 10^4$ years	α	5·14	35 μm	Surface and marrow
^{90}Sr + ^{90}Y	28 years	β	2·18	10 mm	Volume
^{89}Sr	51 days	β	1·46	7 mm	Volume
^{45}Ca	1·65 days	β	0·254	900 μm	Volume

The energies and ranges of the first three nuclides include the alphas emitted by the daughters in the decay chains.
The β energies are the maximum emitted energies.

emitters in their decay chain, if present, have been ignored in this table, since their contribution to a tissue dose is relatively small, but the range of energies tabulated includes the alphas emitted by the daughters in the decay chain. The energy measured in MeV of these four radionuclides is high, ranging from 4·6 MeV to 8·8 MeV when the energy of the daughter radionuclides is included. The range of these alphas in tissue is, however, small, ranging from 31 to 88 μm. ^{45}Ca, ^{90}Sr, ^{90}Y, ^{89}Sr, on the other hand, are beta emitters. They have a much lower energy than the alpha emitters but a longer range in soft tissue. This is particularly true of the daughter product of ^{90}Sr, ^{90}Y; the combined range of these two radionuclides is 10 mm.

3. SITE OF RADIONUCLIDE DEPOSITION

The location of these radionuclides in the skeleton is also important. ^{228}Th and ^{239}Pu both deposit on endosteal surfaces and remain on bone surfaces in adult bone. Plutonium is described as also depositing in marrow and this is probably true of ^{228}Th. Radium and strontium like calcium are found throughout bone mineral and are therefore spoken of as volume seekers. The case of ^{224}Ra however requires special mention. The alkaline earths are all initially taken up on bone surfaces (Rowland 1966, Ellsasser, Farnham and Marshall 1969) and subsequently are distributed throughout bone mineral. ^{224}Ra has, however, a very short half life of 3·69 days and therefore decays markedly on the bone surface before a volume distribution can occur (Spiess and Mays 1970). Since it has been agreed that the majority of the osteogenic cells lie within 10 μm of the mineral matrix surface (Sissons 1970, Vaughan 1970) it appears likely that radionuclides with a short range in tissue such as ^{226}Ra, will irradiate largely osteogenic tissue, whereas radionuclides with a long range in tissue, like ^{90}Sr + ^{90}Y, will irradiate both marrow and osteogenic tissue. Further radionuclides that both deposit on endosteal surfaces and in the marrow, like ^{239}Pu, even though their range is short, may be expected to irradiate both osteogenic tissue and marrow.

4. CHARACTER OF BONE TRABECULATION

It is essential to realize that there are great differences in the pattern of bone trabeculation and the size of marrow cavities in different species. These differences will influence the radiation dose received from the same radionuclide in different species. Spiers and his colleagues (Spiers 1966, 1968; Spiers, Zanelli, Darley, Whitwell and Goldman 1972;

TABLE 2

MEAN PATH LENGTHS IN HUMAN AND ANIMAL TRABECULAR BONE

Species	Bone	Mean path length in μm		Path length ratio trabeculae to marrow spaces
		(a) Marrow spaces	(b) Trabeculae	
Man*	Skull—parietal bone	390	510	1·31
	Rib	1,705	265	0·16
	Iliac crest	905	240	0·27
	Cervical vertebra	910	275	0·30
	Lumbar vertebra	1,230	245	0·20
	Femur—head	1,155	230	0·20
	Femur—neck	1,655	315	0·19
Beagle†	Tibia	490	200	0·41
	Radius	320	305	0·95
Dog‡	Vertebra	425	180	0·42
Pig‡	Vertebra	470	175	0·37
Cow‡	Vertebra	470	375	0·80

* Adult male, aged 44 years.
† Beagle, UCRL, Davis. Calif.
‡ Origin unknown.

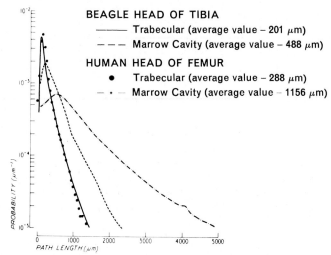

Fig. 1. Path length measurements in the beagle head of tibia and human head of femur (Spiers *et al.* 1972, by courtesy of authors and publishers).

Spiers, Whitwell and Darly 1971) have measured the dimensions of bone trabeculae and of marrow cavities in cross sections of trabecular bone by means of a special scanning device (Darley 1968). Values for certain bones of man, dog and pig are shown in Table 2. Unfortunately there are no such measurements on mouse bones. Finkel gives the diameter of a mouse femur as 1·5 mm (Finkel, Biskis and Scribner 1959). The figures in Table 2, however, indicate at once that path lengths across trabeculae very little in different species, but that path lengths across marrow cavities can vary by a factor of three or four and that variations can occur within different bones of the same species and between different species.

The differences between marrow cavity and trabecular path length distributions in the human and the beagle dog are illustrated in Fig. 1. The curves for path lengths in trabecular bone are almost identical but the marrow cavity path length is much greater in man than in the dog. This means that in the dog a greater proportion of the marrow will be irradiated than in man for the same concentration of radionuclide in the skeleton. There are significant differences in marrow cavity sizes in the same bone at different ages. In Fig. 2 are shown marrow cavity sizes in trabecular bone of the third lumbar vertebra of an adult and a child aged 5 years (Spiers 1966).

These results make it extremely unwise to extrapolate results obtained on one species to another species and one age group to another age group without making precise measurement of bone trabecular pattern.

RESULTS OF EXPERIMENTAL EXPOSURE TO RADIONUCLIDES

In Table 3 is shown in summary terms an analysis of the types of tumour that are recorded following both single and continuous administration of the six radionuclides under discussion. For the purpose of this particular table the column headed "Angiosarcoma" covers a wide variety of tumours including reticulum-cell sarcomas, reticuloendotheliomas and giant-cell tumours. The term "leukaemia" also includes a variety of myeloproliferative disorders.

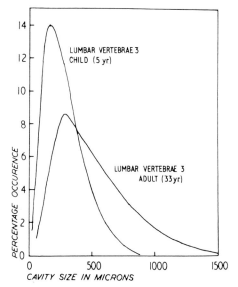

Fig. 2. Marrow cavity sizes in trabecular bone of the third lumbar vertebrae of an adult and a child aged 5 years (Spiers 1966, by courtesy of author and publishers).

TABLE 3

RADIONUCLIDES AND SKELETAL TUMOUR INCIDENCE IN ANIMALS

Radionuclide	Osteo-sarcoma	Chondro-sarcoma	Fibro-sarcoma	"Angio"† sarcoma	"Leukaemia"*
^{228}Th	+++			+	
^{226}Ra	+++		+		
^{224}Ra	+++				
^{239}Pu	++	+	+		+
^{90}Sr + ^{90}Y	+++	+	+	++	+++
^{89}Sr	++	+	+	+	
^{45}Ca	++				

* The term leukaemia here is used to cover any myeloproliferative disorder.
† The term "angio" is used to cover a miscellaneous group of tumours probably arising from marrow mesenchyme tissue. Angiosarcoma, reticuloendothelioma, etc.

It is at once apparent that the two radionuclides ^{226}Ra and ^{224}Ra with the shortest range in tissue, i.e. which might be expected theoretically to irradiate largely osteogenic tissue, do in fact, in animals, induce preeminently osteosarcoma and possibly fibrosarcoma. In 1968 Finkel and Biskis suggested that ^{226}Ra induced tumours with telangiectatic features but in 1969 the same authors stated that this radionuclide produced no more of this type of tumour than occurred in the controls. Spiers and his colleagues

(Spiers, Whitwell and Darley 1971) have calculated that, with the exception of the parietal bone, only about 31% of the total active marrow in man is irradiated by ^{226}Ra. The rest of the high-energy alpha radiation is directed to the osteogenic tissue, hence the high incidence of osteosarcoma. The significant incidence of fibrosarcoma suggests that fibroblast precursors may also be present in this tissue. It is of interest in this connection to note that in the human radium cases there is also a high fibrosarcoma incidence (Finkel, Miller and Hasterlik 1969). Finkel and his colleagues list seven fibrosarcomas and six osteogenic sarcomas in the Chicago radium cases. The other short range alpha emitter, ^{224}Ra, also induces largely osteosarcoma though Russian workers mention fibrosarcoma and chondrosarcoma (Moskalev *et al.* 1969). ^{228}Th which has a rather longer range is recorded to have induced one haemangioendothelioma and 33 osteo-sarcomas in the Utah dogs. ^{239}Pu, a short-range alpha emitter, deposits in marrow as well as on bone surfaces (Vaughan, Bleaney and Williamson 1967; Bleaney and Vaughan 1971). Marrow may therefore receive an appreciable radiation dose. Leukaemia is indeed recorded as occurring in rats with this radionuclide though osteosarcomas predominate (Bensted, Taylor and Sowby 1965; Moskalev *et al.* 1969). In dogs given a single injection of plutonium citrate osteogenic sarcomas predominate, but haemopoietic dyscrasias are recorded (Vaughan, to be published).

TABLE 4

EFFECTS OF A SINGLE INJECTION ^{90}SR OR ^{89}SR

Species	No.	Route	Dose administered μCi/kg	*Received* Average rad dose	Leukaemia myeloid	Leukaemia lympho	Haemo-poietic dyscrasia
Swine	2	intravenous	1,869–6,160				
Dog		intravenous	97·9–63·6	6,435			
		intravenous	10–500				2
		inhalation ^{90}SrCl$_2$	?		1		
Rabbits		intravenous					
2 days old	8		500				
6–8 weeks	7		50–200				
6–8 weeks	13		500–1,000				
old	22		200–1,000				
Rats		intraperitoneal	5–500		+		
Mice							
CFl	810	intravenous	44–2,200		+(c)		
(b) CBA	11	intravenous	20 μCi per mouse μCi/g				
(b) CBA	219		1·6				
	292		0·8		+(c)		
	90		0·4		+(c)		
	8		0·2		+(c)		

(a) Tumours in soft tissues, i.e. sinuses of skull and mucous membranes of mouth, etc.
(b) No tumours in controls.
(c) The mouse leukaemias are not classified.

On the other hand, ^{90}Sr + ^{90}Y, the radionuclide with the longest range, 10 mm in soft tissues, is noted in all species as inducing a wide variety of tumours, included under the heading of "angiosarcoma" and also a range of haemopoietic tumours included under the heading "leukaemia".

Further many observers comment on the mixed character of the osteosarcoma induced by ^{90}Sr. Downie and her colleagues state—"an interesting histological feature of some of the established tumours was the type of regional variation in histological structure" (Downie, Macpherson, Ramsden, Sissons and Vaughan 1959). Skoryna and Kahn (1959) comment—"All the subtypes of osteogenic sarcoma seen in human pathology (osteoid, telangiectatic, undifferentiated) were found. A few tumours with almost pure chondro-sarcomatous or fibrosarcomatous differentiation were observed."

Such comments are not found in connection with the description of tumours produced by other radionuclides. ^{45}Ca, a beta emitter with a short range induces only osteo-sarcoma.

The summarized data presented in Table 3 have made it obvious that ^{90}Sr + ^{90}Y, the radionuclide with the longest range in tissue, and therefore most likely to irradiate marrow as well as osteogenic tissue, is the radionuclide that appears to induce a wide variety of "bone tumours" other than the classical osteosarcoma. An attempt must now

TABLE 4

(CONTINUED)

Osteo-sarcoma (sometimes multiple)	Fibro-sarcoma	Chondro-sarcoma	Osteo-chondro sarcoma	Angio-sarcoma	Giant-cell tumour	Cancer of head(a)	
2					1		Howard *et al.* 1969
6				2		2	Doughtery & Mays 1969
1	3			3		3	Finkel *et al.* 1972
5	3		2	7			McClellan *et al.* 1972
							Vaughan & Williamson
						7	1969
2						6	
20						1	
12							
+							Moskalev *et al.* 1969
++	+	+		+			Finkel, *et al.* 1959
6				5			Barnes *et al.* 1970
expressed as percentage							
87·2	11·0	0·9		0·9		16	Nilsson 1970
68·8	29·8			2·1		3	
24·4	71/1			4·4			
(50·0)	(37·5)			(12·5)			

be made to look more closely at the data available on the histology of tumours induced by the strontium isotopes. To do this, it is necessary to separate tumours induced by a single administration of the radionuclide from those induced by continuous administration. The latter includes repeated injections over varied periods, and continuous feeding. Any such tabulation can only be taken as a rough guide since the doses of ^{90}Sr injected or fed were variable in each experiment. In many cases detailed histology was not available and absolute numbers of tumours seen were not given. Further animals reported on by one author are sometimes included in the report of a colleague. The tabulation does however indicate that, as would be expected, there are differences in the type of tumour induced by single and by continuous administration. The character of the radiation dose received by sensitive tissues is different under the two conditions of administration, since in the first case the distribution of the radionuclide in the skeleton is uneven, so radiation dose will be unevenly distributed, and in the second, the whole skeleton will become labelled with ^{90}Sr in the young and will become more generally labelled in the adult. In Fig. 3 is illustrated the distribution of radiation dose measured by a crude autoradiographic technique in the posterior wall of the upper half of the rabbit tibia 200 days after a single injection of ^{90}Sr (600 μCi/kg) at the age of 6 weeks and 250 days after daily feeding of ^{90}Sr (8·5 μCi/kg) started at the same age. The high dose at the point of maximum uptake at the time of injection is at once apparent, while the dose distribution is much more even throughout the length of the bone in the case of continuous administration.

TABLE 5

Animal	Route of Administration	μCi/kg	Leukaemia myeloid	Leukaemia lympho	Myeloid hyperplasia	Osteosarcoma
Monkey	ingestion gavage 5–10 days	500–1000	1 "monocytic"			1
Dog	ingestion					17
	in utero—540 days		14			
	injection					
	multiple, from birth	150				38
	from 6 months	150	1			24
	from birth	15	1	1		1
	from 6 months	15	2			
	repeated over 2–3 year period	100–200	+			+
Swine	ingestion F$_1$ and F$_2$ generations		23	17	29	7
		μCi/g				
Rats	injection multiple at monthly intervals	4·4 total				+++
	10 consec. daily or monthly	0·1–3·5				+
	fed 10–30 days	330–790 total	+	++		+

*Tumours in soft tissues , i.e. sinuses of skull and mucous membranes of mouth, etc.

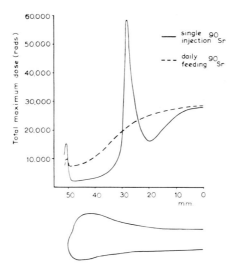

Fig. 3. Variation in the maximum accumulated dose received at different levels in the posterior wall of the upper half of the rabbit tibia 200 days after a single injection $600\mu\text{Ci}/\text{kg}$ ^{90}Sr at the age of 6 weeks and 250 days after daily feeding of $8\cdot5$ $\mu\text{Ci}/\text{kg}$ ^{90}Sr from the age of 6 weeks.

TABLE 5

(CONTINUED)

Fibro-sarcoma	Chondro-sarcoma	Angio-sarcoma	Reticulum cell-tumour	Giant-cell tumour	Cancer of head*	
	1					Casarett, Tuttle & Baxter, 1962
2	1	1			4	Pool *et al.* 1972 ⎱ same group
						Dungworth *et al.* 1969 ⎰ of dogs
1		4			2	Finkel *et al.* 1972
1			1			Finkel *et al.* 1972
1	1	1				Finkel *et al.* 1972
						Finkel *et al.* 1972
						Finkel *et al,* 1972
				3		Clarke *et al.* 1972
+	+	+		+		Skoryna & Kahn 1959
+		+	+		+	Kuzma & Zander 1957
		+	+			Casarett, Tuttle & Baxter 1962

In Table 4 are seen the recorded bone and marrow tumours following a single injection of ^{90}Sr. The mouse data are divided as far as possible, according to strain, since it appears probable that some strains carry a virus that appears to be associated with a bone dyscrasia and high natural "bone tumour" incidence, apparently potentiated by radiation. The high leukaemia incidence in certain strains of mice appears also to be associated with the presence of certain viruses and to be increased by radiation (Kaplan 1967). This association between a bone dyscrasia and a virus is seen in the CFl/Anl mouse (Lisco, Rosenthal and Vaughan 1971, personal communication) and possibly was present in the Simpson strain described by Pybus and Miller (1938). The majority of other strains, except that used by Hug et al. (1969) are not recorded as having a significant natural osteosarcoma incidence. The natural incidence in beagle dogs is extremely low. The natural incidence in pigs is also low though a lymphoproliferative disorder is known to occur.

In Table 4 it is shown that mice given a single injection of ^{90}Sr, in addition to osteosarcoma, develop an appreciable number of angiosarcomas or haemangioendotheliomas. Finkel and her colleagues (Finkel, Biskis and Scribner 1959) record that 13% of their CFl/Anl female mice given ^{90}Sr had such tumours whereas ^{226}Ra given to the same strain by these workers had no effect on the normal incidence of 1·3% of haemangioendotheliomas (Finkel, Biskis and Jinkins 1969). Barnes (Barnes, Carr, Evans and Loutit 1970) in a small series of CBA male mice injected with ^{90}Sr in connection with another experiment induced six osteoblastic tumours and five haemangioendotheliomas. Nilsson (1968, 1970) also using CBA male mice noted a significant number of haemangioendotheliomas and fibroblastic tumours. Again in the case of dogs a wide variety of tumours, myeloid and lymphatic leukaemia, haemopioetic dysplasia, osteosarcoma, fibrosarcoma, chondrosarcoma and angiosarcoma occur (Dougherty and Mays 1969, Howard et al. 1969, Finkel et al. 1972, McClellan et al. 1972). In Table 5 there appears a striking difference from the results shown in Table 4, namely that in the larger animals "leukaemia" appears to dominate the clinical picture in animals fed ^{90}Sr indicating the extreme importance of marrow irradiation from this radionuclide. The leukaemia in these animals, in many cases, is both clinically, haematologically and histologically like human myeloid leukaemia. In the pigs concerned seven small osteosarcomas were found, but only at autopsy, the animals having died as a consequence of their myeloproliferative disease (Howard, Clarke, Karagianes and Palmer 1969). In dogs fed ^{90}Sr continuously there is also a high incidence of a myeloproliferative disorder but there are also a number of osteosarcomas, fibrosarcomas and angiosarcomas (Goldman, et al. 1969; Pool, Williams and Goldman 1972; Dungworth, Goldman, Switzer and McKelvie 1969). Among seven monkeys that ingested ^{90}Sr (500–1,000 μCi by gavage daily for 5–10 days) there was one leukaemia described as monocytic, one chondrosarcoma, and one osteosarcoma (Casarett, Tuttle and Baxter 1962). Rats fed ^{90}Sr in their drinking water over 10–30 days developed osteosarcoma and "leukaemia" (Casarett et al. 1962). The osteosarcoma were described "as all osteogenic in that some osteoid or bone was found. There were fibroblastic types, some that resembled angiosarcoma, others producing relatively mature cancellous bone, other anaplastic types resembling reticulum cell sarcoma, some producing cartilage as well as bone and some mixed types." Both Skoryna and Kahn (1959) and Kuzma and Zander (1957) who gave several repeated injections of ^{89}Sr to rats, describe the same mixed response.

CONCLUSIONS

This survey of the character of bone tumours induced by internal radiation suggests the following conclusions:

1. Radiations with a short range in tissue will induce malignant transformation primarily in the osteoprogenitor cells of the endosteum and result therefore in osteosarcoma.

2. Radiations with a long range in tissue will induce malignant transformation in stem cells both of the endosteum and of all known marrow elements. Since it is only ^{90}Sr + ^{90}Y that induces a significant number of tumours described as angiosarcomas and haemangiosarcomas it is suggested that these tumours arise from marrow rather than osteogenic tissue.

3. The fact that fibrosarcomas are described following irradiation with both long- and short-range particles suggests that the fibroblast stem cell may be present in both marrow and osteogenic tissue.

4. No light is thrown on the origin of the giant-cell tumour by a study of radionuclide induced tumours.

BIBLIOGRAPHY

Barnes, D. W. H., Carr, T. E. F., Evans, E. P. & Loutit, J. F. ^{90}Sr-induced Osteosarcomas in Radiation Chimaeras. *Int. J. Radiol. Biol.*, **18**, 531–537, 1970.

Barnes, D. W. H., Evans, E. P. & Loutit, J. F.   Local Origin of Fibroblasts deduced from Sarcomas induced in Chimaeras by implants of Pliable Discs. *Nature (Lond.)*, **233**, 267–268, 1971.

Barnes, D. W. H. & Khrushchov, N. G.   Fibroblasts in Sterile Inflammation: Study in Mouse Radiation. *Nature (Lond.)*, **218**, 599–601, 1968.

Bensted, J. P. M., Taylor, D. M. & Sowby, F. D.   The Carcinogenic Effects of Americium 241 and Plutonium 239 in the rat. *Brit. J. Radiol.*, **38**, 920–925, 1965.

Bleaney, B. & Vaughan, J. M.   Distribution of ^{239}Pu in the Bone Marrow and on the Endosteal Surface of the Femur of Adult Rabbits following Injection of ^{239}Pu(NO$_3$)$_4$. *Brit. J. Radiol.*, **44**, 67–73, 1971.

Casarett, G. W., Tuttle, L. W. & Baxter, R. C.   Pathology of imbibed ^{90}Sr in Rats and Monkeys. In *Some Aspects of Internal Irradiation*, pp. 329–336, Eds. Dougherty, T. F., Jee, W. S. S., Mays, C. W. and Stover, B. J. Pergamon Press, Oxford, 1962.

Clarke, W. J., Busch, R. H., Hackett, P. L., Howard, E. B., Frasier, M. E., McClanahan, B J., Ragan, H. A. & Vogt. Strontium-90 Effects in Swine: A Summary Up-to-date. In *Biomedical Implications of Radiostrontium Exposure*, Eds. Goldman, M. & Bustad, L. K. Division of Technical Information, U.S. Atomic Energy Commission, Oak Ridge Conference ZONF. 710201, 1972.

Darley, P. J.   Measurement of Linear Path Length Distribution in bone and marrow using a scanning device. In *Proceedings of the Symposium on Microdensitometry*. E.A.E.C. Publication EUR 3747, d–e–f, 509–526, 1968.

Dougherty, T. F. & Mays, C. W.   Bone Cancer Induced by Internally-deposited Emitters in Beagles, pp. 361–367, from *Radiation Induced Cancer*. International Atomic Energy Agency, Vienna, 1969.

Downie, E. D., Macpherson, S., Ramsden, E. N., Sissons, H. A. & Vaughan, J. M.   The Effect of Daily Feeding of ^{90}Sr to Rabbits. *Brit. J. Cancer*, **13**, 408–423, 1959.

Dungworth, D. L., Goldman, M., Switzer, J. W. & McKelvie, D. M.   Development of a myeloproliferative disorder in beagles continuously exposed to ^{90}Sr. *Blood*, **34**, 610–632, 1969.

Ellsasser, J. C., Farnham, J. E. & Marshall, J. H.   Comparative Kinetics and Autoradiography of ^{45}Ca and ^{133}Ba in 10-year-old Beagle Dogs. *J. Bone Jt. Surg.*, **51**–A, 1397–1412, 1969.

Finkel, A. J., Miller, C. E. & Hasterlik, R. J. *Radium induced Malignant tumours in Man.* Sun Valley Symposium *Delayed Effects of Bone-Seeking Radionuclides*, Eds. Mays, C. W., Jee, W. S. S., Lloyd, R. D., Stover, B. J., Dougherty, J. H. and Taylor, G. N. University of Utah Press, Salt Lake City, 1969.

Finkel, M. P. & Biskis, B. O. Experimental Induction of Osteosarcoma. *Progr. exp. Tumor Res.*, **10**, 72–111, 1968.

Finkel, M. P., Biskis, B. O., Greco, J. O. & Camden, R. W. ^{90}Sr Toxicity in Dogs. Status of Argonne Study on Influence of Age and Dose Pattern. To be published in *Biomedical Implications of Radiostrontium Exposure*, Eds. M. Goldman and L. Bustad, Division of Technical Information, U.S. Atomic Energy Commission, Oak Ridge, Conference ZONF, 710201, 1972.

Finkel, M. P., Biskis, B. O. & Jinkins, P. B. Toxicity of Radium-226 in Mice. In *Radiation Induced Cancer*, International Atomic Energy Agency, Vienna, pp. 369–391, 1969.

Finkel, M. P., Biskis, B. O. & Scribner, G. M. The Influence of ^{90}Sr upon Life Span and Neoplasms of Mice. Progress in Nuclear Energy **Series VI, Vol. 2.** *Biological Sciences*, pp. 199–209. Pergamon Press, London, 1959.

Goldman, M., Dungworth, D. L., Bulgin, M. S., Rosenblatt, L. S., Richards, W. P. C. & Bustad, L. K. Radiation-induced Neoplasms in Beagles after Adminstration of ^{90}Sr and ^{226}Ra in *Radiation Induced Cancer*, International Atomic Energy Agency, Vienna, pp. 345–360, 1969.

Howard, E. B., Clarke, W. J., Karagianes, M. T. & Palmer, R. F. ^{90}Sr Induced Bone Tumours in Miniature Swine. *Radiat. Res.*, **39**, 594–607, 1969.

Hug, O., Gössner, W., Müller, W. A., Luz, A., & Hindringer, B. Production of Osteosarcoma in Mice and Rats by Radium 224. In *Radiation Induced Cancer*. International Atomic Energy Agency, Vienna, pp. 393–409, 1969.

International Commission on Radiological Protection. **Publication 11.** *A review of the radio-sensitivity of the Tissues in Bone.* Pergamon Press, Oxford, 1968.

Jaffe, H. L. *Tumors and Tumorous Conditions of the Bones and Joints.* Lea & Febiger, Philadelphia, 1958.

Kaplan, H. S. On the Natural History of the Murine Leukaemias. *Cancer Res.*, **27**, 1325–1340, 1967.

Kuzma, J. F. & Zander, G. Cancerogenic Effects of Ca^{45} and Sr^{89} in Sprague–Dawley Rats. *A. M.A. Arch. Path.*, **63**, 198, 1957.

Lisco, H., Rosenthal, M. W. & Vaughan, J. M. Observations on Skeletal Pathology in Female CF1/Anl Mice Possibly Related to Virus Infection. Personal communication, to be published, 1971.

Loutit, J. F. & Vaughan, J. M. The Radiosensitive Tissues in Bone. *Brit. J. Radiol.*, **44**, 815, 1971.

McClellan, R. O., Boecker, R. B., Jones, R. K., Barnes, J. F., Chiffelle, T. L., Hobbs, C. H. & Redman, H. C. Toxicity of Inhaled Radiostrontium in Experimental Animals. To be published, *Biomedical Implications of Radiostrontium Exposure*, Eds. M. Goldman, and L. Bustad, Division of Technical Information, U.S. Atomic Energy Commission, Oak Ridge, Conference ZONF. 710201, 1972.

Moskalev, Y. J., Streltsova, V. N. & Buldakov, L. A. Late Effects of Radionuclide Damage In *Delayed Effects of Bone Seeking Radionuclides*, Eds. Mays, C. W., Jee, W. S. S., Lloyd, R. D., Stover, B. J., Dougherty, J. H. and Taylor, G. N. University of Utah Press, Salt Lake City, pp. 589–599, 1969.

Nilsson, A. Pathologic Effects of Different Doses of ^{90}Sr in Mice. Development of carcinomas in mucous membranes of the head. *Acta Radiol.*, **7**, 27–41, 1968.

Nilsson, A. Pathologic Effects of Different Doses of Radio Strontium in Mice. Dose Effect Relationship in ^{90}Sr Induced Bone Tumours. *Acta Radiol.*, **9**, 155–176, 1970.

Pool, R. R., Williams, R. J. R. & Goldman, M. ^{90}Sr Toxicity in Beagles. To be published in *Biomedical Implications of Radiostrontium exposure*, Ed. M. Goldman, and L. Bustad, Division of Technical Information, U.S. Atomic Energy Commission, Oak Ridge, Conference ZONF.710201, 1972.

Pybus, F. C. & Miller, E. W. Spontaneous Bone Tumours of Mice. *Amer. J. Cancer*, **33**, 98–111, 1938.

Rowland, R. E. Exchangeable Bone Calcium. *Clin. Orthop.*, **49**, 233–248, 1966.

Sissons, H. A.   Tumours of Bone, pp. 1396–1428, in *Systematic Pathology*, Eds. A. Payling Wright and W. St. Clair Symmers. Longmans, London, 1966.

Sissons, H. A.   *Dimensions of Cells Covering Bone Surfaces.* Medical Research Council(London) Subcommittee on Permissible Levels, PIRC/PL/70/4, 1970.

Skoryna, S. C. & Kahn, D. S.   The Late Effects of Radioactive Strontium on Bone. *Cancer*, **12**, 306–322, 1959.

Spiers, F. W.   Dose to bone from strontium 90: Implications for the Setting of the Maximum Permissible Body Burden. *Radiat. Res.*, **28**, 624–642, 1966.

Spiers, F. W. *Radioisotopes in the human body.* Academic Press, New York and London, 1968.

Spiers, F. W., Whitwell, J. R. & Darley, P. J.   Dose in bone marrow cavities from radium 226. To be published, personal communication, 1971.

Spiers, F. W., Zanelli, G. D., Darley, P. J., Whitwell, J. R. & Goldman, L. M.   Beta Particle Dose Rates in Human and Animal Bone. To be published in *Biomedical Implications of Radiostrontium Exposure*, Eds. M. Goldman and L. Bustad, Division of Technical Information, U.S. Atomic Energy Commission, Oak Ridge, Conference ZONF.710201, 1972.

Spiess, H. & Mays, C. W.   Some Cancers Induced by [224]Ra (ThX) in Children and Adults. *Hlth. Phys.*, **19**, 713–729, 1970.

Vaughan, J. M.   *Note on Character of Cells on Trabecular Bone Surfaces in Adult Human Vertebrae.* Medical Research Council (London) Subcommittee on Protection against Ionizing Radiation PIRC/PL/70/1, 1970.

Vaughan, J. M.   Distribution, Excretion and Effects of Plutonium as a Bone Seeker. To be published in *Handbook of Experimental Pharmacology Series*, Vol. on *Uranium and Transuranium Elements*, Eds. H. C. Hodge and J. N. Stannard, Springer-Verlag, Berlin.

Vaughan, J. M., Bleaney, B. & Williamson, M.   The Uptake of Plutonium in Bone Marrow— a Possible Leukaemic Risk. *Brit. J. Haemat.*, **13**, 492–502, 1967.

Vaughan, J. M., & Williamson, M.   [90]Sr in the rabbit: the relative risks of osteosarcoma and squamous cell carcinoma, delayed effects of bone-seeking radionuclides. *In Delayed Effects of Bone-Seeking Radionuclides* Ed. Mays, C. W., Jee, W. S., Lloyd, R. D., Stover, B. J., Dougherty, J. H. and Taylor, G. N. pp. 337–355. University of Utah Press, Salt Lake City, 1969.

Willis, R. A.   *Pathology of Tumours.* 4th ed., pp. 658–659, 682–685. Butterworths, London, 1967.

Discussion

Dr. Owen I was particularly interested in the leukaemia results in the dog and the pig. I think you said that in the dog they were all myeloid leukaemias and in the pig many different types of leukaemia. It is of interest because in the natural state of things lymphosarcoma in the dog or lymphatic leukaemia is extremely common of course, and myeloid leukaemia you can count up on one hand pretty well, In the pig lymphosarcoma of solid glandular type is what is seen but is not very common. I think that there are perhaps two cases of other sorts of leukaemia.

Dame Janet Vaughan I have seen a lot of both the dog and pig material myself. It is extremely well documented. The references will be found in my bibliography. Some of the experiments I have mentioned are not well documented, but both the dog and pig material is. Some of the work is done in Davis, University of California and some of it is done in the Battelle North West Laboratory, Richland, but the people who are doing the work share their information and are in constant contact with one another. The Davis investigators who work with dogs are quite dogmatic about the myeloid character; and having seen the Richland material I am equally certain they are correct in their description of the very mixed pattern that they obtain in the pigs. Some of these pigs have been fed from a very early age. Some of them have been born to mothers who have been fed, and then as soon as they have been weaned they have been fed. There are a variety of ways in which both the dogs and the pigs were treated. The pattern in both experiments is of the same type. I don't think the differences are dependent on the radionuclide dose administered to the dogs and pigs being different but may be associated with the pattern of bone trabeculation in the two species which of course will alter the dosimetry. At present we are just left with this different haematological picture as an interesting fact.

Dr. Finkel I wonder if you are aware of our ^{90}Sr work in dogs with repeated injections?

Dame Janet Yes.

Dr. Finkel We have had lymphosarcomas in those animals. Quite a few lymphosarcomas appeared in animals that were inoculated five days a week for a whole year with small amounts of ^{90}Sr.

Dame Janet But they were not fed continuously. The administration of radionuclide followed a different pattern: they were given intermittent injections which probably gives you a different picture because of a different distribution of radionuclide in the skeleton. I should have mentioned them I agree.

Dr. Price Would you be able to give us any indication about the ages or age distributions of these various groups of animals included in the tables? Don't you think that the age at which the radiation is applied may well have a significant bearing on the type of tumours produced?

Dame Janet I think I could tell you the important ones. The dogs given single injections of all the radionuclides were injected when they are supposed to have all their epiphyses closed. I think it was found when some animals were sacrificed that one epiphysis, the rib, was not closed, but they were what are described as young adults. With the dogs fed continuously, some of them started feeding when they were young adults and carried their pups, and then the pups were weaned and as soon as they were weaned they were put onto ^{90}Sr. In the published paper there will be a reference to all the experiments for anybody who wants to look up the ages. I don't think that the age makes any difference to the type of tumour produced by short range alpha as compared with the long range beta. I don't think this is the factor. I think it is the range of the particle, though the geometry involved in bone trabeculation may account for some of the differences which at the moment are difficult to explain between the dog and the pig, because the dogs continuously fed with ^{90}Sr also developed a lot of osteosarcomas. There were almost as many osteosarcomas as leukaemias as you may have seen from the chart, while the pigs had only seven very insignificant osteosarcomas. *They were all periosteal* which is very unlike most osteosarcomas induced by internal radiation.

Professor Bonfiglio (Chairman) May I ask if there is a difference between the marrow-containing capacity of the bones of pigs as compared with dogs as they mature?

Dr. Moore While to my knowledge there have been no reports of the induction of tumours resembling Ewing's tumour by radionuclides in laboratory animals, it is perhaps worth noting that tumours composed exclusively of the tissue elements of bone marrow may be induced by intramedullary deposition of a chemical carcinogen (N-hydroxy-2-acetyl aminofluorene-cupric-chelate) in rats. In one series (Stanton[1]) some of the tumours induced were classified as reticulum cell sarcoma because of their predominant tissue characteristics, but areas of myeloblastic cells and plasma cells or cells that were entirely undifferentiated could be found in all. The latter were uniform cells with poorly defined cytoplasm and without supporting reticulum and in this respect resembled Ewing's tumour in man. Indeed, it was suggested that whilst a separate classification was not justified since partially differentiated reticular tissues of one type or another could be found in all these tumours, their study might contribute to knowledge of the histogenesis of Ewing's tumours.

Dame Janet That might make a difference. But I don't think there is a great deal of difference in the marrow distribution in the two groups.

Dr. Friedman Is it possible to deplete the marrow by say X-irradiation or chemically prior to using the nuclides to protect the animals perhaps from developing leukaemia?

Dame Janet Nobody has tried this.

Dr. Price May I please ask you to comment on the obviously extraordinary absence of anything which one would label a Ewing's tumour in your protocol.

Dame Janet   I knew somebody would ask me that. Ewing's tumour, by that name, has not been recorded following internal radiation as far as I know.

Professor Bonfiglio   Weren't you hinting at it when you were talking about the "angio" group?

Dame Janet   No, that didn't include it. Nobody has mentioned Ewing's tumour specifically and a lot of these tumours have been looked at by competent pathologists. It isn't that they were not aware of the existence of Ewing's tumour, it just doesn't appear in the literature of radionuclide tumours.

Dr. Jeffree   In relation to giant-cell tumours, giant cells and reticulum cells have a very similar enzyme content. In a giant-cell tumour you have got quite a number of mono-nuclear cells looking rather like reticulum cells with this intense content of hydrolytic enzymes. I was wondering if they come from a similar stem cell. I notice that you have got a reticulum cell sarcoma in a dog and no giant cell tumours.

Dame Janet   I think there was only one reticulum cell sarcoma in the dog.

Dr. Jeffree   I was just wondering whether this might be species difference starting from the same stem cell?

Dame Janet   I wouldn't know.

Professor Sissons   Isn't it possible Dame Janet that species differences which are based on genetic factors as opposed to anatomical differences in bone pattern are awfully important here? I am thinking again also of the absence of giant-cell tumours generally, and Ewing's tumours absolutely amongst radiation induced tumours. This reflects I think the almost complete absence of most of the spontaneous tumours in species other than man.

Dame Janet   I think this is probably very true. I think that it is important always when you are thinking of radiation tumours, to think of species differences. This only too often is not done by the people who are considering radiation hazards. They lump all these animals together and think they all behave in the same way. I mean the great example of this is the difference between the pigs and the dogs. As far as one knows at present there is no great difference in the dosimetry.

Dr. Owen   I was going to substantiate that. Up to 1969 I have made a pretty extensive review of bone tumours in animals and there are three reports in the veterinary literature of Ewing's tumour in dogs, but I personally don't believe any of them.

Professor Bonfiglio   What about giant-cell tumour?

Dr. Owen   You see giant-cell tumour. I think rare cases exist that are true giant-cell tumours.

Professor Bonfiglio.   Is there a time relationship between various types of tumour formation because these are long term animals; these are not tumours that arise promptly or quickly. Do you suppose that differentiation of a cell line by time and the effect of radiation on it determines the type of tumour that is developing?

Dame Janet   I don't know, I haven't looked at it from that point of view.

Dr. Tudway   I wonder if any one has heard of a radiation induced Ewing's tumour in man?

Dr. Finkel   I don't think there were any in the radium series.

Professor Bonfiglio   There were none in the radium series that I know about.

Dame Janet   I have just been through the radiation induced tumours in man or tried to go through them in the literature. I won't say I haven't missed some: I probably have because I don't read enough languages, but I don't remember a radiation induced Ewing.

Professor Bonfiglio   I recall one patient that had three distinctive types induced by radiation. One was an osteosarcoma and another was a chondrosarcoma and the third was a fibrosarcoma each depending on the area. The fibrosarcoma was in the soft tissue. Parts of that fibrosarcoma were very undifferentiated in the sense that you could not identify cell type, and the question is whether the periphery of that tumour was something of that kind, I don't know—but not a true Ewing's. No, I don't recall seeing one. Hatcher[2] reported a whole series and there were none in his either.

Dame Janet   One of the interesting things about radiation induced tumours in man is that in children you practically never see chondrosarcoma. There are many exostoses, for example in the children treated with radium 224. Treatment with ^{224}Ra in the adult results in many osteosarcomas but in children only exostoses predominate. There were a great many exostoses in the children but no chondrosarcomas, and this again seems to me very fascinating.

Dr. Pizey   I notice you are comparing two isotopes, one is an alpha emitter, and the other a beta emitter. One would expect a quantitative difference in their ability to kill cells. I wonder if there is any difference in the ability to induce malignant changes with different MeV?

Dame Janet   Yes, there is indeed—radionuclides with a high MeV are more carcinogenic than those with a low MeV, but half life and site of deposition are also important. ^{224}Ra with a short half life decays to a large extent on the surface before it has time to be distributed throughout the bone mineral while ^{226}Ra has a long half life and becomes distributed throughout the bone mineral. The MeV of the two radium isotopes, both of

o

them alpha emitters is very similar but [224]Ra appears to be more carcinogenic than [226]Ra The greater carcinogenicty of all alpha emitters compared with beta emitters depends on differences in MeV.

REFERENCES

1. Stanton, M. F. Primary Tumours of Bone and Lung in Rats following Local Deposition of Cupric-chelated N-hydroxy 2-acetylaminofluorene. *Cancer Res.*, **27**, 1000, 1967.--
2. Hatcher, C. H. Development of Sarcoma in Bone Subjected to Roentgen or Radium Irradiation. *J. Bone Jt. Surg.*, **27**, 179, 1945.

Tumours in bone and bone marrow induced in CBA/H mice by ^{90}Sr and ^{226}Ra

by

J. F. LOUTIT,† M. R. BLAND,† T. E. F. CARR, JANET M. SANSOM†
and CHRISTINE SMITH†

SUMMARY

To elucidate the nature of tumours induced by bone-seeking radionuclides, 100 male CBA mice (a strain selected for longevity, i.e. not naturally prone to tumours) were injected intraperitoneally with ^{90}Sr and 100 with ^{226}Ra. The single doses (20 : 13·3 : 6·7 μCi— ^{90}Sr and 500 : 150: 50 nCi ^{226}Ra) were based on previous reports (Finkel, Nilsson—^{90}Sr : Finkel ^{226}Ra).

This preliminary communication of a yet incomplete experiment is offered because the predominant tumours attributable to ^{90}Sr are not osteosarcomas but haemangial and lymphoreticular sarcomas, presumably arising in bone marrow. Furthermore only one tumour within bone of the radium treated mice has been recorded after 2 years.

Many of the "lymphomatous" tumours are notable in being histochemically positive for alkaline phosphatase. The tumours classed as haemangioendothelial sarcomas resemble pictorially some of the "fibroblastic osteosarcomas" illustrated by Nilsson in mice and the human cases described by Dorfman et al. (1971) and Unni et al. (1971).

THE LIMITING HAZARD to man from the deposition of radioactive materials in bone is usually considered to be osteosarcoma. This is based on industrial experience with ^{226}Ra and medical experience with ^{226}Ra and ^{224}Ra. Publication 11 of the International Commission on Radiological Protection (1968) noted as additional hazards leukaemia and carcinoma of cranial sinuses when bone marrow and sinus epithelium are within range of the ionizing particles emitted from bone. The tissue at risk for genesis of osteosarcoma was reckoned to be endosteum and its osteoprogenitive cells.

A recent experiment (Barnes, Carr, Evans and Loutit 1970) was designed to exclude undifferentiated stem cells of bone marrow as the cells undergoing malignant transformation and differentiating to osteosarcoma. Radiation chimaeras, whose marrow was distinctively identifiable from host tissue, were given 20 μCi of strontium-90: as a control of the method normal CBA/H mice were given the same dose of strontium-90. The results of the experiment clearly showed that in chimaeras osteosarcomas arose from host tissue—presumably cells already determined to osteogenesis—and not from donated

† External Staff—Medical Research Council.
From M.R.C. Radiobiology Unit, Harwell, Didcot, Berkshire.

bone marrow. However, in the few animals required for the control a greater variety of tumours was observed (Table 1).

TABLE 1

BONE TUMOURS FOLLOWING ADMINISTRATION OF [90]SR TO CBA MICE OF BOTH
SEXES, PREDOMINANTLY MALE

	Chimaeras	Normal
No. of tumours	15	12
No. of animals	23	14
Osteo- or fibro-blastic sarcoma	15	6
Angiosarcoma + leukaemia	0	5 + 1

Although haemangiosarcoma has been reported in several species of animals (Loutit and Vaughan, 1971), the incidence here was much higher than previously experienced. Therefore, a larger array of normal CBA/H male mice was subjected to either strontium-90 or radium-226 by intraperitoneal injection of soluble salt.

This is a preliminary report of the confirmatory experiment based only on findings at necropsy. More detail is given of the histology of the tumours from the first experiment.

RESULTS

In the second experiment a range of doses was used for both nuclides (Table 2) and 50 similar mice were maintained uninjected.

TABLE 2

CBA MALE MICE, $2\frac{1}{2}$-$3\frac{1}{2}$ MONTHS OLD, INJECTED INTRAPERITONEALLY WITH
BONE-SEEKING NUCLIDES

No. of animals	20	40	40
^{90}Sr μCi (nominal)	20	13·3	6·7
^{226}Ra nCi (nominal)	500	150	50

The times of survival so far are given in the histogram (Fig. 1) with a key to the tumours relevant to skeletal irradiation.

Diagnosis of the tumours rested on appearances, radiological of the whole skeleton and morbid anatomical at necropsy, supported by histology of frozen sections and passage of tumours.

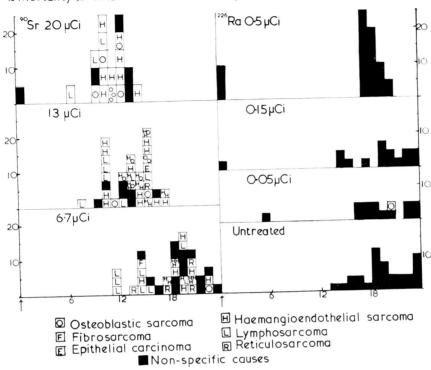

Fig. 1.

SKELETAL TUMOURS

(*a*) *Radiological.* Tumours of the skeleton were basically of two types, osteoblastic and osteolytic.

A florid example of the osteoblastic type is given in Fig. 2. Commonly an increased density in the marrow cavity of shaft or metaphysis of a long bone was the only sign. This might be the early finding in a tumour which subsequently escaped from the confines of the bone, or it might be the late finding in an ageing animal that died with bone tumour rather than from tumour. Most of the osteoblastic tumours were of intermediate size having erupted from the bone. Some of these at first sight were osteolytic, but whereas in growth and expansion the tumour had destroyed bone a deep focus of increased density in the marrow could still be seen.

Basically osteolytic tumours appeared first as an undue translucency, often in a meta-physis of a long bone, and gradually enlarged to give spontaneous fracture and frag-mentation of bone—Fig. 3. In many sites, e.g. vertebrae, the early stages were not visualized radiographically. Most osteolytic tumours were apparently vasoformative, but fibroblastic tumours (one seen in this particular series) give similar appearances and osteoblastic sarcomas with only limited osteoblastic activity can be radiological mimics.

(*b*) *Morbid anatomical. Skeletal disorders.* Just as there are basically two types of radiological appearances, so also there were two anatomical appearances.

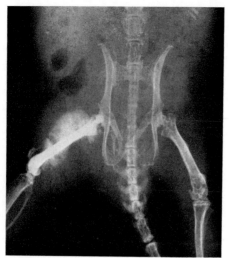

Fig. 2. Radiograph (×1·5) of CBA male mouse with florid osteosarcoma of L. femur "mouse 101" of Barnes *et al.* (1970)—dense opacity of whole femur and "sunburst" calcification outside—histologically chondro-osteoblastoma. Histology also showed osteoblastic sarcoma just erupting from R. ilium, not diagnosed at the time but just visible with hindsight, and probable tumour bud of R. femur (see Fig. 11).

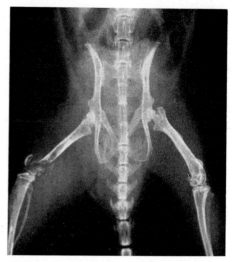

Fig. 3. Radiograph (×1·5) of CBA *T6·T6* male mouse with osteolytic sarcoma of L. femur "mouse 108" of Barnes *et al.* (1970) and pathological fracture in lower metaphyseal region. There is also an intramedullary opacity in R. ilium approximating the sacroiliac joint, which histologically was diagnosed as an early osteoblastic sarcoma (see Fig. 10).

The osteoformative tumours usually presented in long bones either as a pyriform enlargement of metaphysis or roughly fusiform enlargement of shaft. They were a pale biscuit colour like bone (Fig. 4), densely firm and rubbery with a granular cut surface: frequently they were bony hard and either splintered on section or presented a gritty granular surface. Small ones were seen as a localized opacity of the marrow cavity, confirmed on splitting the bone. Some osteoformative tumours occurred in jaws or trunk.

In contrast, osteolytic tumours almost invariably presented as a dark pink or reddish purple mass, the former consisting of soft gelatinous tissue usually with small purple cysts, the latter being almost entirely blood cysts. Most were large (>1 cm diameter) with muscle stretched over them (Fig. 5). Frequently there was evident recent haemorrhage into connective tissue or muscle and yellow staining of former haemorrhage often as gelatinous œdema. These tumours were found frequently in the trunk, especially pelvis, as well as in limb bones.

Lympho-myeloid disorders. In addition to the tumours attributed to the skeletal connective tissue, disorders of the lympho-myeloid complex including tumours were seen. Barnes *et al.* (1970) recorded only one such case, but they have been more frequent in the second series particularly with the reduced doses of strontium-90.

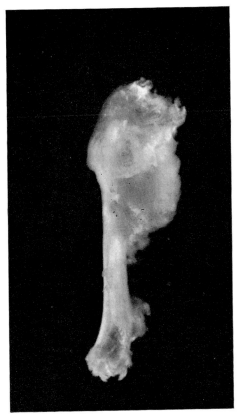

Fig. 4.   Roughly cleaned specimen of osteoblastic sarcoma in long bone.

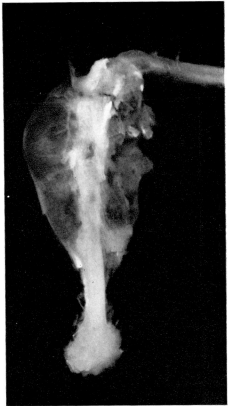

Fig. 5.   Roughly cleaned specimen of osteolytic sarcoma, largely blood-cystic, in upper part of tibia (part removed for histology etc.).

Those arising relatively early, i.e. in the first year, were acute, even fulminating. Mice would lose weight rapidly and had to be killed within a few days of enlarged lymph nodes or spleen becoming visible or palpable. One or two died undiagnosed.

There were no characteristic skeletal radiological signs, though enlarged peripheral lymph nodes often created soft shadows.

At necropsy generalized involvement of the lympho-myeloid complex (enlarged lymph nodes and spleen—often also of liver and kidneys—and pallor of bone marrow) was seen: only rarely was the thymus apparently involved.

Those arising relatively late had either localized involvement (liver and spleen) and a chronic course of some weeks or, if generalized, a less acute progress than those of earlier onset.

Strontium-90 versus Radium-226. So far all tumours of skeletal and lympho-myeloid systems except one have arisen in mice given strontium-90.

400

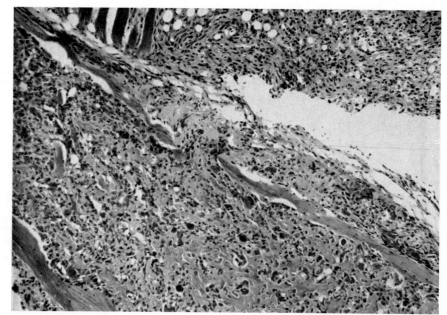

Fig. 6. (H & E × 200) Osteoblastic sarcoma of R. ilium—with intramedullary multiform tumour cells, including giant cells, and trabeculae of atypical bone and osteoid in what normally is a tubular bone. To the left of centre the tumour has eroded cortex and is invading surrounding fibro-muscular tissue—"mouse 110" of Barnes *et al.* (1970).

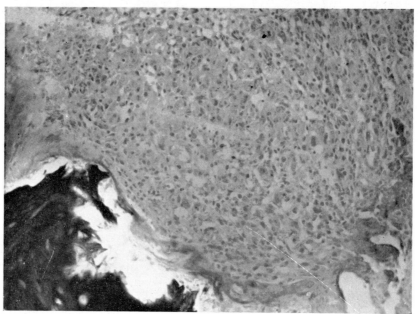

Fig. 7. (H & van G × 180) Angiosarcoma (haemangioendothelial sarcoma) of vertebra prepared to show absence of dark staining collagen fibres except in preformed bone and parosteal fibrous tissue. The spongy tumour tissue with lightly stained nuclei is composed of multiform, but predominantly rather succulent, epitheloid cells and contains many empty capillary vessels "mouse 102" of Barnes *et al.* (1970).

HISTOLOGY OF COMPARABLE MICE IN EARLIER SERIES

Six animals in the right-hand column of Table 1, normal CBA/H or CBA. *T6T6* mice injected with 20 μCi of strontium-90, were recorded as osteoblastic sarcoma according to the criteria of Jaffe (1958). In five of them there was little doubt about diagnosis from routine histology in that typical tumour-bone and osteoid were present as trabeculae within an irregular arrangement of multiform cells, predominantly fusiform but also circular and polygonal, and often with giant forms, only some of which resembled osteoclasts (Fig. 6). One was confined to the bone; the others showed eruption through the cortex, in one instance two separate bones being involved. For the sixth animal the available section showed a small osteoblastic mass within the bone and not all histological criteria of malignancy were satisfied, but a piece of this tumour on passage grew in all four recipients with production of small amounts of atypical bone and osteoid. In all six animals tumour buds (Nilsson 1962) of more than one histological type were also noted in other bones sampled.

In all five animals recorded as angiosarcoma the bloody osteolytic masses found in long bones or vertebrae were comparable histologically. They were composed of loosely knit cells of variable form, from fusiform to polygonal epithelioid. Giant-forms, uni- and multi-nucleate, were common. This non-specific malignant connective tissue was freely supplied with capillary blood vessels (Fig. 7) some of which appeared to be lined by flat endothelium, but not infrequently spaces containing blood were lined by atypical cells of the tumour type (Fig. 8). Whereas in some instances local haemorrhage could have accounted for the appearances, in others the red corpuscles seemed confined to these lacunae. Some of the tumours were freely infiltrated with granular leucocytes and small round lymphoid cells. Pigment phagocytes were common. Material taking van Gieson's stain was rare and could be attributed to stroma or fibrous connective tissue overrun by tumour. Argyrophil fibres were present as a net round clumps of cells but were not dense. This tumorous tissue was seen both within bone and outside it, where it infiltrated muscle and connective tissue. All the tumours took on passage and reproduced bloody tumours in subcutaneous connective tissue. Here the vascular nature seemed histologically to be more prominent with the formation of large blood islands and cysts with large areas of haemorrhage and necrosis (Fig. 9). The five mice bearing the primary vaso-formative tumours also had tumour buds, both osteoblastic (Fig. 10) and non-osteoblastic (Fig. 11) in other bones sampled.

DISCUSSION

The points of special interest in this experiment on CBA male mice are:

1. The paucity of skeletal tumours in mice given radium: lymphomyeloid tumours were not anticipated because of the short range of the α rays of radium. The one tumour so far involving bone (fourth lumbar vertebra) in a radium injected mouse was associated with enlarged aortic lymph nodes which in frozen section were populated by large round cells.

2. Despite the productivity for neoplasia of strontium-90 at all three doses the preponderant tumours were not osteosarcomata but rather angiosarcomata and varieties of lymphoma, both probably originating in bone marrow irradiated by the penetrating β particles of ^{90}Sr and ^{90}Y.

o*

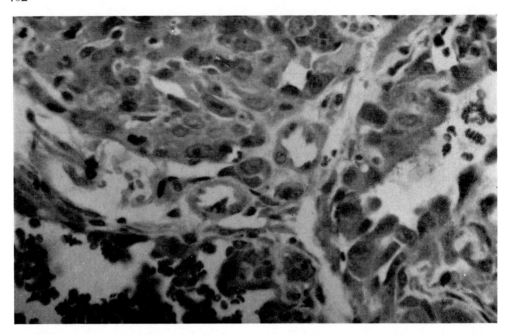

Fig. 8. (H & E ×640) Angiosarcoma (haemangioendothelial sarcoma) of femur (see Fig. 3). Spongy tissue with blood spaces some showing flattened endothelial cells, others lined by succulent tumour cells apparently budding into blood space "mouse 108" of Barnes *et al.* (1970).

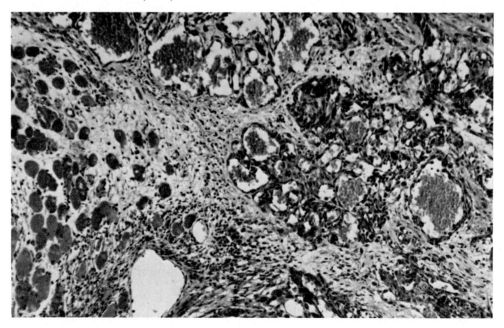

Fig. 9. (H & E ×160) Transplant of angiosarcoma (haemangioendothelial sarcoma) in subcutaneous tissue of syngeneic mouse showing well marked formation of vessels lined and surrounded by tumour tissue, invading muscle and with scattered small round cells and granulocytes both in tumour tissue and stroma "mouse 104" of Barnes *et al.*, (1970) third passage.

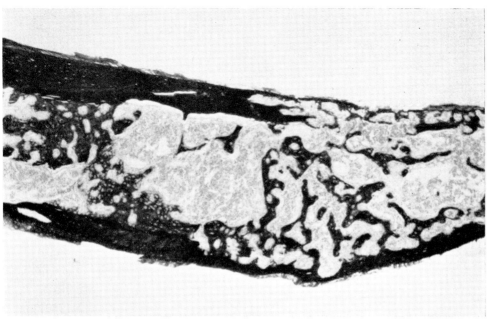

Fig. 10. (H & van G ×70) Early osteoblastic tumour of R. ilium, bone shown black. This may well be interpreted as benign osteoma especially in lower part of figure with dense trabeculae stemming from endosteum. In the upper part the mass spreads across the marrow cavity with finer trabeculae and erodes into cortex; this favours diagnosis of sarcomatous transformation even though at higher power the cells are moderately uniform. No test by transplant was undertaken, "mouse 108" of Barnes *et al.* (1970), see Fig. 3.

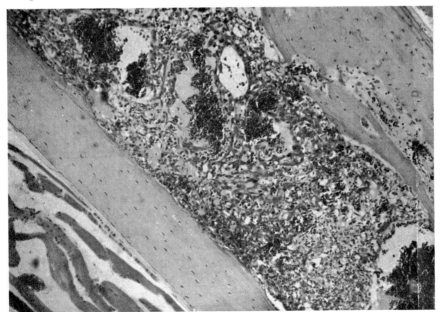

Fig. 11. (H & E ×120) Focal lesion, in aplastic bone marrow of femur shaft, with a net of young stromal cells with some diversification surrounding some of the abnormal vessels. It is postulated that this is a "tumour bud" of the haemangioendothelial sarcomatous type, "mouse 101" of Barnes *et al.* (1970), not identifiable in Fig. 2.

RADIUM

Considerable lip-service is paid in discussions of the toxicity of bone-seeking radio-active materials to the role of ^{226}Ra as a reference-standard. This stems from the knowledge that ^{226}Ra has been toxic in man, and osteosarcoma is the term usually used to describe the tumours of bone which were seen in radium-contaminated subjects. However, although osteosarcomas have been reported, dyscrasias of fibrous tissue in bone may be the more important. Of the earlier and more highly dosed cases Martland (1931) states "differentiation . . . is unusual in the sarcomas occurring among dial painters, most of the tumours being of embryonal or anaplastic types"; and his description of bone marrow suggests "myelosclerosis" (Loutit 1970). In a more recent review Finkel, Miller and Hasterlik (1969) diagnostically label eight patients with osteosarcomas, 12 with 13 fibrosarcomas, three with other sarcomas, together with 16 cranial tumours and seven haematological disorders.

Radium-226 has been used experimentally as a reference standard in dogs (Mays *et al.* 1969) and mice (Finkel and Biskis 1968). From both one forms the impression that osteosarcomas are the malignant sequels: "most of the osteosarcomas consisted of well-differentiated bone-forming osteoblastic tissue" (Finkel and Biskis). However, the CF1 mice (female) used by Finkel and Biskis had a significant incidence of natural osteosarcoma and, it is rumoured, a high incidence of osteosclerotic bone-disease. According to Finkel and Biskis the CF1 mouse is also highly prone to lymphomatous disease and harbours a C-type virus called by them "FBJ" virus.

The CBA/H mouse has not been seen to suffer naturally from bone disease or osteosarcoma; it is prone only to benign hepatoma (which may kill by vascular accident), not to generalized lymphoma, though a small percentage die aged with localized lymphomas usually abdominal and of reticulosarcomatous type. In the experiment now reported it has resisted doses of ^{226}Ra which in CF1 female mice would be expected to produce in the time available 0·5 to two tumours per mouse (Finkel and Biskis, 1968). This might be attributed to absence of FBJ virus (but strontium-90 produced tumours in abundance), or to resistance of male mice (but strontium-90 acts on males; females are under test with ^{226}Ra), or to the fact that in mice like CBA the osteoprogenitive tissue, like much of the marrow, is not within range of the α particle, i.e. not endosteal (but osteoblastic tumour buds in the mice injected with strontium-90 appear to stem from endosteal regions).

We would propound the following hypothesis. The site of election for tumours in the radium-injected mice of Finkel and Biskis was the spine in contrast to the limbs for their strontium-90-injected mice. In CBA/H mice the strontium-90 induced osteoblastic sarcomas also occurred most commonly in limbs and ilia which are tubular bones. Unlike dog and man, the vertebral bones of the CBA/H mouse are also largely of tubular structure with a minimum of cancellation. Although strontium and radium may initially deposit in the limited endosteal surfaces at growing ends of tubular bones of CBA mice, the material is soon translocated to periosteum where circumferential growth occurs. Radium-226, but to a much less extent strontium-90, is thus put out of range of endosteum for most of its life in CBA mice. The same mass of radium-224 (Gössner, Hindringer, Hug, Luz and Müller 1971), however, because of its much shorter half-life could give a much larger dose to endosteal tissue in the limited time available. If the CF1 mouse has a high rate of turnover of vertebral bone, perhaps associated with later osteodystrophy, radium may be translocated less to periosteal sites but rather within endosteum.

STRONTIUM

At the three doses examined the total incidence of tumours was high. The median time to death or killing decreased with increasing dose from the 20th to the 12th month.

The final score of tumours must wait till the experiment is complete and the histological material examined. However, at this preliminary stage it is evident from radiological and morbid anatomical scores that vaso-formative osteolytic bone tumours and lymphomas are likely to be more common than osteosarcomas (see Table 3) particularly at doses 13·3 and 6·7 μCi.

TABLE 3

PROVISIONAL SCORES OF SPECIFIC TUMOURS INDUCED IN MICE UP TO THE AGE OF $2\frac{1}{4}$ YEARS (2 YEARS AFTER INJECTION) BY STRONTIUM-90

(figures in brackets—no. of tumour-bearing mice)

Dose	Died or killed with tumour			Died without specific tumour	Total	
	Osteo-sarcoma	Angio-sarcoma	Lympho-reticular system		Mice	Tumours
20 μCi	7(5)*	8(8)*	3	5	20	18
13·3 μCi	9(8†)	25(20†)	8†	8	38	42
6·7 μCi	2(2§)	15(10†)	12‡	15	38	29
0	0	0	0	28	28	0
Totals	18	48	23			89

* One animal had both osteosarcoma and angiosarcoma when killed.
† Five animals had both osteosarcoma and angiosarcoma when killed.
† One animal had both lymphoma and angiosarcoma when killed.
‡ One animal had both lymphoma and angiosarcoma when killed.
§ One fibrosarcoma of jaw.

The question that presents itself is: are the haemangiosarcomas reported here a peculiarity of the CBA/H mouse. They were not originally reported by Nilsson (1962) in an extensive study of CBA male mice. Many of numerous illustrations given by Nilsson seem compatible with the diagnosis and more recently he (1970) has recorded angiosarcoma in a small percentage of his mice treated with strontium-90. Finkel, Biskis and Scribner (1959) reported up to 13% of them amongst the tumours occurring in their CF1 mice given strontium-90. They have been noted in dogs (Mays *et al.* (*loc. cit*), Goldman, Pool and Williams 1970, and Boecker, Chiffelle, Hobbs, Jones, McClellan,

Pickrell and Redman (1969) given strontium-90 by various routes. There is a rare human equivalent occurring spontaneously (Jaffe, 1958; Dorfman, Steiner and Jaffe, 1971, Unni, Ivins, Beabout and Dahlin, 1971). Jaffe also notes another rare but seemingly benign condition—aneurysmal bone cyst, the histology and general description of which appears to be very similar to some of the murine cases observed in the present series. It seems, therefore, that such angiosarcomas are not confined to CBA mice. It is notable, however, that they have been reported as radiation-induced only after strontium-90, possibly attributable to the hard β rays rather than the particular element. The cells of these tumours were negative for alkaline phosphatase.

Tumours of the lymphoreticular tissue, as noted above not a feature of normal CBA mice, were also induced even at the 6·7 μCi dose by strontium-90. Again this can be attributed to the hard β-rays irradiating the bone marrow. Most of these tumors were generalized and only one or two involved the thymus macroscopically. A few in the middle-aged and senescent mice were localized to the abdomen—the so-called reticulosarcomatous type. Notably, most of the generalized tumours were shown on passage to consist of mononuclear blast cells staining positively for alkaline phosphatase. Those localized to the abdomen—reticulosarcoma—were negative for alkaline phosphatase.

The osteoblastic osteosarcomas of this series ranked only third in order of frequency behind angiosarcoma and lymphoreticular tumours. They were typical in being osteoblastic according to radiological appearance and formed atypical bone and osteoid to a variable degree. Unlike the human equivalent they metastasised rarely, but were strongly invasive locally. Typically, abnormal bone formation was most marked in the marrow cavity and more scanty outside the bone after breakthrough. The growing edges were of flattened cells like fibroblasts and all parts were strongly positive for alkaline phosphatase.

Unlike Nilsson (1969) we have observed cranial carcinoma only rarely—once from strontium-90.

REFERENCES

Barnes, D. W. H., Carr, T. E. F., Evans, E. P. & Loutit, J. F. ^{90}Sr-induced Osteosarcomas in Radiation Chimaeras. *Int. J. of Radiat. Biol.*, **18**, 531–537, 1970.

Boecker, B. B., Chiffelle, T. L., Hobbs, C. H., Jones, R. K., McClellan, R. O., Pickrell, J. A. & Redman, H. C.   Toxicity of Inhaled ^{90}SrCl$_2$ in Beagle Dogs, **III**, pp. 1–7, in *Lovelace Foundation Fission Product Inhalation Program. Annual Report.* LF 41 UC 48, 1969.

Dorfman, H. D., Steiner, G. C. & Jaffe, H. L.   Vascular Tumors of Bone. *Human Pathology*, **2**, 349–376, 1971.

Finkel, A. J. Miller, C. E. & Hasterlik, R. J.   Radium-induced Malignant Tumors in Man, pp. 195–225, in *Delayed Effects of Bone-seeking Radionuclides*, University of Utah Press, Salt Lake City, 1969.

Finkel, Miriam P. & Biskis, Birute, O.   Experimental Induction of Osteosarcoma. *Progr. expl. Tum. Res.*, **10**, 72–111, 1968.

Finkel, Miriam, P., Biskis, Birute, O. & Scribner, Gertrude, M.   The Influence of Strontium-90 upon Life Span and Neoplasms of Mice, pp. 199–209, in *Progress in Nuclear Energy Series VI, Biological Sciences*, **vol. 2**, Eds. J. G. Bugher, J. Coursaget and J. F. Loutit. Pergamon Press, London, 1959.

Goldman, M., Pool, R. R. & Williams R. Jean.   Tumors Involving Bone in Beagles Fed Toxic Levels of Sr-90, pp. 57–63, in *Radiobiology Laboratory, School of Veterinary Medicine, University of California, Davis*, UCD 472–117, Annual Report, 1970.

Gössner, W., Gindringer, B., Hug, O., Luz, A. & Müller, W. A.   Early and Late Effects of Incorporated ^{224}Ra in Mice. Vth International Congress of the French Society for Radio-protection, Grenoble, 1971.

International Commission on Radiological Protection ICRP Publication **11**.   *A Review of the Radiosensitivity of the Tissues in Bone*. Pergamon Press, Oxford, 1968.

Jaffe, H. L.   *Tumors and Tumorous Conditions of the Bones and Joints*. Kimpton, London, 1958.

Loutit, J. F.   Malignancy from Radium. *Brit. J. Cancer*, **24**, 195–207, 1970.

Loutit, J. F. & Vaughan, Janet M.   The Radiosensitive Tissues in Bone. *Brit. J. Radiol.*, **44**, 815, 1971.

Martland, H. S.   The Occurrence of Malignancy in Radioactive Persons. *Amer. J. Cancer*, **15**, 2435–2516, 1931.

Mays, C. W., Dougherty, T. F., Taylor, G. N., Lloyd, R. D., Stover, Betsy J., Jee, W. S. S., Christensen, W. R. & Dougherty, Jean A. Radiation-induced Bone Cancer in Beagles, pp. 387–408, in *Delayed Effects of Bone-seeking Radionuclides*. University of Utah Press, Salt Lake City, 1969.

Nilsson, A.   Histogenesis of Sr^{90}-induced Osteosarcomas. *Acta vet. scand.*, **3**, 185–200, 1962.

Nilsson, A.   Dose-dependent Carcinogenic Effect of Radiostrontium, pp. 173–182, in *Radiation Induced Cancer*. International Atomic Energy Agency, Vienna, 1969.

Nilsson, A.   Pathologic Effects of Different Doses of Radiostrontium in Mice. *Acta radiol. (Stockh.)*, **9**, 155–176, 1970.

Unni, K. K., Ivins, J. C., Beabout, J. W. & Dahlin, D. C.   Hemangioma, Hemangiopericy-toma, and Hemangioendothelioma (Angiosarcoma) of Bone. *Cancer*, **27**, 1403–1414, 1971.

Discussion

Dr. Suit I would like to know whether you have any control data indicating the dose level equivalent of X-radiation producing the same frequency of these various types of neoplasms?

Dr. Loutit No. I haven't done the mathematics on these cases to be able to say that with these various doses by the time of death they had accumulated so many rads, be it of alpha in the case of radium, or beta in the case of strontium-90. But in terms of rems at any rate, it will be of the order of the thousand to ten thousand range. You cannot get a mouse to survive this dose of X-rays unless you do prolonged fractionation which I haven't done.

Immunology: chondrosarcoma

Chairman: Professor R. BARNES

Tumour-associated antigens of experimentally-induced osteosarcomata

by

MICHAEL MOORE

SUMMARY

Studies on tumour antigenicity in four contrasting models of bone oncogenesis in rodentia were undertaken by the attempted induction of tumour specific immunity in hosts syngeneic with the strain of origin of the osteosarcomas. Immunogenic sarcomas were induced by each oncogenic agent but differed significantly in relative antigenic strength and specificity. Osteosarcomas induced by internal irradiation with bone seeking radionuclides (^{90}Sr/^{226}Ra/^{32}P) in mice and rats displayed weak immunogenicity or evoked no detectable immune response, a feature of spontaneous neoplasia in rodentia and sarcomas induced by other physical agents. Mesenchymal sarcomas induced by FBJ virus, an oncogenic RNA virus isolated from a spontaneously arising murine sarcoma were more consistently immunogenic than radiation-induced osteosarcomata and possessed a virus-specified cross-reacting antigen. In marked contrast osteosarcomas arising in rats following intrafemoral deposition of a chemical carcinogen (cupric chelated N-hydroxy-2-acetylaminofluorene) were highly immunogenic and, in common with soft tissue sarcomas induced by classical chemical carcinogens, were characterized by a high degree of antigenic individuality. Mononuclear cell infiltration of primary osteosarcomas and their early generation transplants provided suggestive histological evidence of cell-mediated host resistance reflecting the high immunogenic capacity of these tumours. However, radiation- and virus-induced sarcomata may be more relevant models for the study of the immunological parameters of host–tumour relationships than the chemically-induced osteosarcomas whose high antigenicity may be a secondary feature of their malignancy.

INTRODUCTION

RECENT ADVANCES IN EXPERIMENTAL TUMOUR IMMUNOLOGY

FOLLOWING THE demonstration almost 20 years ago that chemically induced sarcomas in rodentia were capable of inducing resistance to their own transplantation in genetically compatible (syngeneic) hosts (Foley 1953, Baldwin 1955, Prehn and Main 1957, Klein, Sjogren, Klein and Hellström 1960) new and extensive information has emerged from many laboratories. Neoplasms induced by both DNA and RNA viruses were subsequently shown to be susceptible to rejection reactions induced in the syngeneic host by homologous virus or inoculation of tumour cells. Isograft or autograft reactions of varying intensity have now been demonstrated against a large number of chemically and virally induced tumours of widely different histological types in different species (Sjogren 1965,

Klein 1968, Baldwin 1970) and even against spontaneous tumours in inbred animals not exposed to any known oncogenic influence (Hammond, Fisher and Rolley 1967, Baldwin 1966, Baldwin and Embleton 1969). It is well established that the tumour rejection phenomenon is induced by tumour specific transplantation antigens (TSTA)* which, like normal histocompatibility antigens, are localized on the cell surface where they evoke immunological recognition and initiate the mechanism of rejection (Klein 1970).

It is probably true to say that at least weak immune responses have been shown to exist in most tumour–host systems which have been adequately investigated. This general correspondence has given rise to the concept that antigenicity is a necessary and intrinsic part of the neoplastic cellular alteration (Prehn 1967). Although more recent experimentation has shown that other factors such as antigen masking or modulation may modify antigen expression on tumour cells (Currie and Bagshawe 1969, Boyse, Old, Stockert and Shigeno 1968) the only notable exception to this general finding is the situation where immunological tolerance against TSTA prevails. So far this latter phenomenon is restricted to tumours induced by vertically transmitted noncytopathogenic RNA viruses of which the mouse mammary tumour agent (MTV) is the well studied example (Blair 1971).

A second important concept to emerge from these experimental studies was that of immunosurveillance—that is, the process whereby newly developed antigenic malignant cells are the subject of continuous elimination by immune recognition (Prehn 1968, Keast 1970). Theoretically the existence of an immune system which recognizes foreign antigens and effects their removal provides the biological basis of the homograft reaction and contributes to tissue homeostasis. An important limitation of tumour specific immune reactions is their inability to deal with more than a relatively small number of cells. Though the maximum level of resistance induced in terms of cell numbers rejected varies considerably from system to system and often between tumours of the same system, it is in general promptly overwhelmed by excessive cell numbers. For this reason, attempts to control the growth of established tumours solely by immunotherapeutic procedures have been largely unsuccessful. However, from the biological standpoint it is reasonable that a surveillance mechanism operating in the immunocompetent host should protect against small numbers of neoplastic cells localized as incipient clones or disseminated throughout the organism, rather than against large tumours. The emergence of frank neoplasia would then signify the breakdown of the system—for example, by immuno-suppression or alternatively, by senescence (Stjernsward 1966, Celada 1968).

Evidence for the existence of a surveillance mechanism derives from the demonstration that impairment of immune function by neonatal thymectomy or treatment with anti-lymphocyte serum (ALS) increases the incidence of experimentally induced tumours. The effects are particularly marked for tumours induced by the oncogenic DNA viruses such as polyoma or SV40 (Law 1966, Allison and Taylor 1967, Allison and Law 1968). With chemically induced tumours the results are less consistent particularly where ALS is used as the immunosuppressant (Balner and Dersjant 1969, Cerilli and Treat 1969, Wagner and Haughton 1971), although there appears to be little doubt about the effectiveness of thymectomy at least in some systems (Grant and Miller 1965, Johnson 1968). By contrast, oncogenesis by murine leukaemia virus (MLV) and mammary tumour

---

* Alternatively called "tumour rejection antigens".

virus (MTV) is not increased by thymectomy (Law 1966, Blair 1971). These viruses induce tolerance after neonatal exposure, hence thymectomy has no detectable potentiating effect.

Cell mediated anti-tumour immunity against tumour rejection antigens, rather than humoral antibody, is probably the most important mediator of immunological surveillance mechanisms operative against solid tumours. Studies on cell mediated immunity to animal tumours may therefore be potentially indicative of the prospects for immunotherapy of cancer in man. To obtain an overall view of the problem and to evaluate the nature of the tumour–host immune response in relation to osteosarcoma, studies are being currently undertaken on tumour antigenicity in four contrasting models of bone oncogenesis in rodentia, each of which bears some correspondence to the aetiological, morphological or behavioural features of osteosarcoma in man.

Procedures consistently effective for the demonstration of cell mediated immunity to a wide variety of tumour types were employed in these studies—viz. repeated implantation of X-irradiated tumour biopsies and in some tests, excision of subcutaneously developing tumour grafts.

MATERIALS AND METHODS

ANIMALS

Radiation- and virus-induced mouse sarcomas were serially passaged by subcutaneous implantation in young adult male syngeneic CBA or CBA*T6T6* mice; and radiation- and chemically-induced rat osteosarcomas by subcutaneous implantation in young adult female syngeneic AS rats.

The genetic uniformity of each animal strain was regularly checked by skin grafting.

RADIATION-INDUCED MURINE OSTEOSARCOMAS

Bone tumours were induced by a single intraperitoneal injection of ^{90}Sr (20 μCi) or ^{226}Ra (50 nCi) in normal CBA mice and syngeneic or allogeneic radiation chimaeras. Approximate latency periods ranged from 229 to 746 days. All tumours arising in chimaeric mice were confirmed to be of host (CBA) origin by cytological and/or genetic analysis (Barnes *et al.* 1970). With one exception (fibrosarcoma, S27) all primary bone tumours subjected to transplantation immunity tests were classified histologically as osteoblastic osteosarcomas, were strongly alkaline phosphatase positive and as such were distinguished from haemangioendotheliomas which also appeared in mice administered with ^{90}Sr but were not included in this study. Serial transplantation of the osteosarcomas in syngeneic recipients resulted in a gradual loss of bone forming capacity accompanied by transformation to a spindle cell morphology. Although the osteosarcomas were consistently invasive, metastases to the lungs or liver were observed only in a few primary tumour bearers, and occurred even less frequently in mice bearing tumour transplants.

FBJ VIRUS-INDUCED MURINE SARCOMAS

Finkel, Biskis and Jinkins (1966) have described the origin and some of the biological properties of an oncornavirus* (FBJ virus) derived from a 260-day old male mouse of

* Oncornavirus: a designation recently proposed for RNA oncogenic viruses.

the CF1/An1 strain, in which the spontaneous incidence of malignant bone tumours is usually between 1 and 2%. In the present study, sarcomas were induced in CBA mice by inoculation of FBJ virus (Moloney concentrate) i.m. into the right hind limb within a few hours of birth. The latent period varied from 27 to 48 days. Tumours which arose at the site of injection were characterized by slow growth, low-grade malignancy and failure to metastasize. Histologically, the majority were primitive fibroblastic sarcomas which may undergo matrix evolution to form a little metaplastic cartilage, osteoid or bone, usually in areas of hyaline collagen. Their only resemblance to human osteosarcoma is in the parosteal or juxtacortical osteosarcoma which is characterized by a less ominous microscopic structure than those tumours of typical osseous origin (Price, Moore and Jones 1972). Despite this tenuous morphological resemblance the importance of this agent in experimental tumour immunology is emphasized by the fact that FBJ virus is the first murine sarcoma virus to be isolated from a spontaneously occurring sarcoma.

RADIATION-INDUCED RAT OSTEOSARCOMAS

Osteosarcomas were induced in female AS rats by intraperitoneal injection of ^{32}P (total dose 4 μCi/g body weight) in six fractionated dosages according to the procedure of Blackett (1959). The latency periods ranged from 193 to 361 days. With one exception (intramedullary fibrosarcoma, P8) the histology of these tumours was mostly that of well-differentiated malignant osteoblasts rich in alkaline phosphatase which form bone randomly, and the occasional small area of calcified cartilage lattice (Cobb 1970). In common with the clinical disease, metastatic spread of primary tumours, which occurred in 50% of rats treated with ^{32}P, is most commonly to the lungs and infrequently to the lymph nodes. On repeated transplantation in syngeneic recipients the osteosarcomas developed the cellular pleomorphism commonly seen in bone tumours of man, and in general, synthesis of tumour osteoid and alkaline phosphatase activity was observed for more than 12 transfer generations. Only one tumour (P8) in the series consistently metastasized on subcutaneous implantation. Multiple tumour deposits were found in the lungs of 100% of transplanted animals.

CHEMICALLY INDUCED RAT OSTEOSARCOMAS

Injection of the chemical carcinogen cupric-chelated N-hydroxy-2-acetylamino-fluorene into the intramedullary cavity of the rat femur induced primary tumours of bone as well as epidermoid pulmonary neoplasms resulting from embolism of the compound to the lungs (Stanton, 1967). In common with the tumours induced by radio-phosphorus those induced by the chemical carcinogen were consistently invasive and capable of metastasizing. By contrast however, the chemically induced tumours contain many different tissue components and diversities of cell type. In these respects, bone tumours induced by this agent appear to represent the opposite extreme in neoplastic development from that of the virally induced tumours. Apparent deviations in differentiation observed in these tumours are common phenomena in the bone tumours of man.

Tumours studied by transplantation procedures were morphologically osteosarcomas with varying degrees of new bone formation and arose in association with the injected femora in female AS rats. Approximate latency periods varied from 273 to 321 days.

On transplantation in syngeneic recipients tumour outgrowth was initially slow and early generation implants sometimes regressed. Moreover, chemically induced osteosarcomas lost their bone-producing capacity and alkaline phosphatase activity more rapidly than the radiation induced rat osteosarcomas, becoming morphologically pleomorphic non-osteogenic sarcomas.

INDUCTION OF IMMUNITY TO OSTEOSARCOMAS

Two procedures were used for studying the immunogenicities of osteosarcomas passaged in syngeneic mice and rats:

(*1*) *Implantation of irradiated tumour*. Tumour grafts were attenuated by exposure to X-irradiation (15,000 rad) prior to subcutaneous implantation under the dorsal skin (Moore and Williams 1972). The immunization protocol usually comprised a minimum of three implantations of irradiated tissue at intervals of 10 to 21 days.

Controls were similarly treated with irradiated normal tissues (kidney, liver, muscle and spleen). The specificity of induced resistance to individual tumours was confirmed by pretreatment of hosts prior to challenge with irradiated biopsies of other tumours known from comparable transplantation tests to possess TSTA.

(*2*) *Excision of subcutaneous tumour*. In a few examples subcutaneous developing tumour grafts in mice were surgically excised complete with overlying skin when they had attained an average diameter of 8 to 10 mm.

TUMOUR CHALLENGE

Challenge inocula of defined numbers of tumour cells were given 7–14 days after the last irradiated graft or following tumour excision. Tumours were dissociated into single cell suspensions by treatment with 0.25% trypsin (Difco 1 : 250) in Hanks' balanced salt solution. After washing by centrifugation and resuspension in medium 199 the cells were assessed for viability by trypan blue exclusion; low viability preparations were discarded. In each test a group of untreated control animals was included and, in some cases, all animals received total body X-irradiation (400 rad) delivered at a rate of 33·5 rads/min. twenty-four hours prior to inoculation. This treatment suppresses any primary immune response to the tumour inoculum in the course of early latency without markedly affecting the secondary response in previously immunized mice, thereby allowing weak levels of tumour immunity to be detected. In preliminary tests it was necessary to establish the number of cells of each tumour required to sustain progressive growth in at least 50% of untreated or pre-irradiated (400 rad) controls. These threshold cell numbers varied appreciably from tumour to tumour. The first tumour challenge was then usually given at a dose comparable to the threshold inocula; thereafter all animals were examined twice weekly and tumour sizes were taken as the mean of two diameters.

RESULTS

TUMOUR-SPECIFIC ANTIGENICITY OF RADIATION-INDUCED MURINE OSTEOSARCOMAS

Sixteen sarcomas were examined for their capacity to induce resistance to their own transplantation in syngeneic CBA mice by prior treatment with irradiated tumour cells. Of these, six osteosarcomas (40%) were immunogenic in that the number of tumour takes in immunized hosts was reduced compared with normal untreated controls (Table 1). The maximum cell inoculum rejected by immunized hosts was of the order of 10^4 cells indicating that the level of immunity was relatively weak. The remaining nine sarcomas (60%) elicited no level of immunity that was detectable by this immunization-transplantation procedure. The finding that, of the examples studied, total surgical excision of subcutaneous tumour grafts was, with one exception (S20), generally less

TABLE 1

IMMUNE RESPONSE TO RADIATION-INDUCED MURINE OSTEOSARCOMAS

Immunizing tissue	Immunization procedure	Tumour*	Cell dose	Tumour takes in	
				Treated mice	Untreated controls
S1	4 × IR	S1	5 × 10⁴	9/9	8/8
S5	7 × IR	S5	1 × 10⁴	9/9	8/8
S5A	7 × IR	S5A	5 × 10⁴	7/7	6/6
S15	8 × IR	S15	5 × 10³	0/6	3/5
Normal	8 × IR	S15	5 × 10³	6/6	6/6
S16	3 × IR	S16	2 × 10³	6/6	4/6
S17	8 × IR	S17	2 × 10³	4/7 ⎫	4/5
Normal	8 × IR	S17	2 × 10³	5/5 ⎬	
S115	4 × IR	S17	2 × 10³	5/5	5/5
S18	8 × IR	S18	2 × 10³	6/6	4/5
S20	3 × IR	S20	1 × 10⁴	4/8	4/5
MC2	4 × IR	S20	1 × 10⁴	9/9	6/6
S20	Excision	S20	1 × 10⁴	4/8	5/6
S27	4 × IR	S27	1 × 10⁴	6/6	5/6
S38	3 × IR	S38	1 × 10⁴	0/8 ⎫	4/6
Normal	3 × IR	S38	1 × 10⁴	6/6 ⎬	
S39	4 × IR	S39	1 × 10⁴	7/8	6/6
S100	5 × IR	S100	2 × 10³	0/8	2/6
S101	4 × IR	S101	2 × 10⁴	9/9	6/6
S110	3 × IR	S110	2 × 10³	4/5	4/5
S111	4 × IR	S111	5 × 10³	7/7	6/6
S115	3 × IR	S115	1 × 10³	4/8 ⎫	6/6
MC1	4 × IR	S115	1 × 10³	10/10 ⎬	
FBJ7	4 × IR	S115	1 × 10³	9/9	7/8

* Mice received 400 rad whole-body X-irradiation 24 hours prior to challenge.
S = Transplanted radiation-induced osteosarcoma.
MC = Transplanted chemically induced sarcoma of soft tissue origin.
IR = Immunization by implantation of X-irradiated (15,000 rad) tissue grafts.
FBJ = Transplanted fibrosarcoma induced by FBJ virus.
6 weakly immunogenic tumours, Nos. S15, S17, S20, S38, S100, S115.

effective for the induction of resistance than grafting with irradiated tumour (Moore and Williams 1972) makes radiosensitivity of the TSTA an unlikely explanation for failure to induce immunity to a larger number of osteosarcomas.

The pattern of tumour outgrowth in immune hosts compared with controls which was typical of several of the osteosarcomas in this series, is exemplified by transplantation tests with S115. Mice grafted with irradiated tumour were subdivided into groups and simultaneously challenged with tumour-cell inocula ranging from 500 to 5,000 cells. The rate of outgrowth of each inoculum was significantly retarded in all groups, but complete resistance was demonstrable only against the lower challenge inocula, and limited to 50% of immunized mice (Fig. 1).

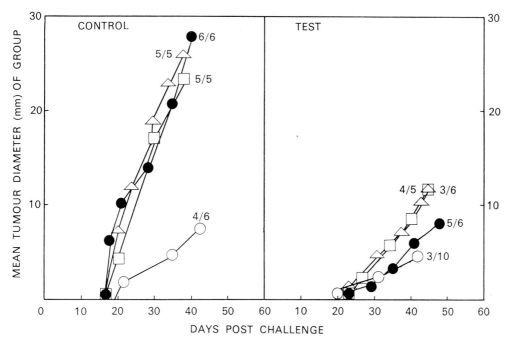

Fig. 1. Outgrowth of radiation-induced osteosarcoma S115 in syngeneic CBA mice pretreated with normal tissue (control) and in mice pretreated with irradiated (15,000 rad) grafts of S115 (test). ●——● s.c. challenge inoculum of 5×10^3 cells. △——△ s.c. challenge inoculum of 2×10^3 cells. □——□ s.c. challenge inoculum of 1×10^3 cells. ○——○ s.c challenge inoculum of 5×10^2 cells.

The weak antigenicity of these tumours could not be attributed to a non-specific increase in immune responsiveness since mice pretreated with irradiated normal tissues or tumours of chemical or viral origin known to possess TSTA did not reject low-cell challenge inocula of five of the immunogenic radiation sarcomas (Table 1). Moreover, in one test pretreatment of mice with one immunogenic radiation sarcoma (S115) failed to protect against challenge with another (S17), suggesting that such weak antigens as these tumours possess do not cross-react. More extensive tests however are necessary to establish this point firmly.

TUMOUR-SPECIFIC ANTIGENICITY OF FBJ VIRUS-INDUCED MURINE SARCOMAS

Eight sarcomas were examined for their ability to evoke immunity in syngeneic CBA mice by pretreatment with irradiated tumour cells, or total surgical excision of developing subcutaneous tumour grafts. Of these, at least six tumours (75%) were immunogenic, the number of tumour takes being reduced in mice pretreated with irradiated FBJ tumours compared with untreated controls (Table 2). The induction of resistance in preimmunized mice which had received whole-body irradiation (400 rad) prior to tumour challenge indicated that pretreatment had exerted a specific immunizing effect and not merely non-specific potentiation of host resistance. This was confirmed in tests where preimmunization with normal tissue, an antigenically unrelated osteosarcoma

TABLE 2

IMMUNE RESPONSE TO FBJ VIRUS-INDUCED MURINE SARCOMAS

Immunizing tissue	Immunization procedure	Tumour	Cell dose	Tumour takes in	
				Treated mice	Untreated controls
FBJ1	4 × IR	FBJ1*	1×10^4	1/6	4/10
FBJ1	4 × IR	FBJ1*	5×10^4	7/8	5/5
FBJ2	Excision	FBJ2*	1×10^3	2/7	7/10
FBJ3	4 × IR	FBJ3	1×10^4	2/10	8/8
Normal	4 × IR	FBJ3	1×10^4	6/9	6/10
FBJ3	3 × IR	FBJ3	5×10^3	2/10	7/9
FBJ4	3 × IR	FBJ4	Graft	8/8	9/9
FBJ5	Excision	FBJ5	Graft	5/9	5/5
FBJ6	Excision	FBJ6	1×10^4	4/8	8/8
FBJ6	4 × IR	FBJ6*	1×10^5	5/10	8/10
FBJ7	4 × IR	FBJ7*	1×10^4	1/4	7/7
FBJ7	3 × IR	FBJ7	5×10^3	2/10	5/9
FBJ7	4 × IR	FBJ7*	1×10^3	0/4	9/10
FBJ9	4 × IR	FBJ9	1×10^4	7/7	5/6
MC3	4 × IR	FBJ2	1×10^4	11/11	7/7
Normal	4 × IR	FBJ7*	5×10^3	5/5	5/5
FBJ7	4 × IR	S115*	1×10^3	9/9	7/8
S115	5 × IR	FBJ6*	5×10^3	9/9	7/8
FBJ2	4 × IR	FBJ4*	1×10^4	4/9	9/10
FBJ3	4 × IR	FBJ7*	5×10^3	2/5	5/5
FBJ7	4 × IR	FBJ4*	1×10^4	1/6	5/5

* Mice received 400rad whole body X-irradiation 24 hours prior to challenge.
IR = Immunization by implantation of X-irradiated (15,000 rad) tissue grafts.
MC = Transplanted chemically induced sarcoma of soft tissue origin.
FBJ = Transplanted fibrosarcoma induced by FBJ virus.
S = Transplanted radiation-induced osteosarcoma.
6 immunogenic tumours, Nos. FBJ1, FBJ2, FBJ3, FBJ5, FBJ6, FBJ7.

(S115), or soft tissue sarcoma (MC3) failed to protect against subsequent challenges with FBJ sarcoma cells. Although in one example (FBJ5) viable grafts of FBJ sarcoma were rejected by immunized hosts, the level of resistance evoked in terms of cell numbers rejected was generally between 10^4 and 10^5 cells. FBJ virus-induced sarcomas thus appear to possess weak-to-moderate immunogenic capacity in syngeneic hosts. In three independent tests pretreatment with irradiated grafts of three FBJ sarcomas (FBJ2, FBJ3, and FBJ7) conferred resistance to challenges by two different tumours in the series (FBJ4 and FBJ7). FBJ virus-induced sarcomas thus possess a virus specified cell surface antigen which is shared by all the tumours induced by this agent.

TUMOUR SPECIFIC ANTIGENICITY OF RADIATION-INDUCED RAT OSTEOSARCOMAS

The immunogenic properties of six sarcomas were studied by implantation of X-irradiated tumour in syngeneic hosts and subsequent challenge with different inocula of viable tumour cells. In a series of tests, summarized in Table 3, only one osteosarcoma

TABLE 3

IMMUNE RESPONSE TO RADIATION-INDUCED RAT OSTEOSARCOMAS

Immunizing tissue	Immunization procedure	Tumour challenge		Tumour takes in	
		Tumour	Cell dose	Treated rats	Untreated controls
P1	$3 \times$ IR	P1	5×10^4	7/7	4/4
P1	$5 \times$ IR	P1	1×10^4	2/6	2/4
P2	$4 \times$ IR	P2	5×10^4	5/5	5/5
P2	$4 \times$ IR	P2*	2×10^4	5/5	4/4
P7	$4 \times$ IR	P7	1×10^5	3/5	5/5
P7	$4 \times$ IR	P7	5×10^4	3/5	5/5
P7	$4 \times$ IR	P7*	2×10^4	5/5	4/4
P8	$4 \times$ IR	P8*	5×10^3	3/5	3/5
P7	$4 \times$ IR	P8	1×10^4	5/5	5/5
P8	$4 \times$ IR	P8	1×10^4	3/5	5/5
Normal	$4 \times$ IR	P8	1×10^4	5/5	5/5
P8	$4 \times$ IR	P8*	5×10^4	5/5	5/5
P9	$4 \times$ IR	P9*	5×10^3	5/5	3/5
P9	$4 \times$ IR	P9*	1×10^4	4/4	5/5
P9	$4 \times$ IR	P9	5×10^4	5/5	2/4
P10	$4 \times$ IR	P10*	5×10^4	5/5	4/4
P10	$4 \times$ IR	P10*	1×10^4	1/5	2/4
P10	$4 \times$ IR	P10	2×10^5	1/5	2/5
P10	$4 \times$ IR	P10	1×10^6	4/5	5/5

* Rats received 400 rad whole-body X-irradiation 24 hours prior to challenge.

P = Osteosarcomas induced by radiophosphorus (^{32}P).

IR = Immunization by implantation of X-irradiated (15,000 rad) tissue grafts.

(P7) was moderately immunogenic, 4/10 immunized rats rejecting challenges of up to 10^5 cells, while the remainder exhibited significant growth inhibition compared with controls but no ultimate protection. The transient nature of the immune response to this tumour was emphasized by the finding that rechallenge with comparable cell numbers of rats initially showing signs of immunity invariably overcame the resistance. In tests on a second tumour (P8), tumour outgrowth was prevented in 2/5 immunized rats, while in two of the remaining three rats the subcutaneous challenge inoculum was resisted although rats succumbed to multiple metastases principally in the lungs and liver. In controls, tumour outgrowth was local in 5/5 rats at the site of subcutaneous inoculation and widely disseminated tumour metastases were also present. These observations on the inconsistency of induction of tumour immunity and the failure to control disseminated tumour cells may all be reflections of the weak antigenicity of this tumour. For the remaining tumours in this series, no resistance was evoked and in some examples tumour growth was even enhanced in immunized hosts compared with controls. These tests therefore underline the relatively weak nature of TSTA associated with radiophosphorus induced rat osteosarcomas as studied by these procedures.

TUMOUR SPECIFIC ANTIGENICITY OF CHEMICALLY INDUCED RAT OSTEOSARCOMAS

Three transplantable osteosarcomas were examined for their ability to evoke immunity in syngeneic AS rats by pretreatment with irradiated tumour grafts. All three sarcomas were highly immunogenic, resistance being consistently induced against inocula of 1 to 2×10^6 cells and, in at least one instance (CC8), against viable grafts of tumour. These challenges grew progressively in rats similarly treated with irradiated normal tissue and also in untreated controls (Table 4). Rats which rejected challenges with 1 to 2×10^6 cells almost invariably resisted further challenges with comparable tumour-cell inocula and in all three examples this number of tumour cells could be repeatedly implanted at regular intervals without any breakdown of protection. Resistance could however, be overcome by inoculation of larger cell doses of the order of 10^7 cells or large trocar grafts. The specificity of the resistance evoked against the osteosarcomas was examined by rechallenging rats which were resistant to one osteosarcoma with cells derived from another tumour of the same group. There was no cross-resistance to grafts of the second osteosarcoma which developed in all treated rats and at rates comparable with those in untreated rats or controls pretreated with irradiated normal tissues (Table 4). These tests thus established a high degree of antigenic individuality for the osteosarcomas induced by the chemical carcinogen.

DISCUSSION

Tumour specific antigenicity defined as that property of neoplastic cells which evokes immunity to the transplantation of tumour cells in syngeneic hosts has been reported for many experimentally induced neoplasms of different aetiology and histological type (Klein 1968).

In this study on tumour antigenicity in four contrasting models of bone oncogenesis, immunogenic tumours were induced by each agent but differed widely in respect of relative antigenic strength and specificity. Thus, osteosarcomas induced by internal irradiation with bone seeking radionuclides (^{90}Sr/^{226}Ra/^{32}P) in mice and rats were in

TABLE 4

IMMUNE RESPONSE TO CHEMICALLY-INDUCED RAT OSTEOSARCOMAS

Immunizing tissue	Immunization procedure	Tumour	Cell dose	Tumour challenge	
				Tumour takes in	
				Treated rats	Untreated controls
CC5	$3 \times$ IR	CC5	1×10^5	0/6	5/5
CC5	$4 \times$ IR	CC5*	1×10^5	1/5	5/5
CC5	$4 \times$ IR	CC5*	5×10^5	1/5	5/5
CC5	$4 \times$ IR	CC5	1×10^6	0/4	4/5
CC8	$4 \times$ IR	CC8	Graft	0/6	8/10
Normal	$4 \times$ IR	CC8	Graft	5/5	5/5
CC5	$4 \times$ IR	CC8	Graft	4/5	5/5
CC10	$4 \times$ IR	CC8	Graft	4/5	5/5
CC10	$4 \times$ IR	CC10	2×10^6	0/5	4/5
Normal	$4 \times$ IR	CC10	1×10^6	4/5	5/5
CC5	$4 \times$ IR	CC10	1×10^6	5/5	5/5
CC8	$4 \times$ IR	CC10	1×10^6	4/5	5/5

* Rats received 400 rad whole-body X-irradiation 24 hours prior to challenge.

CC = Osteosarcomas induced by a chemical carcinogen (cupric-chelated-N-hydroxy-2-acetylamino-fluorene).

IR = Immunization by implantation of X-irradiated (15,000 rad) tissue grafts.

general weakly immunogenic or nonimmunogenic by the criteria adopted in this investigation. The weak antigenicity of these neoplasms was further emphasized by failure to detect humoral antibody in the serum of syngeneic hosts immunized with radiation-induced osteosarcomas by indirect immunofluorescence tests on tumour cell suspensions (Moore and Williams 1972). The latter technique has been widely applied to the detection of TSTA with sera from specifically immunized syngeneic donors on tumours of several types including a weakly immunogenic spontaneous neoplasm (Baldwin *et al.* 1971). However, tumour antigen expression may be influenced by other factors including masking by sialomucins (Currie and Bagshawe 1969), enhancing antibody (Hellström *et al.* 1969) or serial passage in incompetent hosts (Globerson and Feldman 1964, Woodruff and Symes 1962) so that antigenic deficiency in these tumour systems may be a quantitative rather than a qualitative phenomenon.

Mesenchymal sarcomas associated with bone induced by FBJ virus were more consistently antigenic in syngeneic hosts than osteosarcomas induced by internal irradiation, although in studies conducted to date, only moderate levels of resistance were evoked by excision of subcutaneously developing tumour or repeated implantation of X-irradiated biopsies. In common with DNA and RNA virus induced neoplasms which carry a virus-determined surface antigen shared by all tumours induced by the same virus (Sjögren 1965, Klein 1968) cross-resistance studies revealed an antigen common to

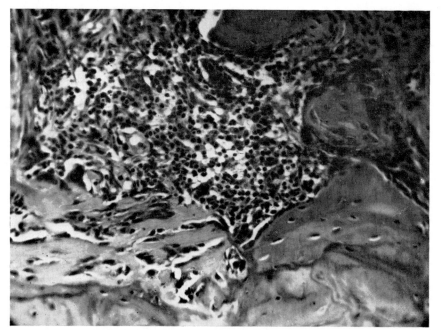

Fig. 2. (H & E ×185) Chemically induced primary osteosarcoma of rat femur (CC8), showing marked periosteal reaction which is predominantly lymphocytic, and to a lesser degree fibroblastic in character.

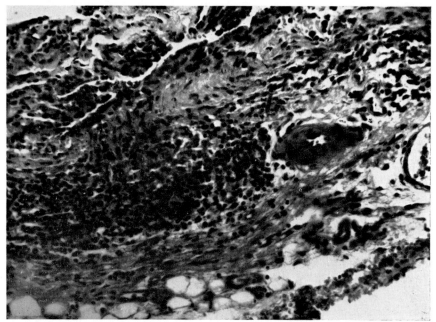

Fig. 3. (H & E ×185) Primary osteosarcoma of rat femur (CC8). Marked lymphocytic reaction adjacent to blood vessel in parosteal soft tissue at the growing edge of the tumour.

FBJ virus-induced sarcomas. Since transplanted FBJ tumours are known to release infectious virus by a process of budding from the cell membrane (Biskis and Finkel 1969), these tests do not discriminate between new virus determined cellular antigens and those of the virion. Studies with other murine sarcoma viruses have similarly revealed cross-reactivity of virus specified cell surface antigens (Chuat, Berman, Gunvén and Klein 1969) but whether these have any relationship to those expressed on FBJ sarcoma cells is not yet known.

By contrast with sarcomas induced by radiation and oncornavirus, chemically induced osteosarcomas in rats elicited very strong immune reactions such that high inocula of transplanted tumour cells (in excess of 2 million) were rejected by immunized hosts; moreover, these tumours revealed a high degree of antigenic individuality, such that immunization with one tumour failed to protect against another of similar morphology and induced by the same agent. Thus chemically induced osteosarcomas elicit comparable immune reactions to soft tissue sarcomas induced by the classical chemical carcinogens with respect to intensity and unique antigenic specificity (Baldwin 1970).

A significant histopathological feature of the chemically induced tumours was marked inflammatory reaction in the periosteum of primary osteosarcomas (Fig. 2) and in parosteal muscle of the growing edge of the tumours (Fig. 3), as well as to varying degrees in tumour tissue. Patchy necrosis was evident in most of the primary tumours even in well vascularized areas and was associated with an inflammatory reaction principally involving lymphocytes. Mononuclear cell infiltration was also observed in early generation transplants of tumours in immunocompetent hosts (Fig. 4). The absence of comparable inflammatory reactions to primary osteosarcomas induced by radiophosphorus in the same strain suggests that these phenomena may be related to the antigenic status of the chemically induced bone tumours. Although inflammatory responses of a non-specific nature cannot be excluded, this suggestion would be in line with the observation that early generation transplants of chemically induced osteosarcomas in immuno-competent hosts may actually regress, presumably by an immunological mechanism in view of their high immunogenicity (unpublished observations). Whether such reactions may be considered to represent cell-mediated immunity by the autochthonous host reflecting possible immune surveillance mechanisms would require further detailed histological study early in the latency period in these tumour systems as Lappé (1971) has undertaken for chemically induced murine skin papillomas.

It is possible that the radiation induced osteosarcomas are antigenically deficient on account of immunoselection against antigenic neoplastic cells during the latency period. However, it is difficult to conceive of an immune surveillance mechanism which would not be equally efficacious against antigenic osteosarcomas induced by irradiation and chemical carcinogens. In the absence of comparative information on secondary factors such as immunosuppression by these respective agents which may contribute to their oncogenic potential in the autochthonous host (Stjernsward 1969), this interpretation cannot be substantiated. Moreover, absence of antigenicity is not necessarily a conse-quence of immunoselection since cells transformed *in vitro* by a chemical carcinogen and maintained in tissue culture apart from an immune environment may also be deficient in TSTA (Prehn 1970, Embleton and Heidelberger 1972).

The antigenicity of radiation induced rodent osteosarcomas assessed by the level of resistance to tumour challenge induced in hosts previously exposed to the same tumour

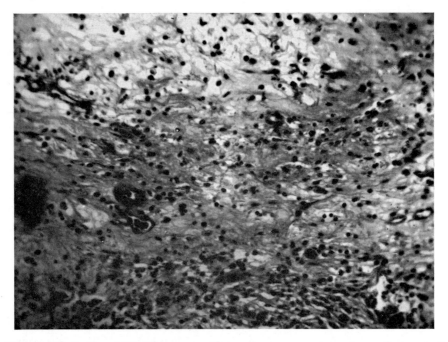

Fig. 4. (H & E ×185) First generation subcutaneous transplant of chemically induced osteosarcoma CC5, showing an area of oedematous fibrous tissue adjacent to viable tumour, with several blood vessels and uniform mononuclear round-cell infiltration.

quantitatively corresponds more closely to that of spontaneously occurring murine and rat sarcomas (Prehn and Main 1957, Hammond, Fisher and Rolley 1967, Baldwin 1966) and sarcomas induced by other physical agents (Klein, Sjögren and Klein 1963) than the chemically induced sarcomas which are in general highly antigenic. In this respect, a similar correlation with spontaneous neoplasms exists for sarcomas induced by FBJ virus identified as the aetiological agent of spontaneously arising malignant bone tumours in CFl mice. One possible conclusion from this correspondence is that sarcomas induced by irradiation or FBJ virus may have greater relevance for the study of the immunological parameters of tumour-host interactions in sarcoma of man, than those induced by chemical carcinogens. However, it is at least questionable whether expression of TSTA is an essential requirement in bone tumourigenesis initiated by radiation, since sensitive transplantation tests failed to reveal significant immunity to the majority of tumours so studied. Furthermore, the apparent obligate association of strong TSTA with chemically induced sarcomas of bone and soft tissues may be a secondary feature of their malignancy produced by cell and carcinogen interaction at the macromolecular level.

It is often claimed that the relative nature of tumour specific rejection reactions may have some important practical consequences in relation to immunotherapy (Alexander 1968). Radiotherapy and chemotherapy act by single hit kinetics and the same dose of therapy is required for each 10-fold decrease of the tumour cell population, irrespective of whether the population is large or small. This imposes very severe limitations on attempts to eradicate entire populations of tumour cells since risks of toxicity and other side effects will increase with each 10-fold unit of population decrease. An immune reaction that can act against 10^5 cells will have minimal effectiveness against a population of 10^9 cells but is potentially important when the population has been reduced down to 10^5 cells by other forms of therapy. The high degree of specificity of the immune rejection mediated by TSTAs, its ubiquitous action in the host, and its nontoxic nature are other important facets. The potential contribution of immunotherapeutic approaches thus lies in the protection against recurrence and metastases in conjunction with other forms of therapy (Mihich 1969, Currie and Bagshawe 1970, Fefer 1971, Glynn and Kende 1971).

ACKNOWLEDGEMENTS

I wish to thank Dr. J. F. Loutit, F.R.S., MRC Radiobiology Unit, Harwell, Berkshire, who provided the radiostrontium-induced murine osteosarcomas for immunological study and Dr. C. H. G. Price, Bristol Bone Tumour Registry, for histological advice throughout the investigation.

In addition, the contribution of my colleagues, Mr. N. W. Nisbet, Mrs. Dorothy E. Williams and Mr. D. B. Jones to this work is gratefully acknowledged.

This work was supported by grants from the Medical Research Council, Cancer Research Campaign and the Research Subcommittee of the Birmingham Regional Hospital Board.

REFERENCES

Alexander, P.   Immunotherapy of Cancer: Experiments with Primary Tumours and Syngeneic Tumour Grafts. *Progr. exp. Tumor Res.* **10**, 22, 1968.
Allison, A. C. & Law, L. W.   Effects of Antilymphocyte Serum on Virus Oncogenesis. *Proc. Soc. exp. Biol. & Med.*, **127**, 207, 1968.
Allison, A. C. & Taylor, R. B.   Observations on Thymectomy and Carcinogenesis. *Cancer Res.*, **27**, 703, 1967
Baldwin, R. W.   Immunity to Methylcholanthrene-induced Tumours in Inbred Rats following Atrophy and Regression of the Implanted Tumours. *Int. J. Cancer*, **9**, 652, 1955.
Baldwin, R. W.   Tumour-specific Immunity Against Spontaneous Rat Tumours. *Int. J. Cancer*, **1**, 257, 1966.
Baldwin, R. W.   Tumor specific antigens associated with chemically induced tumors. *Rev. Europ. Études Clin. et Biol.*, **XV**, 1, 1970.
Baldwin, R. W., Barker, C. R., Embleton, M. J., Glaves, D., Moore, M. & Pimm, M. V.   Demonstration of Cell-surface Antigens on Chemically-induced Tumours. *Ann. N.Y. Acad. Sci.*, **177**, 268, 1971.
Baldwin, R. W. & Embleton, M. J.   Immunology of Spontaneously Arising Rat Mammary Adenocarcinomas. *Int. J. Cancer*, **4**, 430, 1969.
Balner, H. & Dersjant, H.   Increased Oncogenic effect of Methylcholanthrene after Treatment with Antilymphocyte Serum. *Nature (Lond.)*, **224**, 376, 1969.
Barnes, D. W. H., Carr, T. E. F., Evans, E. P. & Loutit, J. F.   ^{90}Sr-induced Osteosarcomas in Radiation Chimaeras. *Int. J. Radiat. Biol.*, **18**, 531, 1970.
Biskis, B. O. & Finkel, M. P.   *Electron Microscopy of the FBJ Osteosarcoma Virus.* 27th Ann. Electron Microscopy Society of America Meeting p. 384. Ed. C. J. Arceneaux, 1969.
Blackett, N. M.   An Effect of Dose Fractionation on the Incidence of Bone Tumors using Radioactive Phosphorus. *Nature (Lond.)*, **184**, 565, 1959.

P

Blair, P. B.   Immunological Aspects of the Relationship between Host and Oncogenic Virus in the Mouse Mammary Tumor System. *Israel J. Med. Sci.*, p. 161. In *Immunological Parameters of Host Tumour Relationships*. Ed. David W. Weiss. Academic Press, 1971.

Boyse, E. A., Old, L. J., Stockert, E., & Shigeno, N.   Genetic Origin of Tumor Antigens. *Cancer Res.*, **28**, 1280, 1968.

Cerilli, G. J. & Treat, R. C.   The Effect of Antilymphocyte Serum on the Induction and Growth of Tumor in the Adult Mouse. *Transplantation*, **8**, 774, 1969.

Celada, F.   The Immunologic Defence in Relation to Age. In *Cancer and Aging*, Engle, A. and Larson, T. (Eds.)., Stockholm, Thule International Symposium, p. 97, 1968.

Chuat, J.-C., Berman, L., Gunvén, P. & Klein, E.   Studies on Murine Sarcoma Virus: Antigenic Characterization of Murine Sarcoma Virus Induced Tumor Cells. *Int. J. Cancer*, **4**, 465, 1969.

Cobb, L. M.   Radiation-induced Osteosarcoma in the Rat as a model for Osteosarcoma in Man. *Brit. J. Cancer*, **24**, 294, 1970.

Currie, G. A. & Bagshawe, K. D.   Tumour Specific Immunogenicity of Methylcholanthrene-induced Sarcoma Cells after Incubation in Neuraminidase. *Brit. J. Cancer*, **23**, 141, 1969.

Currie, G. A. & Bagshawe, K. D.   Active Immunotherapy with Corynebacterium Parvum and Chemotherapy in Murine Fibrosarcomas. *Brit. Med. J.*, **1**, 541, 1970.

Embleton, M. J. & Heidelberger, Ch.   Antigenicity of Clones of Mouse Prostate Cells Transformed *in vitro*. *Int. J. Cancer*, **9**, 8, 1972.

Fefer, A.   Adoptive Chemoimmunotherapy of a Moloney Lymphoma. *Int. J. Cancer*, **8**, 364, 1971.

Finkel, M. P., Biskis, B. O. & Jinkins, P. B.   Virus Induction of Osteosarcomas in Mice. *Science*, **151**, 698, 1966.

Foley, E. J.   Antigenic Properties of Methylcholanthrene-induced Tumors in Mice of the Strain of Origin. *Cancer Res.*, **13**, 835, 1953.

Globerson, A. & Feldman, M. Antigenic Specificity of Benze-pyrene-induced Sarcomas. *J. nat. Cancer Inst.*, **32**, 1229, 1964.

Glynn, J. P. & Kende, M.   Treatment of Moloney Virus-induced Leukemia with Cyclophosphamide and Specifically Sensitized Allogeneic Cells. *Cancer Res.*, **31**, 1383, 1971.

Grant, G. A. & Miller, J. F. A. P.   Effect of Neonatal Thymectomy on the Induction of Sarcoma in C57B1 Mice. *Nature (Lond.)*, **205**, 1124, 1965.

Hammond, W. G., Fisher, J. C. & Rolley, R. T.   Tumor-specific Transplantation Immunity to Spontaneous Mouse Tumours. *Surgery*, **62**, 124, 1967.

Hellström, I., Hellström, K. E., Evans, C. A., Heppner, G. H., Pierce, G. E. & Yang, J. P. S.   Serum-mediated Protection of Neoplastic Cells from Inhibition by Lymphocytes immune to their Tumour Specific Antigens. *Proc. nat. Acad. Sci. (Wash.)*, **62**, 362, 1969.

Johnson, S.   The Effect of Thymectomy and of the Dose of 3-Methylcholantrene on the Induction and Antigenic Properties of Sarcomas in C57B1 mice. *Brit. J. Cancer*, **22**, 93, 1968.

Keast, D.   Immunosurveillance and Cancer. *Lancet*, **2**, 710, 1970.

Klein, E.   The Cell Surface in Immune Response. *Europ. J. Cancer*, **6**, 15, 1970.

Klein, G.   Tumor-specific Transplantation Antigens: G. H. A. Clowes Memorial Lecture. *Cancer Res.*, **28**, 625, 1968.

Klein, G., Sjogren, H. O., & Klein, E.   Demonstration of Host Resistance against Sarcomas induced by Implantation of Cellophane Films in Isologous (Syngeneic) Recipients. *Cancer Res.*, **23**, 84, 1963.

Klein, G., Sjogren, H. O., Klein, E. & Hellström, K. E.   Demonstration of Resistance against Methylcholanthrene Induced Sarcomas in the Primary Autochthonous Host. *Cancer Res.*, **20**, 1561, 1960.

Lappé, M. A.   Evidence for Immunological Surveillance during Skin Carcinogenesis. Inflammatory foci in Immunologically Competent Mice. *Israel J. Med. Sci.*, **52**. In *Immunological Parameters of Host-Tumour Relationships*, Ed. David W. Weiss. Academic Press, 1971.

Law, L. W.   Studies of Thymic Function with Emphasis on the Role of the Thymus in Oncogenesis. *Cancer Res.*, **26**, 551, 1966.

Mihich, E.   Modification of Tumor Regression by Immunologic Means. *Cancer Res.*, **29**, 2345, 1969.

Moore, M. & Williams, D. E.   Studies on the Antigenicity of Radiation-induced Murine Osteosarcomata. *Brit. J. Cancer*, **26** 90, 1972.

Prehn, R. T.   The Significance of Tumor distinctive Histocompatibility Antigens. In *Cross-reacting Antigens and Neoantigens*. Ed. John J. Trentin. The Williams and Wilkins Co., Baltimore, p. 105. 1967.

Prehn, R. T.   Tumor-specific Antigens of Putatively Non-viral Tumors. *Cancer Res.*, **28**, 1326, 1968.

Prehn, R. T.   In *Immune Surveillance*. Ed. R. T. Smith and M. Landy. Academic Press, London p. 454, 1970.

Prehn, R. T. & Main, J. M.   Immunity to Methylcholanthrene-induced Sarcomas. *J. nat. Cancer Inst.*, **18**, 769, 1957.

Price, C. H. G., Moore, M. & Jones, D. B.   FBJ Virus-induced Tumours in Mice. *Brit. J. Cancer*, **26**, 15, 1972.

Sjogren, H. O.   Transplantation Methods as a Tool for Detection of Tumor-specific Antigens. *Progr. exp. Tumor Res.*, **6**, 289. Karger, Basel/New York, 1965.

Stanton, M. F.   Primary Tumors of Bone and Lung in Rats following Local Deposition of Cupric-chelated N-hydroxy-2-acetylaminofluorene. *Cancer Res.*, **27**, 1000, 1967.

Stjernsward, J.   Age-dependent Tumor-host Barrier and Effect of Carcinogen-induced Immunodepression on Rejection of Isografted Methylcholanthrene-induced Sarcoma Cells. *J. nat. Cancer Inst.*, **37**, 505, 1966.

Stjernsward, J.   Immunosuppression by Carcinogens. *Antibiotic & Chemotherapia*, **15**, 213, 1969.

Wagner, J. L. & Haughton, G.   Immunosuppression by Antilymphocyte Serum and its Effect on Tumors induced by 3-Methylcholanthrene in mice. *J. nat. Cancer Inst.*, **46**, 1, 1971.

Woodruff, M. F. A. & Symes, M. O.   Evidence of Loss of Tumour Specific Antigen on repeatedly transplanting a Tumour in the Strain of Origin. *Brit. J. Cancer*, **16**, 484, 1962.

Discussion

Dr. Price   In normal physiological circumstances what is it which limits the number of reacting lymphocytes in the circulating blood or in tissue? There is some mechanism obviously which produces homeostasis as with other forms of cells and tissues.

Dr. Moore   I think on that score we might just make the observation that the number of lymphoctyes committed to reacting with antigenic cells, either in a homograft context or in a tumour immunity context, is a relatively small proportion of the total lymphocyte population.

It has been argued that the primary function of the lymphocyte is to mediate control of growth and morphostasis (Burwell 1963)[1] as well as the recognition and eventual elimination of foreign cells. We cannot now embark upon a discussion of this hypothesis. Suffice it to note that as far as tumour rejection is concerned, it appears that the number of lymphocytes committed to reaction with antigenic tumour target cells is a relatively small proportion of the total population. This appears to be reflected in investigations *in vitro* where the ratio of lymphocytes to target tumour cells has to be large, e.g. 500 or 1,000 to 1 or more, in order to achieve tumour cytotoxicity.

Dr. Tudway   I would like to enquire if you think there is any place for passive immunity in the treatment of tumours. For example, Professor Riddell, our Professor of Surgery in Bristol, has immunized pigs against melanoma, then injected their pulped spleen into the patient. There has been temporary regression in large tumour masses, but if this could be done at the late stage of reduction of cell population that you mention, could this be helpful?

Dr. Moore   The model used by Symes and Riddell[2] is based essentially on an earlier animal model in which xenogenic lymphocytes from sheep were transfused into rats bearing primary sarcomas and found to produce significant inhibition of growth rate, so there may well be a clinical application of treatment by passive transfer of immuno-competent cells in certain clinical cases. Other possibilities might include the passive administration of antibody coupled to radioisotopic agents or chemotherapeutic agents, but these have not yet been explored in a clinical context and one must always be aware of the inherent dangers involved in passive administration of antibody.

Dr. Suit   In your study of the radiation induced sarcomas did you use only one technique to investigate antigenicity? I want to know if you employed any other; particularly, have you investigated the action of neuraminidase to expose antigens on these tumour cells? I am sure you are aware that this has been claimed to be a very attractive way to assist in the treatment of established tumours.

Dr. Moore   You are not entirely correct Dr. Suit in saying that we used only one method. I spoke of only one method because this is the one we have used most extensively, but we have used other methods of immunization including chemical treatment of cells and also excision which I did not say much about this morning. All with similar results. We have in fact shown minimal antigenicity by several techniques, which answers that point. Regarding the action of neuraminidase, I think this should be investigated. We have currently got two experiments on looking at this but I have no data to report yet. In a previous laboratory I was able to enhance slightly the antigenicity of a chemically induced sarcoma by neuraminidase treatment as others have done before; but I know of no instance where a non-antigenic tumour has been made antigenic in the host of origin by neuraminidase treatment.

REFERENCES

1. Burwell, R. G. The role of Lymphoid Tissue in Morphostasis. *Lancet*, **2**, 69, 1963.
2. Symes, M. O., Riddell, A. G., Immelman, E. J. & Terblanche, J. Immunologically Competent Cells in the Treatment of Malignant Disease. *Lancet*, **1**, 1054, 1968.

Immunologic aspects of Osteosarcoma

by

W. F. ENNEKING and B. MARSH

SUMMARY

Experience has shown that osteosarcoma does contain demonstrable tumor-specific antigens. Passive immunization with xenogenic humoral antibody is ineffective. Active immunization with tumor-specific antigens as described may cause enhancement Passive transfer of allogenic cell-bound antibodies in a statistically insignificant group of patients suggests that this may be a useful adjunct to surgery and warrants further investigation.

THE 5-YEAR SURVIVAL RATES for osteosarcoma have remained 5 to 22% during the past 40 years, despite various methods of treatment. Recent reviews of overall results indicate that radical early surgery remains the treatment of choice.

Research in tumor biology during the past 10 years has well established that tumor specific immunity constitutes but one of several factors in the tumor-host relationship, this being unequivocally demonstrated in the experimental animal. Recently, both cellular and humoral antibody have been demonstrated in patients with varying histologic types of tumor, notably, colonic adenocarcinoma and neuroblastoma.

An approach to immunologically influencing the tumor–host relationship is dependent upon determining the degree of antigenic difference between the neoplasm in question and its normal counterpart. This determination classically involves the immunization of animals with saline extract of the tissues and the appropriate immunologic determinations. When a neoplasm possesses strong tumor-specific antigens, injections of a susceptible host with saline homogenates leads to an alteration of the host's response when subsequently challenged with that tumor. Such active immunization may lead to heightened resistance or conversely to the still poorly understood phenomenon of immunologic enhancement with a more aggressive growth of tumor. Whether one gets heightened resistance or enhancement appears, in some cases, to be related to the dose of immunizing material used or to the manner in which the antigen has been prepared. It is now thought by many people that the so-called enhancement is caused by humoral antibody which attaches to the antigenic sites on the tumor cell and masks or protects it from the more efficient cytotoxic effects of the cell-bound antibodies on the sensitized lymphocytes.

The initial objectives of this study were: (a) to determine if osteosarcoma contains identifiable tumor-specific antigens, and (b) to determine the effect of immunizing patients actively with such antigen, or passively with antiserum prepared against them.

431

THE METHOD OF PREPARATION OF TUMOR-SPECIFIC ANTIGENS

Immediately following amputation the fresh tissue from the tumor bone and normal bone was extracted in saline. The saline-soluble proteins were then migrated electrophoretically in pevikon blocks. By dividing the blocks into slices and eluting the protein from them, the antigenic material was fractionated. Various fractions were then used to immunize animals and the sera of these animals was examined by gel diffusion techniques for the presence of precipitating antibodies (Fig. 1).

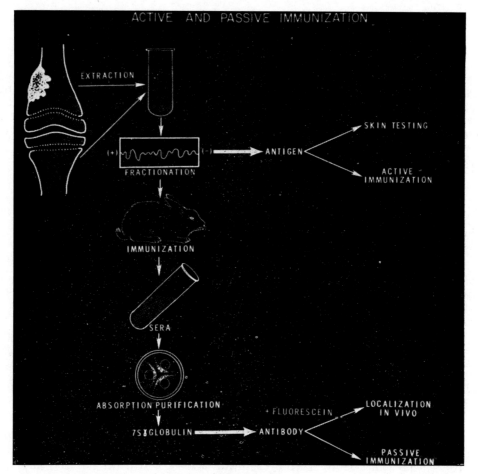

Fig. 1.

ANTIBODY IDENTIFICATION

This was carried out in gel diffusion plates, the zone of precipitation being seen only around the well containing the sera of the immunized animals. The specificity of the reaction was confirmed by the inability to absorb the precipitating antibody with extracts of normal tissue antigens. Electrophoretically, the fraction used to produce this zonal reaction was in the albuminoid range.

Localization of this antibody *in vivo* was sought by conjugating the purified antibody with fluorescein-isothiocyanate. This tagged antibody was then injected intravenously into patients with metastatic osteosarcoma just prior to either thoracotomy or autopsy. Under conditions using UV light it was possible to demonstrate characteristic fluorescence of the tumor tissue but not of the adjacent reactive bone. Microscopically with high magnification the fluorescing antibody was seen surrounding the neoplastic cells. With this evidence of a tumor-specific antigen and the ability of its antisera to localize selectively, the clinical effect of these substances was investigated.

All patients who took part in this study did so with the full knowledge of the procedures involved and were patients of the Clinical Research Center during these studies.

Two patients with early pulmonary metastases were passively immunized with purified tumor-specific antibody. Both died of metastatic disease without any demonstrable effect of the immunization. Four patients were then actively immunized with tumor-specific antigens. The immunization schedule followed was 0·1 mg protein injected intramuscularly beginning 2 weeks after the amputation and continuing for 10 consecutive days. All four patients died of pulmonary metastases, some following an aggressive course of the neoplasm.

One of the patients developed acute intestinal obstruction from an arterial embolus of the tumor to the inferior mesenteric artery. He subsequently died of widespread metastases in a rather bizarre distribution. Another patient followed a similar course.

Patients with osteosarcoma who die of their metastatic disease usually die more or less of suffocation by the continued growth of the tumor in their lungs and the resultant effusion. It is unusual in most recorded experience to find such widespread metastases in these patients.

These few observations indicated that passive immunization with animal humoral antibody was unlikely to affect the course of the disease after pulmonary spread, and that active immunization was not only ineffective in the prevention of metastasis, but possibly enhanced it.

In 1966, Nadler and Moore (1965),[1] at the Roswell Park Institute in New York, published their experience with the cross transplantation of histologically similar tumors between two patients. Two weeks later, white cells were harvested from each of these patients and transfused back into their so-called partner. Although these studies were by necessity poorly controlled and all patients had far-advanced disease, there was some evidence that the patients' clinical situation was improved as a result of these procedures. A similar study was reported from the Tulane Medical Center (1967)[3]. Following this experience, an attempt was made by us to stimulate cell-bound rather than humoral antibodies and assess their effectiveness.

Figure 2 is the protocol of this portion of the study. Immediately following amputation, slices of fresh tumor were implanted subcutaneously in volunteer human recipients. The remainder of the tumor was extracted with saline to obtain tumor-specific antigens for testing purposes. Two weeks following implantation, when the rejection process was well advanced, the implanted tumor was excised and studied histologically. The recipients were skin tested for cutaneous hypersensitivity with tumor-specific antigens One to three billion sensitized white cells were obtained by leukophoresis from the implant recipient and suspended in the recipient's serum. They were immediately transfused into the implant donor. Forty-eight to seventy-two hours following this

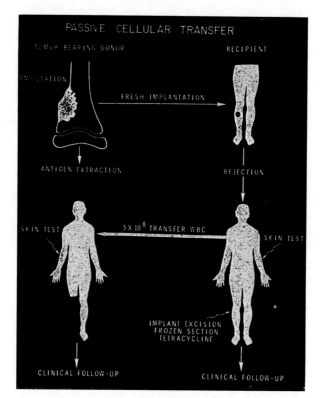

Fig. 2.

passive transfer, the patients were tested for cutaneous hypersensitivity and both patient and donor were clinically followed. These skin tests were done in an attempt to find some manner in which we could measure the success of our transfer of immunity.

A boy with a recently amputated leg may be cited as an example of this routine. Multiple slices of his freshly removed tumor were implanted into the subcutaneous tissues of the recipient. Shortly after this procedure a lymphangiogram demonstrated numerous lymphatic channels forming "pools" at the implantation site, and when removed two weeks later the slices had fused into a solitary mass histologically infiltrated by pyroninophilic immunologically active inflammatory cells. The implant donor was then infused with the recipient's leucocytes amongst which were presumably such sensitized cells. The patient's skin test following the infusion showed a delayed positive reaction to the tumor-specific antigens, whilst the control test was quite negative to extracts of his normal bone. This boy remains well more than 3 years after amputation

Although this patient did all the right things, and did develop a cutaneous hypersensitivity to his tumor-specific antigens following the infusion of the sensitized white cells from his partner, in general, it has not been possible to show any correlation between the skin testing procedures and the clinical course of the patient. The ability to measure the degree or presence of recognition or immunity to a tumor is certainly an area which needs more attention.

Patient	Age	Interval metastases	Interval death	Length of follow-up
TC	14 years	4 months	11 months	—
MU	16	8	12	—
BE	16	6	20	—
KR	14	6	21	—
DB	16	5	—	15 months
SG	8	None	—	10
EL	19	None	—	12
CD	22	None	—	30
HW	17	None	—	43
JH	17	None	—	52

Fig. 3.

Twenty-two patients have been managed by this method. In eight the follow up is less than 1 year although they are clinically free of disease. Another four had pulmonary metastases prior to treatment and all died with no detectable alteration in the clinical course of their disease. All patients have been children or adolescents with histologically confirmed osteosarcoma about the knee. All recipients have been volunteers with metastatic malignant disease. There have been no complications from the implantations. Histologic study of the excised implants has shown evidence of rejection in all instances, although as measured by tetracycline incorporation, in some cases the interval has been delayed beyond that for normal bone.

There have been no complications in the patients from the white cell transfer, despite the fact that major blood groups have been crossed in some instances. Three of nine patients so tested demonstrated passive transfer of cutaneous hypersensitivity to tumor-specific antigens. Five implant recipients have died and come to autopsy. In none has there been evidence of localized or distant recurrence of the implanted sarcoma.

The ten patients with a potential 1-year follow-up and who were free of metastases at the time of treatment are presented in Fig. 3. Four have died of pulmonary metastases, one is alive with metastases and five patients are alive without evidence of metastases.

Figure 4 shows the expected interval of survival for patients with osteosarcoma treated surgically who were free of metastases at the time of treatment. This curve was determined by Marcove *et al.* (1970)[2] from a series of 145 juvenile patients. At 1 year only 45% of cases remain alive and at 2 years it has dropped to 22%. However, at 5 years, 18% remain alive and free of disease suggesting that in this disease a 2-year survival is meaningful.

It also compares the cases with supplementary immunologic therapy with this curve (VAH, Gainesville).

The failure to alter the clinical course of the patients who had small but definite pulmonary lesions at the time of treatment may be due to several factors—not the least of which may be an insufficient number of allogeneic cells.

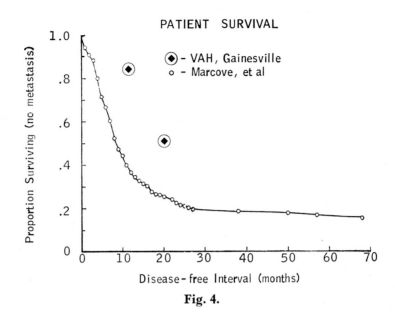

Fig. 4.

It is apparent that this type of immunologic intervention is based upon several requisites to influence favorably the course of the disease:
1. The implant must contain tumor-specific antigens.
2. A satisfactory quantity of tumor must be implanted.
3. The recipient must be immunologically competent.
4. The sensitized cells must survive transplantation.
5. Each tumor cell in the donor must be "available" to a sensitized lymphocyte(s).
6. An adequate transport system must convey the sensitized cells to all the donor's tumor cells prior to the donor rejecting these transfused cells.
7. The quantitative relationships between tumor cells and cell-bound (presumably cytotoxic) antibody must be optimal.

Many if not all of these factors represent as yet unsolved problems and will require further attention in the future. The work presented in this paper has been well put into perspective in a recent review of tumor immunobiology by Richard T. Smith (1971)[4] as but one of many ways in which the current data obtained from animal experiments may be applied to human cancer. He has also pointed out that this modest apparent increase in the survival rate from this tumor may be due to several non-specific factors related to these procedures as opposed to any tumor-specific immunity which may be transferred.

ACKNOWLEDGEMENTS

The presentation is a resumé of both laboratory and clinical work done in the investigation of immunity as related to osteosarcoma.

Under the direction of Dr. W. F. Enneking, the following have worked on this project in its various stages: Mr. Thomas Moore, Dr. Leo Flynn, Mr. Hans Burchardt. Dr. Richard Smith, and Dr. Burton Marsh.

REFERENCES

1. Nadler, S. H. & Moore, O. E. Clinical Immunologic Study of Malignant Disease: Response to Tumor Transplants and Transfer of Leucocytes. *Ann. Surg.* **164**, 482, 1965.
2. Marcove, R. C., Miké, Valerie, Hajek, J. V., Levin, A. G. & Hutter, R. V. P. Osteogenic Sarcoma under the Age of Twenty-one. *J. Bone Jt. Surg.*, **52 A**, 411, 1970.
3. Krementz, E. T. & Samuels, M. S. Tumor Cross-transplantation and Cross-transfusion in the Treatment of Advanced Malignant Disease. *Bull. Tulane Med. Fac.*, **26**, 263, 1967.
4. Smith, R. T. Potentials for Immunologic Intervention in Cancer. Fifth Annual Brook Lodge Conference, April 26–28, 1971.

Discussion

Dr. Moore   I would like to endorse Professor Enneking's conclusions about the use of passive antibody in the treatment of osteosarcoma in man. All the indications from animal experiment work are, that passively administered antibody will not have any effect on an established disease, and may even cause enhancement. I think there are one or two indications from his cases suggesting that this might have happened: so I endorse that caution. I have two questions for him. The first one, I notice that he described one of his recipients as a patient with metastatic carcinoma, I wonder whether his allogeneic lymphocytes might have been more active had he used a more healthy recipient? I realize that there are ethical problems here of course. Perhaps he could comment on that. Were all his recipients in fact patients with advanced malignancies of other types? Secondly, had he considered the deployment of non-specific immuno-stimulants such as BCG or corynebacterium parvum with or without irradiated autologous tumour cells as a possible immunization procedure?

Professor Enneking   In regard to the first question, the first nine recipients all had metastatic carcinoma of some type for the obvious reason of an ethical consideration. All however were tested with DNCB* to ensure that they would have a degree of immunocompetence. It is quite obvious that healthy patients would be better. The following eleven recipients have been survivors who had previously themselves received sensitized lymphocytes, who were at the time of receiving the implant, clinically free of disease and ostensibly healthy patients. Presumably then these eleven recipients may be more immunocompetent than the original nine. On one of the patients immunized we did employ Freund's adjuvant at that time, although other than that we have not used cells non-specific stimulants.

Professor Van Rijssel   I want to comment about the survival curve of patients with osteosarcoma. Professor Enneking yesterday made a remark about the natural history of osteosarcoma that after 2 years only 20% of the patients are living and it remains nearly constant after that. In the Dutch records after 2 years the survival was 35% or 40% and then 1 year later fell to 20%. I think that the slides you demonstrated now give the explanation because your 20% are patients living *without any signs of metastases*. Ours are just survival figures, so that patients with metastases or recurrence who are living after 2 years are included as survivors in our series.

Professor Enneking   I follow you. Basically the kinds of experiments we are doing have no demonstrable end-point other than freedom of disease. There is nothing you can measure that tells you objectively what the effect of the manipulation is other than a statistically significant prolongation of the disease-free interval or survival rate. Survival rates, to be meaningful, I think most people would accept, they have to go 5 years. In

---

* Dinitrochorobenzene.

order to get some quicker assessment of a method of treatment, I think disease-free interval is more meaningful than crude survival figures, because there is a fairly close agreement on this in the various studies published.

Professor Van Rijssel I quite agree but just wanted to explain the difference between the two curves, which I think are otherwise identical.

Dr. Loutit In these clinical cases did you find any evidence of a common antigen between cases or could you not demonstrate the specificity of the individual tumour antigens?

Professor Enneking The immunologic work suggested that between six different tumours there was common recognition by any of the sera, although it could be quantitated in a rough way by serial dilutions and they were of various strengths. In the clinical material we have skin tested two of the patients who demonstrated hypersensitivity following the transfer with material from theirs as well as other patients' tumours. These patients do react to other patients' tumours as manifestation of subcutaneous hypersensitivity; but I think everyone is aware of the non-specificity of such a test. This is the only test that we have carried out.

Detection of a concanavalin A-induced reactive serum factor in patients with osteogenic sarcoma

by

J. T. MAKLEY, A. KANAIDE, A. E. POWELL and A. SLOSS

SUMMARY

Lymphocytes obtained from patients with osteogenic sarcoma stimulate poorly with concanavalin A in the presence of autologous plasma, but stimulate to a greater degree in plasma from normal donors. The plasma effect rarely is seen in the transformation of lymphocytes from normal persons. The mitogenic action of phytohemagglutinin is independent of the plasma employed. Patients with non-malignant disease had normal plasmas so far as the ability to support concanavalin A-induced blast transformation is concerned.

Allogeneic stimulation of patient's cells (mixed lymphocyte reaction) was plasma-sensitive and apparently not specific for plasmas of tumor patients.

As a first approximation, it appears that the action of the active substance is directed at some structure of the responding cell.

RECENT STUDIES HAVE demonstrated that serum from a variety of disease states can inhibit the ability of autologous lymphocytes to undergo blast transformation when stimulated with phytohemagglutinin (PHA). Elves in 1966[1] found that plasma from uremic donors had a suppressive effect on PHA-stimulated lymphocytes. A similar phenomenon was demonstrated by McFarlin and Oppenheim[2] in serum from patients with ataxia telangiectasia. These sera also had elevated levels of alpha$_2$-globulin. Cooperband, *et al.*[3] prepared a serum alpha-globulin which they found inhibited PHA-induced transformation of human lymphocytes. This material was similar to that described by Kamrin[4] and by Mowbray.[5] The materials are known to possess immunoregulatory alpha-globulins.[6] Ribonuclease activity is associated with the preparations isolated by Mowbray[7] and conjugates of ribonuclease are known to inhibit *in vitro* lymphocyte stimulation.[8]

Whittaker and his associates[9] demonstrated that lymphocytes from breast cancer patients showed impaired responses to PHA in autologous serum but responded normally in normal serum. Patient's sera had a similar depressive effect on normal cells. They suggested that the transformation response *in vivo* is regulated, at least in part, by a substance in the circulation. Sample *et al.*[10] made the point that concentrations of PHA which are optimal for transformation of one lymphocyte population, often are

TABLE 1

EFFECT OF PLASMA ON MITOGEN-INDUCED TRANSFORMATION ON PATIENT'S

	Patient and diagnosis		Age	Date of test	Date of biopsy	Status of tumor
1	DH	Osteosarcoma	18	10/5/71	8/68	Died 11/71 Metastatic
2	WC	Osteosarcoma	16	10/2/71	8/19/71	Metastatic Amputation
3	AR	Osteosarcoma	17	10/5/71	10/5/71	No evidence of disease
	AR	Osteosarcoma		12/10/71	2 mo. post-op.	No evidence of disease
	AR	Osteosarcoma		2/4/72	4 mo. post-op.	No evidence of disease
4	CA	Osteosarcoma	45	11/5/71	7/10/70	No progression
5	BA	Osteosarcoma	38	12/9/70	1967	Metastatic
	BA	Osteosarcoma		12/10/71		
6	JC	Osteosarcoma	18	12/10/71	9/71	No evidence of disease
7	PH	Osteosarcoma	12	10/20/70	10/20/70	No evidence of disease
	PH	Osteosarcoma		11/7/70		
8	GO	Chondrosarcoma	48	10/14/71	4/27/71	Progressive disease
	GO	Chondrosarcoma		11/5/71		Progressive disease
	GO	Chondrosarcoma		2/4/72		Progressive disease
9	SM	Rhabdomyo-sarcoma	81	12/14/71	12/14/71	No evidence of disease
10	KO	?Hemangio-pericytoma	52	1/31/72	1/31/72	Disease present
11	WY	Chondrosarcoma	51	2/25/72	2/25/72	Local resection presumed no tumor
12	SB	Undifferentiated sarcoma	59	1/4/72	9/71	Amputation No evidence of disease
13	JM	Reticulum cell sarcoma	28	2/18/72	1970	Progressive disease

Note: Date—Month/Day/Year.

TABLE 1 (CONTINUED

CELLS IN MALIGNANT CONDITIONS OF THE MUSCULOSKELETAL SYSTEM

Cells Alone		PHA			Con A		
P	N	P/Plasma	N/Plasma	100 × P/N	P/Plasma	N/Plasma	100 × P/N
252	248	18,197	20,336	89	1,068	1,470	73*
436	338	64,425	33,830	190†	5,047	13,395	38*
346	480	45,020	47,030	96	2,940	12,830	23*
790	360	56,960	61,170	93	19,910	37,290	53*
349	405				40,740	32,450	125
295	267	19,236	17,108	112	3,630	3,531	103
210	180	6,987	4,540	152†	513	1,508	34*
415	280	34,670	50,160	69*	3,520	10,101	35*
555	380	67,490	40,290	168†	35,709	29,360	122
624	688				1,001	3,706	27*
718	610	2,751	6,189	44*	820	1,059	77
298	260	25,638	24,666	103	1,680	7,154	23*
672	378	30,900	41,860	74*	5,840	4,290	136†
299	243	49,503	34,721	143†	11,675	18,511	63*
267	288	39,940	41,530	96	16,488	22,651	73*
223	296	25,080	32,276	78	3,587	7,279	49*
566	462	28,425	28,559	96	4,802	4,318	90
262	242	41,831	34,728	120	3,647	5,805	63*
291	293	48,276	43,989	110	8,608	16,395	53*

*, †—See text p. 445.

inhibitory for another, possibly reflecting the differing carbohydrate contents of the sera. They showed that the dose level of PHA required for peak responses shifted towards a higher value in experiments done in cancer patients' sera. Although their data seems significant, the sample was quite small and no sera from non-cancer patients was used for comparison.

The purpose of this paper is to describe a similar inhibitory activity of plasma to concanavalin A-stimulated lymphocytes. The plasma was obtained from patients with a variety of connective tissue tumors as well as from several non-tumor patients.

METHODS

Lymphocytes were prepared from blood taken from normal donors or patients who were known to have been free of drug therapy for at least 30 days. Samples were collected by venopuncture using lightly-heparinized syringes and sterile glass screw-capped tubes containing herapin. The plasma and buffy coat was removed following centrifugation at $400 \times g$ for 10 minutes. The cells were permitted to settle at $37°C$, increasing the angle of their tubes every 15–20 minutes over a period of about 90 minutes. The lymphocyte-rich plasma was transferred and centrifuged at $500 \times g$ for 10 minutes. The sediment was resuspended in Minimum Essential Medium (Grand Island Biological Co.) supplemented with antibiotics and fresh L-glutamine ($0·29$ mg/ml) and the appropriate plasma at a final concentration of 20%. The cells were then counted in a hemocytometer and viability was determined by dye exclusion using erythrosin B. They were finally diluted to a concentration of 1 million mononuclear cells *per* ml. The cell population generally consisted of from 70 to 90% mononuclear cells and viability was around 95% or better.

Culture tubes were charged with $1·5$ ml of the cell suspension in the appropriate test plasma. Phytohemagglutinin P (Difco) was added in $0·1$ ml quantities using $1 : 20$ dilution of the original solution. Concanavalin A (con A) was prepared by Dr. M. A. Leon and stored in the cold in the lyophilized state. Solutions were made in phosphate-buffered saline and $0·1$ ml, containing 20 μg, was added to the appropriate tubes. Reciprocal one-way mixed lymphocyte cultures were done according to Bach and Voynow.[11]

All transformation experiments were done in quadruplicate if possible. Data was recorded only if the replicates agreed within 15%. If the decision was critical or a close one, a coefficient of variation of not greater than 10% was required for acceptance.

Five hours prior to harvest, the cells were treated with 2 μCi of ^{3}H-thymidine. They were harvested by quantitative transfer to glass fiber filters (Whatman GF/C) supported on a 30-place filter manifold (Millipore Corp.). They were washed with saline and then soaked with ice-cold 5% trichloroacetic acid twice and with absolute methanol twice. The discs were dried under infrared bulbs and placed in counting vials with 2 ml of toluene-based scintillation fluid.

Comparisons of groups were done by the "t" test for matched pairs using counts per minute (CPM) data. We used the Wilcoxon Signed Rank Test where a question arose as to normality of the distribution. The two tests corresponded very closely. The "t" test was performed on an Olivetti Programma 101 computer.

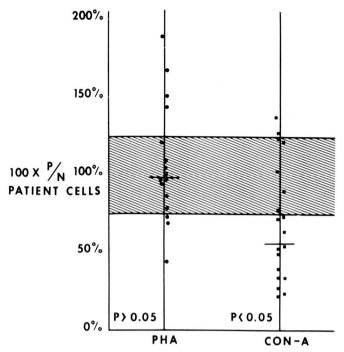

Fig. 1. Effect of plasma from patient with osteosarcoma or chondrosarcoma on mitogen-induced lymphocyte transformation. Each point represents CPM of ^{3}HTdR incorporated by stimulated lymphocytes. The CPM obtained when cultures were made in patients' plasmas were divided by CPM obtained in normal plasmas. The normal range of variation is contained within the horizontal dashed lines. P values relate to differences between plasmas. The horizontal bars show the median values for each group.

RESULTS

Table 1 summarizes the effect of plasma on mitogen-induced stimulation of patients lymphocytes. Counts *per* minute of ^{3}H-thymidine incorporated in the presence of patient plasma were divided by counts obtained in normal plasma and the result was expressed as a percentage. In general, this ratio was not significantly different from 100% in the case of PHA-induced transformation ($p > 0.05$). Four instances of apparent stimulation(†) and 3 cases of apparent inhibition(*) by patient plasma were observed. No consistent pattern was evident.

In the case of con A-induced stimulation, 13 cases of inhibition(*) were observed from 19 possible (Table 1 contd.). Three of the non-inhibitory plasmas were obtained from patients who previously had shown inhibition but whose post-operative plasmas were taken while they were in clinical remission (Patients AR, GO and PH). Patient GO's plasma was inhibitory at the time of surgery, lost its inhibitory character during post-operative remission(†), and regained it as the disease was re-established. Patient JC was examined 6 months post-operatively and Patient CA had undergone amputation 2 years previous to the time of testing. Patient WY was unique only to the extent of presenting

Q

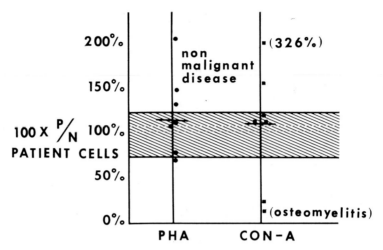

Fig. 2. Effect of plasmas from patients with non-malignant disorders on blast transformation induced by plant mitogens. For explanation of graph, see legend under Fig. 1.

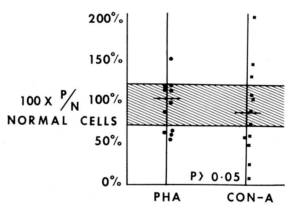

Fig. 3. Effect of pathological plasma on mitogen-induced blast transformation of lymphocytes from normal donors. The P value indicates no significant differences between plasmas and also no significant differences between results obtained with the two mitogens. For further explanation of the graph, see legend under Fig. 1.

a well-localized lesion. Otherwise this group of patients was uniform in exhibiting an inhibitory factor which related to their disease status. The data is presented graphically in Fig. 1.

Figure 2 shows the results of testing cells from a few patients with non-malignant disorders. Significant differences due to plasma or due to mitogen could not be detected. Thus, the factor whose effects were seen clearly in Table 1 and Fig. 1 seems to be specific for autologous cells.

The body of data contained in Table 1 indicate the existence of a peculiarity in the plasmas of our patient population. The distinction between patients and normal plasmas was not evident when PHA was employed as a stimulant. The data in Fig. 3 indicate that con A-stimulated normal cells are not in general responsive to the factor. Of 13 cases, there were five instances of apparent inhibition, four instances of apparent stimulation, and four instances of indifference due to plasma.Effects of PHA treatment were about the same.

The effect of inhibitory plasma on the mixed lymphocyte reaction also was studied. Peripheral blood lymphocytes from normal donors were mixed with equal numbers of patients' lymphocytes and incubated for a week. The medium contained 20% of normal plasma, 20% of patient's plasma or 20% of an equal mixture of the two plasmas. The mixed lymphocyte reaction (MLR) proved to be sensitive to the plasma employed (Table 2). Where inhibition occurred, a dose-response effect was noted in a few cases. In two cases, inhibition was found not to occur. Both involved patients in apparent remission. One patient (PG) was suffering from a non-malignant disease, osteomyelitis, and his plasma possessed inhibitory properties.

In one instance, a reciprocal one-way analysis of the reaction was done. Lymphocytes from each donor, in turn, were treated with mitomycin C and mixed with untreated cells of the other donor. Since mitomycin C-treated cells can stimulate the untreated population but are unable to metabolize thymidine, the contribution of the untreated

TABLE 2

EFFECT OF PLASMA SOURCE ON THE MIXED LYMPHOCYTE REACTION*

Donors		Date of test	Source of plasma		Uptake by the cells ³HTdR†			% Inhibition $1 - \dfrac{\text{CPM (mixed) in P/Plasma}}{\text{CPM (mixed) in N/Plasma}} \times 100$
Patient	Normal		Patient %	Normal %	Patient	Normal	Mixed	
PH (osteosarcoma)	HE	10/20/70 (pre-op.)	0	100	3,056	3,104	7,208	—
			50	50	—	—	5,440	25
			100	0	2,983	2,557	3,275	55
PH (osteosarcoma)	MS	11/4/70	0	100	302	490	1,263	—
			100	0	432	561	799	37
BA (osteosarcoma)	AP	12/9/70 Active	0	100	—	—	44,146	—
			100	0	—	—	24,179	45
BA (osteosarcoma)	JM	2/4/72 Active	0	100	286	477	15,942	—
			100	0	136	230	8,934	56
AR (osteosarcoma)	JM	2/4/72 No disease	0	100	419	477	28,901	—
			100	0	410	569	23,457	19
GO (chondrosarcoma)	JM	2/4/72 ? active	0	100	359	477	21,603	—
			100	0	262	432	25,510	18+
JM (reticulum cell sarcoma)	EA	2/18/72 active	0	100	775	351	14,581	—
			100	0	560	218	16,916	16+
PG (osteomyelitis)	SL	1/27/71	0	100	320	2,538	11,228	—
			50	50	—	—	8,827	21
			100	0	186	615	5,140	54

Reciprocal one way					PHm + MS	PH + MSm	% Inhibition	
							PHm	MSm
PH (osteosarcoma)	MS	11/4/70	0	100	1,036	609	—	—
			100	0	171	68	84	89

* Cells were cultivated in medium 199 containing a final concentration of 20% of the appropriate plasma or plasma mixture.
† Tritiated thymidine.

donor can be isolated and evaluated. When this was done, a strong plasma effect was seen. Patient plasma was inhibitory for either the normal or abnormal cell population.

It has been reported several times that cancer patients exhibit diminished lymphocytic responses to mitogens. According to our cumulative experience, only patients DH, CA, BA and PH showed responses to PHA significantly lower than was to be expected. This result was supported by a similar finding using con A as mitogen. The data indicate that impaired responsiveness to mitogens is an irregular finding and probably is related to many factors other than neoplasia, such as debilitation and age.

DISCUSSION

No single serum factor characteristic of malignant disease has been reported. It is known however, that seromucoid glycoprotein may be elevated considerably.[12] Snyder and Ashwell[13] have shown that alpha$_1$-acid glycoprotein, ceruloplasmin and alpha$_1$-antitrypsin were elevated in cancer patients and in certain chronically ill individuals while hapto-globin and hemopexin were elevated in their cancer group but not in their non-malignant controls. It is possible that some related material accounts for the inhibitory factor(s) described in the present report.

If the inhibitory material were a simple glycoprotein, its action could be ascribed to its ability to interact with con A but not with PHA. This cannot be the whole explanation however, since the material had no effect on stimulation of normal cells and also inhibited the mixed lymphocyte reaction. Thus, the interaction must be directed in part towards a cellular constituent.

It is possible that the material has a non-specific metabolic effect on the responding cells, but if this were true, then normal cells and PHA-induced transformation ought to be affected as well. Perhaps the effect is directed at a metabolic peculiarity of cells from tumor patients.

Other possibilities exist. For example, the material might be directed towards con A binding sites at the cell surface, or towards receptor sites for allogeneic recognition, these not being mutually exclusive possibilities. There was only one reciprocal one-way MLR done, but if the data proves to be representative, it might be that the material reacts with the stimulating site of a given cell, with the receptor site of a given cell, or with both.

The inhibitory factor appears quite regularly in plasma of patients with osteogenic sarcoma in the active phase. We have noticed that occasionally the plasma will inhibit normal cells, but as a rule (cf. Fig. 3) it does not. Frequently we find plasmas obtained from other kinds of patients which inhibit blastogenesis, but none has been so regular in this respect as the osteosarcoma group. The mixed lymphocyte data, particularly that obtained with plasma from patient PG, indicate that plasma factor must not yet be considered diagnostic for osteosarcoma or any other malignant disease. However, it may be of value in assessing patient status in view of the fact that its presence seems to be related to disease activity. Further work is required to establish this point.

Preliminary experiments show that activity to be heat stable (56°C for 45 minutes). It seems to survive storage at −60°C for 24 hours or more rather poorly. This fact, and the infrequency with which the factor is active against cells from normal donors, will impede the rate of progress of its characterization.

ACKNOWLEDGEMENT

This work was supported by the Cuyahoga County Chapter of the American Cancer Society and the Health Fund of Greater Cleveland.

REFERENCES

1. Elves, M. W., Israels, M. C. G. & Collinge, M. An Assessment of the Mixed Leucocyte Reaction in Renal Failure. *Lancet*, **1**, 682, 1966.
2. McFarlin, D. E. & Oppenheim, J. J. Impaired Lymphocyte Transformation in Ataxia Telangiectasia in part due to a Plasma Inhibitory Factor. *J. Immunol.*, **103**, 1212, 1969.
3. Cooperband, S. R., Bondevik, H., Schmid, K. & Mannick, J. A. Transformation of Human Lymphocytes: Inhibition by Homologous Alpha Globulin. *Science*, **159**, 1243, 1968.
4. Kamrin, B. B. Successful Skin Homografts in Mature Non-littermate Rats treated with fractions containing Alpha Globulins. *Proc. Soc. Exp. Biol. Med.*, **100**, 58, 1959.
5. Mowbray, J. F. Effect of Large Doses of an Alpha$_2$-glycoprotein on the Survival of Rat Skin Homografts. *Transplantation*, **1**, 15, 1963.
6. Mannick, J. A. & Schmid, K. Prolongation of Allograft Survival by an Alpha globulin isolated from Normal Blood. *Transplantation*, **5**, 1231, 1967.
7. Mowbray, J. F. Immunosuppressive Action of Ribonucleases. *J. Clin. Path. (suppl.)*, **20**, 499, 1967.
8. Mowbray, J. F., Boylston, A. W., Milton, J. D. & Weksler, M. E. Studies on the Mode of Action of Immunosuppressive Ribonucleases. *Antibiot. et Chemother.*, **15**, 384, 1969.
9. Whittaker, M. G., Rees, K. & Clark, C. G. Reduced Lymphocyte Transformation in Breast Cancer, *Lancet*, **1**, 892, 1971.
10. Sample, W. F., Gertner, H. R. & Chretien, P. B. Inhibition of Phytohemagglutinin-induced *in vitro* Lymphocyte Transformation by Serum from Patients with Carcinoma. *J. nat. Cancer Inst.*, **46**, 1291, 1971.
11. Bach, F. H. & Voynow, N. K. One-way Stimulation in Mixed Lymphocyte Cultures. *Science*, **153**, 545, 1966.
12. Winzler, R. J. & Smyth, I. M. Studies on the Mucoproteins of Human Plasma. II. Plasma Mucoprotein Levels in Cancer Patients. *J. Clin. Invest.*, **27**, 617, 1948.
13. Snyder, S. & Ashwell, G. Quantitation of Specific Serum Glycoproteins in Malignancy. *Clin. Chim. Acta*, **34**, 449, 1971.

Discussion

Prof. Enneking At the first glance it would seem that whatever this substance is it is loosely analogous to what Good has termed "blocking antibody". I would like to have the author's and Dr. Moore's comments.

Dr. Makley I don't think I am prepared to say that this may well be "blocking antibody" —I really don't know. If we think that the "blocking antibody" may be a specific thing for tumours involved, particularly for osteosarcoma, I find it hard, particularly in these results to say that this might be it, simply because other patients demonstrated this, and also the fact that the osteomyelitis patients did (and there were 2 patients with osteo-myelitis who demonstrated this thing). Some of our results were on burn patients all of whom are presented here, and they showed similarly an inhibitory substance. We are really dealing with a fairly non-specific substance here—whatever it is. Also in some instances it would react with normal cells although it wasn't significant. So I don't know how to answer this question: maybe Dr. Moore will have some comments.

Dr. Moore I think you can exclude a "blocking antibody" here because it does not have the degree of specificity you would expect. The Hellströms[1] have looked at "blocking antibodies" in human sarcomas using the colony inhibition technique. Where patients were clinically free from disease the titres of "blocking antibody" were observed to fall. So I do not think there is any direct correlation between the results which you have reported in your very elegant study and those of the Hellströms.

Prof. Dahlin This isn't directed at Dr. Makley but it occurred to me when I heard the rather optimistic reports of Enneking and Marcove on the use of newer methods of treatment of osteosarcoma, that perhaps there are hidden some similar paths that have been unsuccessful by other workers and hence have not been published. I wonder if Dr. Enneking and Dr. Marcove know of any people who have tried this kind of work and abandoned it?

Prof. Enneking Yes, cross transplantation has been done by Nadler and Moore[2] in patients who had more advanced disease without any demonstrable effect on the course of the disease. We interpret this as being related to the fact that Dr. Moore was expressing in terms of quantitative relationships. I wouldn't want to leave an impression that our report was presumably optimistic. I think it is very prematurely characterized by that word.

REFERENCES

1. Hellström, I., Sjogolen, H. O., Warner, E. & Hellström, K. E. Blocking of Cell-mediated Tumor Immunity by Sera from Patients with Growing Neoplasms. *Int. J. Cancer*, **7**, 226, 1971.
2. Nadler, S. H. & Moore, O. E. Clinical Immunologic Study of Malignant Disease: Response to Tumor Transplants and Transfer of Leucocytes. *Ann. Surg.*, **164**, 482, 1965.

Cartilaginous tumours of the pelvic girdle

by

J. M. THOMINE

SUMMARY

A report is given of fifteen cartilaginous tumours of the pelvis. Seven were histologically confirmed chondrosarcomas; eight were chondromas, of which seven were subject to prognostic reservations. No significant correlation was found between the microscopic structure and the aetiology, the radiographic appearances and the final behaviour. Even those which are not histologically malignant may more slowly recur, eventually proving fatal from local extension of active growth. The relatively late presentation and somewhat different manifestations of tumours inside the pelvic cavity is described and the resulting delay in diagnosis and treatment. Three tumours were associated with multiple exostoses and these patients were long-term survivors. For these radio-resistant cartilage tumours, a "correct" surgical ablation avoiding spillage of tumour cells in the operation area is emphasized, but this has only been possible in about one-quarter of the cases.

THE PRESENT PAPER is a retrospective study of the cartilaginous tumours of the pelvic girdle, observed and treated at the Orthopaedic Clinic of the Cochin Hospital in Paris.

In view of the difficulties in establishing the prognosis of cartilaginous tumours of the pelvis, the group reported has been histologically classified. The cases included here are all those histologically diagnosed as chondroma or chondrosarcoma by pathologists experienced in bone tumours. Chondromas and chondrosarcomas have been studied together, particularly for their clinical features and their behaviour in attempting to correlate these aspects with pathological data (see Table 1).

HISTOLOGICAL DEFINITION

From a histological point of view the present series is composed as follows:

In 11 cases the microscopic diagnosis was *chondrosarcoma* (or malignant chondroma). In the remaining eight cases the diagnosis was *chondroma* (most of them described as active, suspect or invasive chondroma). But in fact, the group of clear-cut malignant tumours must be divided. Indeed four of the 11 cases appear to be on the borderline of conventional chondrosarcoma.

One patient had a mesenchymal chondrosarcoma. This was the only case in which we had the opportunity of observing pulmonary metastasis. These were apparent during the

TABLE 1.

No.	Initials	Age at onset	Sex	Primary site	Histological diagnosis	Previous treatment and duration of symptoms	
1	FR..	16	Female	Sacral canal	Chondrosarcoma	0	3 months
2	LER.	20	Female	Ischiopubic ramus	Chondrosarcoma	0	4 months
3	DE..	37	Male	Iliac wing	Chondrosarcoma	0	36 months
4	AV..	23	Male	Iliac wing	Chondrosarcoma	0	4 months
5	AD..	36	Male	Iliac wing	Chondrosarcoma	Radiotherapy (12,000 R)	24 months
6	BA..	55	Male	Iliac bone	Chondrosarcoma	0	24 months
7	HA..	31	Male	Ischium	Chondrosarcoma	1. Local removal 2. Local removal 3. Local removal	16 months
8	DU..	24	Male	Unknown	Chondroma	0	48 months
9	RA..	4	Female	Ischium	Chondroma	0	6 months
10	BL..	31	Female	Unknown	Chondroma	0	96 months
11	MO..	37	Male	Iliac wing	Chondroma	1. Local removal 2. Local removal 3. Radiotherapy	228 months
12	OL..	29	Male	Ischiopubic ramus	Chondroma	1. Local removal 2. Radiotherapy	120 months
13	VA..	36	Male	Ischiopubic ramus	Chondroma	0	24 months
14	LEC.	38	Male	Iliac wing	Chondroma	1. Partial removal 2. Partial removal 3. Betatron 4. Partial removal 5. Betatron	72 months
15	GA..	48	Male	Iliac wing	Chondroma	1. Radiotherapy 2. Endoxan	84 months

first examination and their discovery was followed by rapid death, without any treatment being possible. In two other patients histological features were of a highly cellular sarcoma with scanty matrix but some patches of cartilaginous differentiation; the presence of osteoid in some areas separated them from the typical chondrosarcomas. The fourth case was a very peculiar tumour made up of two macroscopically distinct parts.

TABLE 1 (CONTINUED)

Surgical treatment at Cochin Hospital	Other treatments	Follow up after treatment	Total duration of tumour evolution (when not apparently cured)
Partial removal	0	Dead After 5 months With tumour	8 months (death)
Resection (correct)	0	Alive Without tumour signs After 60 months	
Resection (correct)	0	Alive Without tumour signs After 60 months	
Resection (incorrect)	0	Alive Without tumour signs After 4 months	
Partial removal	0	Recurrence at 4 months Dead after 24 months With tumour	48 months
Hind-quarter amputation (correct)	0	Alive Without tumour signs After 5 months	
Hind-quarter amputation (incorrect)	0	Recurrence at 12 months Alive with tumour After 60 months	78 months
1. Palliative removal 2. Palliative removal 3. Translumbar amputation (incorrect)	0	Recurrence at 18 months Surgical removal Alive without tumour signs After 30 months	
0	Radio-cobalt	Dead after 12 months With tumour	18 months
Resection (incorrect)	0	Dead from septic complication of surgery After 3 months	
Resection (correct)	0	Alive Without tumour signs After 120 months	
Hind-quarter amputation (incorrect)	0	Recurrence at 84 months Alive with tumour After 84 months	204 months
1. Partial removal 2. Partial removal 3. Partial removal	0	Dead after 36 months With tumour	60 months
0	Radioactive sulphur	Dead from acute pulmonary oedema After 4 months	76 months
Hind-quarter amputation (incorrect)	0	Alive Without tumour signs After 5 months	

One was a central chondromatous tumour of the ischium. Recurrence after limited surgery led to a hindquarter amputation. Examination of the amputation specimen demonstrated the existence of two different and independent tumours. The intra-osseous one was a typical chondrosarcoma; but there was another mass inside the pelvis which proved to be a typical osteosarcoma. In consideration of these pathological

Q*

features, these four cases have been discarded from the study. Thus, 15 cases remain to be reviewed.

Seven tumours were regarded as chondrosarcomas. The diagnosis of malignancy was based on the following features: frequency of nuclear and cellular atypism with high cellularity; but the presence of mitoses was noted in only one tumour. *In the eight remaining* cases malignancy was not affirmed by the pathologist and *the diagnosis was chondroma.* But in seven cases this diagnosis was coupled with prognostic reservations based on the following features: Some cellular atypism (e.g. binucleated chondrocytes), mesenchymatous aspect of the tumour in its peripheral part, and invasion of the adjacent bone or muscle by the tumour. As previously known the diagnosis of malignancy in cartilaginous growths may be based on subtle histological differences. Further difficulty arises from variation within the same tumour. Twice in the present series, the diagnosis of chrondroma based on the biopsy specimen has been changed to chondrosarcoma after examination of the whole tumour.

AETIOLOGY

SEX

Four patients were female and 11 were male. This 1 to 3 ratio is a little lower than usually stated for chondrosarcoma.

AGE

At the first presentation of the tumour, the age of the patients ranged from 4 to 57 years. Eleven of the 15 tumours however appeared between 20 and 40 years, most patients being in their forties (7 cases, nearly half of the total). No significant difference can be shown to exist between chondromas and chondrosarcomas.

PRE-EXISTING LESIONS

In three patients multiple exostoses associated with the cartilaginous growth could be demonstrated (one out of five). The age of these patients did not differ from the average. Twice the cartilaginous tumour was, as expected, diagnosed as a chondrosarcoma by the pathologist. But in the third case, despite resection of the whole tumour after recurrence, microscopic examination failed to find convincing proof of malignancy, and the diagnosis remained "invasive chondroma".

SYMPTOMS

In most cases, the first symptom was the appearance of a painless tumour mass. This was observed in nine out of the 15 cases. The second symptom, in order of frequency, was radiating pain, mainly of sciatic distribution. This obtained in four of the 15 cases. In the two remaining patients pain at the site of the tumour was the first sign of the disease. Tumefaction is mainly encountered in extra-pelvic growths. Thus in six of seven tumours growing mainly out of the pelvic girdle, the first symptom has been a palpable mass.

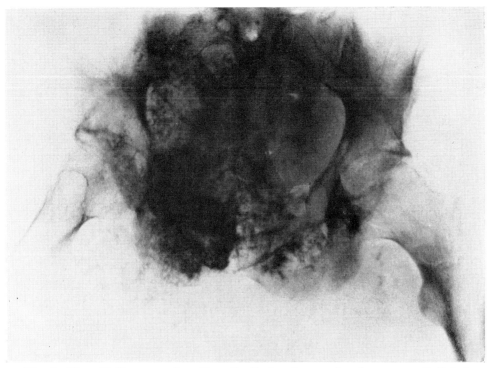

Fig. 1. (Case 8) Features of an "invading" chondroma after four years of clinical evolution; pain, ureteral and rectal compression led to a translumbar amputation.

On the other hand, if the growth is mainly inside the pelvic cavity, pain due to nerve compression (sciatic, femoral or obturator nerve) has been more frequently the first symptom. This was observed in four cases out of eight; less frequently the palpable tumour mass was the first symptom (three patients out of eight). Such tumours are discovered very late because they remain for a long time hidden in the pelvic cavity; they cannot be detected until they are big enough, either by becoming palpable through the abdominal wall or by causing nerve compression. It is in such cases that huge tumours have been encountered (Fig. 1) sometimes as big as a rugby football. It must be here emphasized that this clinical behaviour (slow growth of a usually painless tumour) leads in itself to a delayed diagnosis and so to delayed and more difficult treatment. Indeed, after clinical discovery, these tumours have usually been quickly identified by X-ray examination. In three-quarters of the present cases, the tumour has been recognized within the 3 months following the first clinical manifestation. Twice only, diagnosis has not been suggested by the first X-ray examination. Finally, no correlation appears between clinical symptoms and microscopic evaluation.

RADIOLOGICAL FEATURES

Anatomical and embryological characteristics of the pelvic bones may explain why *all the observed tumours were of the peripheral type*. As a rule the lesion appears as a mass arising from a pelvic segment which is usually either normal or hidden by opacities

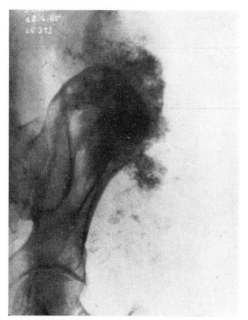

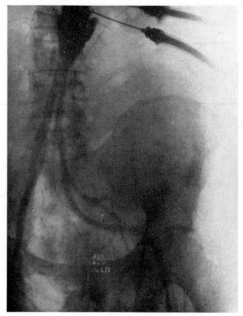

Fig. 2. (Case 3) The usual features of a chondrosarcoma of the iliac wing. Notice radiolucency of the peripheral part of the tumour, which presents only a few calcified areas.

Fig. 3. (Case 5) Mainly radiolucent chondrosarcoma of the iliac wing. Actual volume of the tumoral mass is shown by arteriographic modifications.

within the tumour. Only twice was some destruction of normal bone observed at the base of the tumour. The iliac wing was the commonest site of such tumours (seven cases); the ischium and ischio-pubic ramus were the origin of most of the remaining cases. In one case, the tumour had arisen inside the sacral canal.

The tumour shadow itself has the usual features of a cartilaginous mass, with more or less lobulated contours and a mixture of radiolucent and calcified or ossified radiopaque areas (Fig. 2). There is a great deal of variation in density and the extent of radiopaque areas in different tumours. Some are massively calcified; in others, calcification appears as a few dots in a mainly radiolucent mass. Such variation can also be observed inside the same tumour; radiolucency may be complete in the peripheral part of the tumour or in an outlying part which thus remains indiscernible. From a practical point of view, clinical appreciation of the tumour's size is a better guide than a conventional X-ray film in anticipating operative difficulties. But frequently contrast radiography of neighbouring organs has been used to determine the exact size of the cartilaginous mass (Fig. 3).

We have not been able to find consistent correlation between radiological features and histological conclusions. Nevertheless, one can roughly state the following points: tumours diagnosed as chondromas appeared more likely to show a radiopaque shadow. Conversely, a radiolucent mass with scanty calcification occurs a little more frequently in chondrosarcomas; but a chondrosarcoma can also be heavily calcified; bone destruction has been observed in each group.

BEHAVIOUR AND PROGNOSIS

It must be first stressed that such tumours, even untreated or incorrectly treated, can have a very protracted course. So only four tumours have been seen at the Cochin Hospital in the first year following their discovery (eight in the first two years). On the contrary, nearly half of the patients had their tumours for more than two years when referred to the Orthopaedic Clinic; five of them had their tumours for between 6 and 19 years. During this period six of the 15 patients were subjected to ineffective treatment. Two had radiotherapy only (radiocobalt in one, and conventional 200 kV therapy in one) without being cured. Four had limited surgical procedure—such as local excision, usually followed by multiple recurrences and multiple surgical attempts at removal (nine operations in four patients). In three of these four patients irradiation has been associated with surgery with no noticeable benefit. Slow growth is also shown by the appearance of late recurrences after surgery (up to 7 years in the present series) and by the duration of its overall course when the tumour has been left *in situ* (up to 5 years). A certain correlation does appear between histological grading and the speed of growth. Indeed, most of the tumours diagnosed as chondrosarcoma had been referred to the Orthopaedic Clinic of the Cochin Hospital in the first 2 years of their progress (six cases out of seven). On the contrary, all the tumours (five cases) referred after 4 years have been classified as "chondromas" by the pathologist.

EFFECT OF TREATMENT

The following point must first be stressed: after admission to the Orthopaedic Clinic a surgical attempt at radical removal has been considered possible in *only 10 cases out of 15*.

In one-third of the cases local extension was important enough to contra-indicate any surgical procedure. These five patients had have the following treatment:
One had radiocobalt treatment, followed by death from the tumour within 1 year.
One had radioactive sulphur, but died from intercurrent pulmonary oedema after the fourth month.
Three patients had partial removal of the tumour aiming at decompression. All three died with persistence of local growth in 6 months, 2 years and 3 years.
In no patient did we have the opportunity of observing the appearance of pulmonary metastasis, but no post-mortem examinations were carried out.

In 10 patients, an attempt at total eradication of the tumour was made by the following means:
In five cases local conditions permitted resection to be performed. It must be here emphasized that resection of pelvic bones carries a specifically high septic risk; deep infection was observed in two of these patients, with one death from general infection in the earliest case.
In four patients hindquarter amputation was required to remove the tumour.
Finally, in one case (a huge tumour with atrociously painful nerve compression, bilateral ureteral compression, and rectal compression with colostomy), a translumbar amputation was performed, after unsuccessful partial excisions.

However, reviewing the operation notes and the pathologist's reports it was evident that removal of the tumour was correctly done in only four out of 10 cases.

Sometimes the pathologist has detected microscopic invasion at the level of the surgical section. More frequently, although the ablation has been macroscopically, and microscopically complete, the surgeon noticed that the tumour had been cut open during dissection.

An adequate follow-up is available for six of these 10 patients. All three patients with correct removal are, at the time of writing, apparently cured, 5 years, 5 years and 10 years after surgery. All the three patients with incorrect removal have developed local recurrence 18 months, 2 years and 7 years after surgery. There is no parallelism between correctness of the ablation and the extent of surgical procedure; indeed the three cured patients have had resection, while a recurrence has been observed after the translumbar amputation, during which the tumour was opened.

SIGNIFICANCE OF PATHOLOGICAL FEATURES

RESULTS OF CHONDROMAS (EIGHT PATIENTS)

Three cases have insufficient follow-up (less than one year) (Cases 10, 14, 15).

Each time the tumour has not been correctly removed, that is in two patients, recurrence has been observed (Cases 8, 12), but the latest recurrence has been observed in this group (7 years after surgery).

Each time the tumour has been left in place (palliative surgery or irradiation), that is in two cases, the patients have died from their tumours (Cases 9, 13).

One patient remains apparently cured 10 years after correct removal by resection (Case 11).

RESULTS OF CHONDROSARCOMAS (SEVEN PATIENTS)

Two cases have insufficient follow-up (less than one year) (Cases 4, 6). When the tumour has not been correctly removed, i.e. in one patient, recurrence has been observed (Case 7).

Each time the tumour has been left in place (palliative surgery or irradiation), the patients (two in number) have died from their tumours (Cases 1, 5).

Two patients have apparently been cured 5 years after correct removal by resection (Cases 2, 3).

INFLUENCE OF AETIOLOGICAL FACTORS

One can only state that the three long-term survivors have presented a cartilaginous growth complicating multiple exostoses.

CONCLUSIONS

1. In no case of this series has radiotherapy (either as radiocobalt, conventional 200 kV irradiation or betatron radiation) led to the cure of a chondroma or chondrosarcoma.

2. Correct surgical removal, that is to say total ablation of the tumour without opening or even seeing it during dissection appears able to cure such tumours, whatever the surgical technique is used for. Conversely, "incorrect" removal, mainly by opening the tumour during surgery, regularly leads to local recurrence, probably by seeding of tumour cells.

3. The predominance in prognosis of correct removal appears so strong as to mask more or less all other correlations. Nevertheless, the study of recurrence and fatal evolution demonstrates that, whatever the histological prognosis, a cartilaginous growth in the pelvis behaves as a locally malignant tumour killing the patient from local progression.

4. No practical difference can be made between chondrosarcomas and so-called chondromas, which have to be treated in the same way.

5. But it must be emphasized that correct surgical removal has rarely been possible (four out of 15 cases in the present series). The reasons appear to be:
   (a) Location of tumour.
   (b) Clinical behaviour of the tumour, which allows it to reach considerable size.
   (c) Prognostic underrating of chondromas, leading to limited surgical procedures, recurrences and increased difficulties for further radical surgery.

Discussion

Prof. Barnes Can I just say that I agree entirely with your view that no useful distinction can be made between chondroma and chondrosarcoma amongst cartilaginous tumours of the pelvis. I believe that in an adult where the tumour is increasing in size and is giving rise to symptoms, and can be shown to be cartilaginous, it should be regarded as being malignant. I know that some pathologists may argue with me about this, but this is my belief. I would be interested to hear what some of the pathologists think on this particular aspect of the cartilaginous tumours of the pelvis.

Prof. Schajowicz First of all I want to know what your pathologists call a chondroma in bone because I believe that some of your chondromas are really chondrosarcoma. Often you find in a typical chondrosarcoma some cells and you cannot decide about them at the biopsy and you take it out and it is a typical chondrosarcoma. I think that all of your chondromas are what we call low-grade chondrosarcomas. I am sure Prof. Dahlin and Prof. Ackerman would say the same. But we want to know exactly what you call a chondroma—and what you call a chondrosarcoma?

Prof. Thomine Most of these cases were studied by André Mazabraud using the criteria generally accepted for skeletal cartilaginous tumours.

Prof. Schajowicz What does he call a chondroma or a chondrosarcoma?

Prof. Thomine That is a question for André Mazabraud. Nevertheless, the practical point is that the series includes all our cases of cartilage tumours which show unequivocal evolution whatever may be the prognosis assessed by histology.

Dr. Murray I am very interested in this paper which showed some beautiful cases. I am going to recall one error I made in the past and I learnt a bitter lesson from it. We had a woman who appeared with pain in the hip, and I overlooked at that time the lesson I was trying to stress the other day—the presence of a smoothly-defined very small soft tissue mass projecting from the acetabulum. She was given physiotherapy and her symptoms regressed. She went away after 6 weeks and returned $2\frac{1}{2}$ years later with an absolutely established chondrosarcoma of the acetabulum. The clue was there on the original film, and one missed it because one didn't recognize this soft tissue asymmetry. Since that occasion I have seen such an appearance (including medico-legal cases) more than once. I think that one should always assess the soft tissue shadows in relation to the acetabulum; a tumour may be suspected long before the actual bone destruction is evident.

Mr. Eyre-Brook I would entirely agree with Prof. Thomine. I am interested in one feature, this is quite a large follow-up and so many of the cases which you say were incompletely removed have died. Our pathologist once told me, "But it is not malignant

—it hasn't produced metastases." Well, that is rather late to make the diagnosis, but I would like to know how many of your fatal cases died from local causes and whether you have got any chondromas that had metastases?

Prof. Thomine As far as I know all are dead from local progression; but as I said we didn't carry out systematic autopsy so I can't say how many had metastases.

Dr. Hadden You didn't tell us whether the patient who had the hemicorporectomy survived or not?

Prof. Thomine Yes, he is alive.

Dr. Hadden And well?

Prof. Thomine No. Not well at all. He has had a recurrence, but the recurrence has been excised. He is still alive but not in good psychological condition. He had a very nice rehabilitation and he began to walk with crutches and so on, and to come back to his student work, but progressively he could not sustain his infirmity and in the end he became quite mad.

Prof. Ackerman I would like to make a few remarks about the pathology. I think that in the past pathologists were greatly in error in this group of cases in that they looked at cells but they didn't look at X-rays. I think that there is nothing more treacherous than a cartilaginous tumour from a stand point of looking at it and saying whether it is good or bad. I think that in those cases where a pathologist said it was a chondroma and then changed his mind later to chondrosarcoma—that only meant he didn't realize what he was seeing the first time and not that anything changed. So I think that the pathologist who sees a cartilaginous tumour in the pelvis by X-ray and it is over 8 cm in size and has the blotchy configuration which you have shown so well, if you put a needle in that and get cartilage cells—I really don't care what they look like—I would have to call it a chondrosarcoma. I don't think you should say that chondroma and chondrosarcomas are the same thing, they aren't the same. Osteochondromas that we see so frequently with the cartilaginous cap which is invariably thin, do not become malignant. If they do it is extremely rare, I think that the pathologist has to work in these things, and he will not make an error except rarely if he takes into consideration the clinical aspects and the radiographic features.

Prof. Bonfiglio This paper I think points up very nicely the wide variation in biological behaviour of cartilaginous tumours. They go from the various slow-growing low-grade chondrosarcomas which behave as locally aggressive to the extremely fast metastasizing varieties. I would recall one patient just to throw something out here that might be heretical in saying it. We followed a patient for 40 years with a large chondromatous tumour, large enough to be two rugby balls, which he lived with symbiotically all of his 40 years and died of renal disease. A complete autopsy showed only involvement of the tumour at the site, nothing in the lungs, nothing in the abdomen or in the pelvis itself. It was fortunate it did not invade any important structures. It stayed in the sacrum and the posterior ilium but nowhere else. It was a huge mass, but he lived with it for 40 years. We had a biopsy early on when he was about 36 and he lived to 74 and no surgery was done. So under certain conditions these low-grade tumours may provide the patient better function if you don't remove them, but that is rather rare.

Prof. Thomine   But this is the reason for our amputation. The tumour was unable to kill the patient. He had the tumour for 5 years; it was atrociously painful and he didn't die. So we had to do something to relieve him.

Prof. Bonfiglio   This patient had minimal symptoms from it other than the size?

Prof. Thomine   Yes.

Prof. Dahlin   I think that most of us in pathology would disagree with my friend André Mazabraud on the diagnosis of chondroma in those eight cases. However, I think the workers are to be complimented in excluding mesenchymal chondrosarcoma, this de-differentiated sarcoma that van Rijssel has described and chondroblastic osteogenic sarcoma. So their group was indeed rather homogenous.

Dr. Price   This is not a question Mr. Chairman, it is a comment. I would just like to mention apropos of Prof. Bonfiglio's remarks, in the records of the Bristol Registry there is a man who hailed from Gloucester who started with a large cartilaginous tumour of his shoulder which we thought was of scapular origin in 1944. When originally excised I believe it was the size of a coconut. Since then he has had at least six or seven recurrences with 16 operations. He has grown, I belive, about 5 kilograms of cartilage. He is now alive and well and there has never been any metastasis. It recurred repeatedly in the shoulder and the Registry regards it as a low-grade chondrosarcoma.

Rehabilitation after hemicorporectomy for chondrosarcoma[†]

by

BERTIL STENER,* ÅKE MAGNUSSON, TORSTEN SUNDIN,
OLLE HÖÖK, GUNNAR GRIMBY and MARGARETA NORDIN

SUMMARY

A ciné film with a commentary described the surgical treatment and successful rehabilitation of a young man of 19 with an immense recurrence of a chondrosarcoma of the pelvis. Following hemi-corporectomy, a cup prothesis was fitted which permitted bending of the trunk, and the convalescent patient rapidly learned to walk with two crutches.

Additional to the patient's youth, mental stability and co-operation, other factors contributing to the satisfactory results have been good muscular development, mobility of the trunk and participation in sports and intellectual persuits. Re-adjustment of cardiac and respiratory function has occurred.

Leading an active life as a student, the patient is now able to drive a motor-car.

IN 1968, A 17-YEAR-OLD BOY presented with swelling and pain in the left groin. Radiography revealed a large tumour originating in the left pelvic bone (Fig. 1). An extended left hemipelvectomy was done with transection of the right pubic bone 2 cm from the symphysis. Microscopic examination showed a chondrosarcoma. The patient was fitted with a Canadian prosthesis and did well to begin with. One year and a half later, however, he had swelling and pain in the right groin, and radiography showed a large tumour involving the remaining part of the pelvis (Fig. 2).

It was decided to do a hemicorporectomy. In fact, having a realistic insight of his own personal and medical situation, the patient suggested this solution himself. Other factors regarded as favourable in the psychological evaluation before the operation were the patient's very good emotional stability and intellectual capacity as well as his age (19 years) and sex.

The operation was done in two stages. On March 13, 1970, an ileal urinary conduit and a colostomy were done. Two months later, on May 13, a lumbosacral amputation was performed. The disc between the fifth lumbar vertebra and the sacrum was transected, and the abdominal wall was divided above the symphysis (Fig. 3(a)). The abdominal muscular wall was sutured to the annulus fibrosus of the transected disc. A sacrospinal musculotendinus flap was spared behind the sacrum (Fig. 3(b)). This flap

*From the Department of Orthopaedic Surgery II, the Department of Urology, and the Institute of Re- habilitation Medicine, Sahlgren Hospital, University of Göteborg, Sweden.
† Synopsis of film.

464

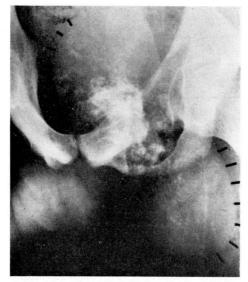

Fig. 1. Radiography in May, 1968. Chondrosarcoma originating in left pelvic bone.

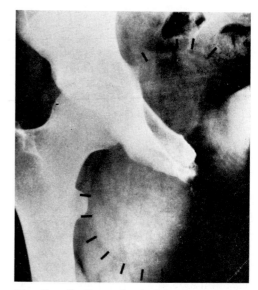

Fig. 2. Radiography in March, 1970. Recurrent tumour indicated.

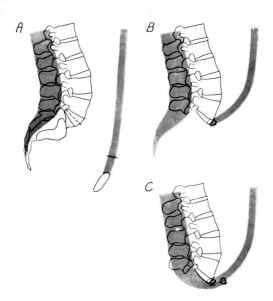

Fig. 3. (a) Transection through disc between LV and sacrum. Abdominal muscular wall divided above symphysis. (b) Abdominal muscular wall sutured to annulus fibrosus. Sacrospinal musculotendinous flap spared. (c) Sacrospinal musculotendinous flap sutured to anterior muscular wall. Active muscular function preserved both anteriorly and posteriorly.

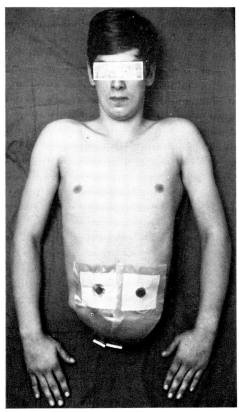

Fig. 4. Patient after hemicorporectomy. Bags for ileal urinary conduit and colostomy.

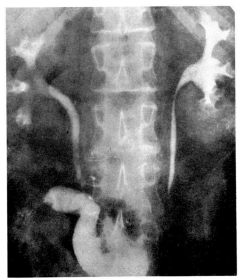

Fig. 5. I.V.P. in June, 1971, showing normal upper urinary tract, and ileal conduit.

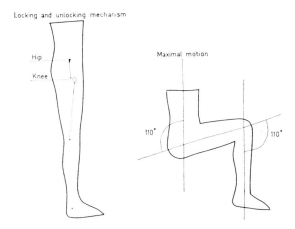

Fig. 6. Prosthesis.

was then sutured to the abdominal muscular wall, thus providing cover for the spinal canal and the transected disc (Fig. 3(c)). Thereby, too, active muscular function was preserved both anteriorly and posteriorly.

The post-operative course was uneventful with primary healing of the wound. The patient soon learned to change the bags for the ileal conduit and the colostomy (Fig. 4) himself. Several intravenous pyelographies after the operation have shown a normal upper urinary tract (Fig. 5).

After the operation the patient was fitted with a prosthesis, the upper part of which is formed as a cup enclosing the trunk. Below, the prosthesis substitutes the removed pelvis and serves as an anchorage for the hip joints. The hip and knee joints are locked synchronously and automatically in the extended position, but can be unlocked manually for flexion up to 110° in each joint (Fig. 6). Using the swing-through technique and two crutches the patient learned to walk with the prosthesis already after 1 week (2 months post-operatively). Later it was found that the spinal stump, covered by the sacrospinal musculotendinous flap and skin with unimpaired sensibility, can take full axial load. The cup of the prosthesis could therefore be reduced in height giving the patient more freedom to bend the trunk. The patient soon learned to get into and out of the prosthesis unaided. He can also independently climb into a bath-tub and get up from it. His mobility outside the prosthesis as well as the good function with the prosthesis depends probably to a large extent on his ability to move the stump actively in all directions. Lying on his back he can lift the stump with good force (Fig. 7), as he can also do in the prone position (Fig. 8).

Continuous physical conditioning training has been of great importance for his successful rehabilitation. His weekly programme includes several sports activities. one being wheel-chair basketball (Fig. 9). He can let himself fall forward to the ground on his hands and is then able to resume the standing position himself. He can walk upstairs and downstairs providing there is a hand-rail.

During the period of 4–11 months after the operation the patient was submitted to several physiological tests.

His circulation was studied repeatedly by exercise test using an arm ergometer. Following conditioning training, good physical performance could be demonstrated (Fig. 10).

The respiration was studied during exercise test and by spirometry. The total lung capacity, the vital capacity and the functional residual capacity were reduced to 63, 60 and 48% respectively of calculated normal values (Fig. 11). Studies of the regional lung function using 133-Xenon showed relative hypoventilation of basal lung regions leading to uneven distribution of the ventilation in relation to the blood flow. The alveolo-arterial oxygen difference was increased, and the carbon dioxide tension decreased indicating hyperventilation. The arterial oxygen tension was normal.

The temperature regulation was influenced by the reduced body surface and the reduced capacity to store heat, e.g. in resting muscles. It was found that the patient adequately regulated his body temperature during exercise using the sweating mechanism.

Driving his own car the patient is largely independent (Fig. 12). During the summer of 1971 he made a four weeks tourist trip (4,300 miles) visiting several European countries. He is now successfully studying to become an engineer.

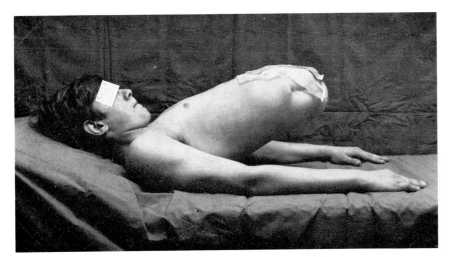

Fig. 7. Lifting the stump in supine position.

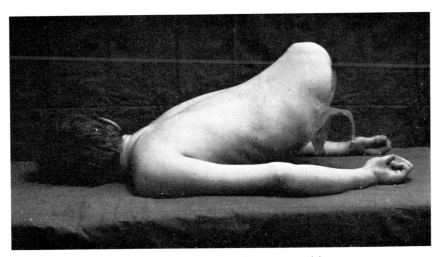

Fig. 8. Lifting the stump in prone position.

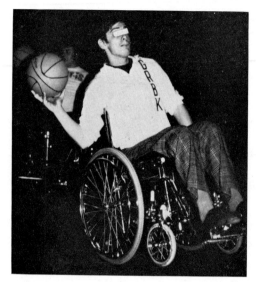

Fig. 9. Patient playing wheel-chair basketball.

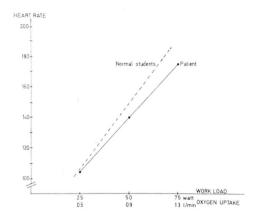

Fig. 10. Exercise test with arm ergometer 11 months after operation.

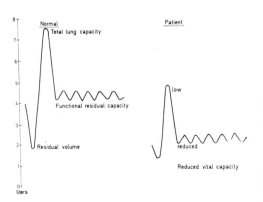

Fig. 11. Spirometry 6 months after operation.

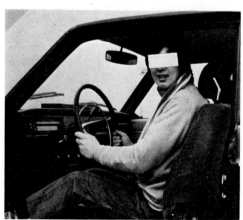

Fig. 12. Patient driving own car.

Discussion

Prof. Barnes (Chairman)   Thank you Prof. Stener for giving us the opportunity of seeing that remarkable film. I think it is a tribute to surgical ingenuity and the fortitude of your patient.

Prof. Duthie   I too would like to congratulate you on a superb description illustrating many of the problems. Of course the bilateral paraplegic, or even the odd polio patient is very much in the same category that you have rehabilitated so well. Though the actual photograph of the individual may have horrified many of the audience, this is not a unique problem from the point of view of rehabilitation. I would like to ask one simple question—Why did you make his legs so long?

Prof. Stener   I didn't make the prosthesis of course. The patient was tall before and I think he likes it like this. You should perhaps make it smaller, but he is doing very well as it is and looks about the right proportions now.

Prof. Schajowicz   Two years ago I saw a very similar film by Prof. Merle d'Aubigné but the patient was not so completely studied as your patient. But I want to know what happens to this man now? The people from Hôpital Cochin could tell me perhaps how he is after 2 years?

Prof. Thomine   He is still alive, although he has had a recurrence and another operation. He is able to walk and drive a car. However he has never been rehabilitated from a psychological point of view.

Mr. Eyre-Brook   When was the amputation done?

Prof. Thomine   About 4 years ago.

Mr. Merryweather   Could I ask Prof. Stener about the problem of the blood volume and how you have to adjust it?

Prof. Stener   The blood volume has been studied. It is 3·3 litres—the total volume of the blood cells 1·1 litres. I may add that this patient has never shown any signs of depression. He is a happy man. He is a remarkable fellow—very intelligent. As a matter of fact he suggested this solution himself. When he was quite sure himself that he had a recurrence he came to me and had this solution. He asked me to do it.

Dr. Hale   I am not quite sure if you said how many operations of this nature you had performed.

Prof. Stener   I haven't done any before.

469

Dr. Hadden   Before I saw this film I was rather prejudiced against this operation, but I think that now I have to change my mind.

Prof. Stener   I think that in many respects this patient is functioning better than a man with paraplegia because he is so light. He can move around much more easily.

Chondrosarcoma of the long bones of the extremities

by

R. MÉARY and A. ROGER

SUMMARY

The surgical treatment and results are described for 27 examples of chondrosarcoma of long bones. Following wide excision all three patients had local recurrence, two sustaining fatal metastases. Of 16 patients treated by resection followed by bone grafting or prosthetic replacement, eight developed recurrences which in three have so far been successfully excised. Secondary ablation of the limb in four patients is to the present date curative: one patient declined amputation and died of metastases. Seven of eight patients with primary amputation are now alive and well, the fatality being a child. The surgical technique and reasons for amputation are briefly discussed.

THIS STUDY CONCERNS the surgical treatment of 28 cases of chondrosarcoma of the long bones of the extremities (representing the total number of cases observed during the past 20 years in the Orthopaedic Department of Hôpital Cochin, in Paris, France*).

One patient, after having a biopsy, refused treatment. The other 27 patients underwent surgery; in three cases by extensive excision of the tumour, in 16 cases by resection, eight cases were amputated.

A. EXTENSIVE EXCISION OF THE TUMOUR

Extensive excision of the tumour, without sacrificing the bone continuity, was performed in three cases. This decision was taken because the malignancy of the cartilaginous tumours had been misjudged and because we were dealing with peripheral tumours developed mostly in the soft tissues. In all three cases there was recurrence of the lesion and all three required amputation: one of them is still alive, the other two died of metastases. This form of treatment, therefore, must be rejected.

B. RESECTION

Resection, sacrificing the bone continuity, was effected in 16 cases. It is admitted today that such resections should be made in one single block removing all the tissues likely to have been contaminated in any previous operation without breaking into the

---

* Prof. Robert A. Merle d'Aubigné, Prof. R. Méary and M. Postel.

tumour at any point. The manner of reconstituting the bone continuity varies according to the site of the tumour and is open to debate.

In tumours of the diaphysis the problem is simple. The two epiphyses are united by means of a Küntscher nail and the loss of substance is filled with graft (autograft or homograft). In the great majority of cases, however, the site of the tumour makes it necessary for the surgeon to sacrifice one of the bone extremities and do an epiphyseal–diaphyseal resection.

AT THE UPPER END OF THE HUMERUS

In two cases we did only a simple resection of an intra-articular tumoral extension which necessitated the removal of the glenoid cavity of the scapula. From an aesthetic viewpoint the result was poor, but the functional result was not bad and both patients can use their hand without the aid of an external appliance. In one case the upper half of the humerus was replaced by homograft taken from the humerus of a cadaver mounted on a nail. After 10 years the result is excellent both from the aesthetic and functional viewpoints.

Nowadays we use a steel or reinforced acrylic prosthesis made to measure. These are easy to manufacture; they become firmly fixed in the diaphysis provided a small antirotation step is put in and the length and width of the intramedullary axis are precisely calculated. We have not observed any fracture of the prosthesis or loosening on rotation, but the small number of cases treated in this manner and the time elapsed since the operation are insufficient for us to exclude the possibility of such complications. Naturally the patients thus treated have no active control of the passive mobility of their shoulder joint. We do not believe this can be obtained with a total prosthesis because when doing the resection one is always forced to sacrifice practically all the periarticular shoulder muscles.

AT THE UPPER END OF THE FEMUR

In two former cases we replaced the upper third of the femur by a homograft mounted with an intramedullary nail, interposing a cup between the cotyloid and the graft to correct the difference in diameters. In one case the functional result was very good and 6 months after the operation, the patient who is light in weight, could walk easily with a cane, almost without limping. Unfortunately the malignant process soon recurred. In the second case the result was poor, the hip remained stiff and painful, making weight-bearing difficult, so that an arthrodesis had to be done secondarily.

At present we use a steel prosthesis made to measure, as we do for the upper end of the humerus. The diameter of the femoral head is measured precisely by teleradiography, using a scale placed along the outer aspect of the thigh and making the diameter of the head of the prosthesis 2 mm smaller. No muscle is reinserted in the prosthesis since the muscles have to be removed over some distance for the resection to be effected without seeing the tumour. The passive mobility obtained is excellent, but its active control is poor; in abduction in lateral decubitus, the lower limbs cannot be kept in a horizontal position. The degree of flexion obtained is sufficient to climb one step, but the lower limb cannot be raised straight from the level of the table. The patients can walk with one cane, almost without limping, without pain, and over quite long distances. We have not noted any fracture or curving of the prosthesis, nor any loosening at the junction of the prosthesis and of the diaphysis or deterioration of the cotyloid. But here again, the number of cases is too small, and the follow-up period too short for us to assess the results (the first case was treated 4 years ago).

AT THE LEVEL OF THE KNEE (LOWER END OF THE FEMUR AND UPPER END OF THE TIBIA)

We do not try to preserve the mobility of the joint with a prosthesis or a homograft. We sacrifice the knee and restore the bone continuity by following Juvara's technique modified by Merle d'Aubigné. When successful this technique gives a stable, painless lower limb. But the operation is difficult and entails important septic risks as well as a lesser risk of non-consolidation (as happened to one of our four patients, forcing us to resort to amputation).

Out of 16 cases, eight had a recurrence, seven of them during the first 10 post-operative months.

In three cases, the tumour recurred subcutaneously in the scar and was smaller than a wheat grain: the scar and tumour were excised and to date all three patients are apparently cured.

In the other five cases, the recurring tumour lay deeper. One patient refused amputation and died of pulmonary metasases. The other four were either amputated or disarticulated and they are doing well.

C. AMPUTATION

Amputation was performed immediately in eight cases, and constituted the ultimate treatment in 16 cases.

The indication to amputate immediately was based on the following arguments:

In four cases the considerable extension of the tumour made resection either too risky or impossible.

In three cases the patient's age or poor physical condition prohibited a major operation, especially on the knee.

All seven patients are now in good condition, 2 to 8 years after the operation.

We have classified in a separate category a case of tumour of the upper tibial metaphysis in a 9-year old child, because this is such an atypical age. This patient died one year after amputation.

Eight cases were amputated secondarily for the following reasons:

Three of them for recurrence following extensive excision of the tumour: two died of pulmonary metastases which developed rapidly.

Five of them for recurrence following resection. One of them has not been seen again. The other four are apparently cured, 1 to 11 years after operation. It would appear therefore that secondary amputation does not carry too adverse a prognosis.

D. CONCLUSIONS

Of a total of 27 cases

    4 died because of their tumour, (15%)
    23 remain cured,   (85%)
    13 following amputation,
    10 having kept their limb.

This series confirms the favorable results of the surgical treatment of chondrosarcoma. Resection is acceptable only when it can be performed without seeing the tumour since it saves the limb in more than 50% of cases, and since in the event of a recurrence secondary amputation affords an important percentage of cures. These conclusions, however, can be only temporary on account of the limited number of cases observed and of the insufficient time elapsed since the operation, i.e.,

1 to 3 years in 6 cases,
3 to 5 years in 10 cases,
5 to 15 years in 7 cases.

Discussion

Prof. Schajowicz   I would like to ask you if you graded histologically your tumours as a means of deciding whether you would treat them by resection or by amputation?

Prof. Méary   No.

Prof. Schajowicz   I think this is the reason for the failure of your cases with resections because as you know in our country Ottolenghi is the champion of resection followed by homograft. But before he undertakes a resection for chondrosarcoma, first we do a puncture biopsy to ascertain if it is a low-, medium- or high-grade malignant chondrosarcoma. If the tumour is highly malignant or a medium-grade chondrosarcoma this is a contraindication to segmental resection—he performs an amputation. Even if the tumour is a low-grade chondrosarcoma that has perforated the cortex and invaded the soft tissues—this again contraindicates resection, it requires either amputation or some more radical treatment. This is the result of our experience. In several resections done by Ottolenghi in cases which are of high-grade malignancy or with cortical perforation, there was always local recurrence. In one of our cases a resection was done in a medium- to high-grade malignant chondrosarcoma with recurrence after 6 years: we have another similar case now with recurrence 3 years after resection.

Prof. Barnes   Could I ask how you determine the degree of the intramedullary extension of tumours which you are proposing to treat by resection?

Prof. Méary   This a problem. Just in one case we have been rather surprised at operation to see at the level where we went in to do the resection that there was tumour tissue. However, I never do a resection without already having the written consent of the patient to do an amputation during the same procedure if necessary. If he refuses, I refuse to operate.

Mr. Wilson   We have done a large number of resections for low-grade tumourous conditions as I think I have mentioned before. Our number is now about 32, replacing with long bone prosthesis. Of these there were 11 chondrosarcomas. I think certain of them were in the upper femur and the others were divided between the humerus and the lower femur. I couldn't agree more with what Professor Schajowicz says about picking the tumour. If it has broken through the bone there is no reaction around it to form a localizing cover—such a case is not suitable and we have had recurrences from this. Secondly, we have run into trouble from not appreciating the aggressive nature of the tumour histologically. I think that from our own practice the resection of the knee has been one of the most successful that we've had. You were saying you were doubtful about it, but I am sure it is well worth while. We have taken up to about half a femur away and got a result which is almost indistinguishable from normal. It is by far the best resection of the whole lot.